# Life and Death Decision Making

# Life and Death Decision Making

Baruch A. Brody, Ph. D.

*New York    Oxford*
OXFORD UNIVERSITY PRESS
1988

Oxford University Press

Oxford   New York   Toronto
Delhi   Bombay   Calcutta   Madras   Karachi
Petaling Jaya   Singapore   Hong Kong   Tokyo
Nairobi   Dar es Salaam   Cape Town
Melbourne   Auckland

and associated companies in
Beirut   Berlin   Ibadan   Nicosia

Copyright © 1988 by Oxford University Press, Inc.

Published by Oxford University Press, Inc.,
200 Madison Avenue, New York, New York 10016

Oxford is a registered trademark of Oxford University Press

**Library of Congress Cataloging-in-Publication Data**

Brody, Baruch A.
  Life and death decision making.

  Includes index.
  1. Medical ethics—Decision making.   2. Life
and death, Power over—Decision making.   3. Medical
ethics—Decision making—Case studies.   4. Life and
death, Power over—Decision making—Case studies.
I. Title.
R725.5.B76      1988      174'.24      87-23965
ISBN 0-19-505007-X

10 9 8 7 6 5 4 3 2 1

Printed in the United States of America
on acid-free paper

# Preface

For the last four and a half years, I have had the unusual opportunity of simultaneously teaching moral philosophy in the setting of an outstanding university and medical ethics in the clinics of a leading medical school and its teaching hospitals. Each of these teaching experiences has taught me something. I have learned at the university the shortcomings of standard clinical thinking about practical issues in medical ethics. I have learned at the clinics the shortcomings of standard moral theories and their practical implications. This book grows out of those teaching experiences and attempts to offer an approach that will be satisfactory in both settings.

Clinicians often approach issues in medical ethics by appealing, explicitly or implicitly, to nontheoretical principles of bioethics. These range from such traditional statements as "Above all, do no harm" and "Further care is inappropriate because it is futile" to more contemporary statements such as "We need to respect the autonomy of the patient" and "That expenditure of health-care resources is inappropriate in light of current fiscal realities." There is some truth to each of these midlevel principles, and good clinicians often acquire an intuitive ability to apply the right principle at the right point. But hard cases, which probe the precise meanings of these principles and their relative priorities, do not work out very well. Lacking any theoretical framework, clinicians often flounder when confronting hard cases. The university has taught me that a theoretical framework is necessary to clarify the meaning, scope, and significance of nontheoretical principles in all areas including medical ethics.

Moral theorists focus on the structure and content of their theoretical systems and on attempts to establish their fundamental principles as true. The questions they consider range from metaethical questions such as "Are basic moral truths derivable from nonmoral truths?" and "Are moral truths objective or subjective?" to substantive questions such as "Are moral rules justified by the consequences of their being followed?" and "Are there any universal moral rights?" All of these questions are perfectly appropriate, but answering them seems to shed little light on hard cases, because little if any attention is paid to the logic of the move from the theory to solutions of concrete moral problems. Moral theories, as they have developed in the university, seem remarkably silent in response to clinical questions. The clinics have taught me that moral theories are useless unless they are developed in a way that illuminates and helps resolve real problems faced by inquiring moral agents.

This book, then, is an attempt to integrate theory and practice. This is one way in which it differs from many other books I have used in the settings in which I teach. But there is another way in which it is different. The approach of this book is that of a pluralistic casuistry. It is pluralistic in that it supposes that there are many different moral appeals that are irreducible to each other, often in conflict with each other, and yet necessary to complement each other. It is casuistrical in that it attends to the range of differences among particular cases and attempts to apply appropriately the different moral appeals to particular cases in different ways. The resulting theory, therefore, has a far more complex basic structure than most traditional theories, which regard all moral appeals as reducible to one basic appeal. The resulting theory is also far more complex in application than most traditional theories; one needs to attend carefully to many subtle complexities in assessing how these varying appeals apply in different ways to different cases. I hope to convince the reader that these complexities are a virtue of my theory, since complex issues require complex theories for their resolution.

The book begins with a presentation of my basic orientation. The next three chapters present my theory. The last three chapters show how it can be used by applying it to the resolution of forty difficult cases. A word about the case presentations: These are composites drawn from several hundred real cases I have encountered in teaching rounds and/or in consultations. No real case in which I have been involved corresponds exactly to the facts in the composite presentations. Each of the facts in these forty case presentations, however, is drawn from a real case. Similarly, the arguments presented by the team in each presentation are drawn from arguments actually offered by sensitive and talented clinicians in several hundred real cases. In that way, I have tried to present the flavor of a real debate in a clinical setting. But these are composite debates, not transcripts of an actual discussion in an actual case.

I have been fortunate to have been aided in my work by many very helpful colleagues. Drs. Michael E. DeBakey, William T. Butler, and Bobby R. Alford have provided administrative support for my activities at Baylor College of Medicine. Similar support has been provided by presidents Norman Hackerman and George Rupp, provosts William E. Gordon and Neal F. Lane, and dean Allen J. Matusow at Rice University, and by directors Ron Sunderland, David Stitt, and J. Robert Nelson and presidents Caroline Clark and David Mumford at the Institute of Religion at the Texas Medical Center. The Center for Ethics, Medicine, and Public Issues, which I head, is a joint project of all three of these institutions. In the Department of Medicine, Drs. Antonio M. Gotto, Edward C. Lynch, Robert J. Luchi, David A. Sears, and H. Irving Schweppe have encouraged their staffs and residents to attend ethics conferences, and Drs. Eugene V. Boisaubin, Fidel Davila, Nelda P. Wray, Mary Ann Zubler, James Young, and their colleagues have welcomed me into their services. In the Department of Pediatrics, Drs. Ralph D. Feigin and Martin I. Lorin have also encouraged their staffs and residents to attend ethics conferences. Dr. Joseph A. Garcia-Prats, Susan Scoggins, R.N., and their colleagues at Jefferson Davis Hospital, and Drs. Larry S. Jefferson and Donald J. Fernbach and their colleagues at Texas Children's Hospital have likewise welcomed me into their services. I have also been helped by Drs. Timothy L. Bayer, Joseph Devance Hamilton, and Norman Decker of Psychiatry, Dr. Raymond H. Kaufman of Obstetrics and Gynecology, Dr. Martin Grabois of Physical Medicine, Dr. Peter T. Scardino of Urology, and Dr. Robert E. Rakel of Family Medicine. Special thanks are due to Dr. Harold B. Haley of the VA Medical Center for his help in opening many opportunities to me and to my old friend and chairman of the Department of Philosophy at Rice University, Professor Richard E. Grandy, for being so patient. As always, my colleague Dr. H. Tristram Engelhardt, Jr., has been immensely helpful in discussing so many of the cases. This is a very long list, but it is incomplete since it leaves out the many chief residents who have carried the burden of organizing ethics conferences and the many house officers who have been willing to present their cases. To all of these people, I can only say thank you. It is hard to imagine how any group could have been more helpful. Finally, special thanks to Drs. Joseph A. Garcia-Prats, Nelda P. Wray, and James B. Young for reading and commenting on all of the case descriptions, to Professor Larry Temkin, my philosophy colleague at Rice, for commenting extensively and helpfully on many points in the theoretical section, and to Jay Jones and Becky White, my research assistants, for their many helpful suggestions on the entire manuscript.

I have not listed Delores Smith, my administrative assistant, among the people to be thanked. Doing so could not adequately acknowledge her indispensable contributions both to this project and to my entire professional life. I will find another way to thank her. I am merely acknowledging here her special contributions.

*Houston*                                                                                           B.B.
*May 1987*

# Contents

# Life and Death Decision Making

# 1

## The Need for a Moral Theory

The tremendous scientific and technological advances of the second half of the twentieth century have given physicians and other health-care providers the ability to keep patients alive who would have died relatively quickly in the past. Successful techniques for resuscitating patients whose cardiopulmonary functioning has ceased, for monitoring and responding to major organ failures in the intensive care unit, and for transplanting kidneys, livers, and hearts all exemplify the advances in medical knowledge and technology that have enabled patients to survive for a considerable period of time.

The initial response to these new capabilities was to use them in all cases with the hope of extending life, even if the underlying problems of the patients could not be resolved.[1] Experience with this fully aggressive approach eventually led many to the conclusion that it was excessive. Physicians and other health-care providers, patients and their families, and the general public eventually came to accept the idea that the technological imperative which urges the use of these techniques on all occasions should be resisted.[2] Out of that recognition arose one of the fundamental problems of modern biomedical ethics; when to strive to preserve the life of the patient and when to simply allow the patient to die.

This book is an attempt to present a moral framework in which such questions can be analyzed and, it is hoped, resolved. The moral framework will be presented in chapters 2 through 4. It is called the model of conflicting appeals, and it is put forward as an alternative to various other models which have been proposed. In chapters 5 through 7, forty very difficult cases will be presented. Each presentation begins with a statement of the facts about the case; then there is a summary of the various questions raised by the health-care providers who were dealing with that case, along with their opinions; finally, the model of conflicting appeals is applied

3

to the case in question in the hope of obtaining greater insight into how the case should be resolved.

This chapter first presents in a brief fashion some of the cases that will be discussed far more extensively in chapters 5 through 7. My aim is to illustrate the great difficulty reflective people have in making decisions in such cases. Then, in sections 1.2 through 1.4, the theoretical background to the model of conflicting appeals is sketched. This chapter thus serves to introduce the reader to the sorts of problems with which we will be concerned throughout the book and to the theoretical framework which will serve as the foundation for our approach to dealing with them.

## 1.1   Some Illustrative Cases

The first case deals with a wish, expressed by a patient who may be competent, to be allowed to die. Mrs. A is an 84-year-old woman who was widowed in her early thirties. She was left with three small children whom she raised on her own. Raising these children was very difficult because of her lack of education and vocational experience, but she did it, never asking for any help, either from family and friends or from social agencies. In general, Mrs. A was a very independent lady who always did things on her own. Her health had always been good. She had no significant history of illness and had not been hospitalized previously. She was admitted to the hospital after sustaining a compound fracture of the tibia in an automobile accident because people weren't quite sure that a woman of her age in a cast could handle her daily needs. Since entering the hospital, she has clearly been depressed. She doesn't like the nurses caring for her because she resents the dependent role in which she is placed, and she has become progressively withdrawn. Her family reports that she is listless and nonresponsive and spends most of her time lying in bed and staring out the window. From the beginning she ate very little and has therefore become progressively weaker. Recently she stopped eating. While she speaks very rarely, Mrs. A has said on more than one occasion something like the following: "I am old and tired. I am ready to die. If you will just let me alone, I will stop eating and die. I am ready to go to God." Psychiatry was called for a consultation concerning her mental status. They report that she is clearly oriented, has good short-term recall, understands what she is doing, and has made a decision to die. They therefore evaluate her as competent, although they recognize that she is also showing significant symptoms of a reactive depression, presumably caused by her hospitalization and dependency. The medical and nursing staff like this woman, although she is making life hard for them, and they are very ambivalent in their feelings about whether they should respect her wish and let her die or whether they should restrain her and force-feed her. Her three daughters have equally ambivalent feelings. It is clear that they love and respect their mother and are reluctant to go against her wishes. At the same time, they don't want her to die, and they think that if she eats and gets stronger, she will be able to go home to live on her own. What should be done about Mrs. A's refusal to eat?

Our next case deals with a much younger patient, Ms. T., who is in much worse shape. She is 28 years old and has been a patient either in the hospital in question or in an affiliated nursing home for the last two and a half years. When she was 25 she sustained extensive head injuries in a motorcycle accident. Since then she has been totally comatose and unresponsive. She has been able to breathe on her own, and she shows evidence of some brain-stem reflexes, so we know that she is not brain dead. In the last two and a half years, however, she has shown no evidence of higher brain functioning. Most of the time she receives only nursing care. She needs to have her airway suctioned to prevent secretions from blocking it, and she is regularly turned in bed to avoid bed sores. She is fed through a tube. Her major medical needs arise from intermittent infections that require careful workups and extensive antibiotic treatment. In severe episodes she is transferred from the nursing home, where she normally lives, to the hospital. That happened two days ago. The family of Ms. T has been heartbroken since her accident. She is her parents' only child, they took great pride in all of her achievements, and they cannot bring themselves to accept the fact that she will never again be able to function normally. They know that if she is treated carefully she can survive for a long time. They hope for a miracle or for some medical advance that can cure her. Many unsuccessful attempts have been made to explain the futility of this. The team treating her has spoken to the family again, now that she has been transferred back to the hospital, and the parents have reiterated their desire that her infection be treated. How should the team respond to this unrealistic but strongly held desire?

Next is the case of a newborn baby with severe problems. Baby D was born to a 16-year-old woman who is unsure of the father's identity. None of the more likely candidates has expressed any interest in the baby. The course of the pregnancy was normal, and the infant seemed normal at birth. However, it was noted by the nurses that the baby was excessively sleepy, cried continuously when awake, and fed poorly because of poor sucking ability. A neurology consult revealed that the child suffered from hydranencephaly, a congenital anomaly in which nearly all of the cerebral hemispheres and the corpus striatum are reduced to a sac covered by intact meninges but filled with clear fluid. This condition is easily detectable; a high-intensity light held up to the skull on one side transilluminates the entire upper skull (since all that is present in the skull is fluid). All of this has been explained to the mother and the maternal grandmother. In order to be sure that they understood the baby's condition, the staff showed them the transilluminated skull. The staff would simply like to keep Baby D comfortable, not providing any nourishment, until the baby dies. They feel that if they use more aggressive treatment there is a chance that the infant will survive for some time and that these poor people will be required to take home a child who has no chance for any neurological functioning. The maternal grandmother, who would probably have the responsibility for providing most of the infant's care, totally agrees. Baby D's mother does not. She insists that the baby is alive, that she wants to take Baby D home and give the child as much love as she can. Whose wishes should be followed?

Finally, we have the case of an adolescent. K was diagnosed at the age of 12 as having nasopharyngeal carcinoma. He was treated with local radiation and chemotherapy, and he initially responded very well. Within a year, however, his condition worsened, and he required radical neck surgery followed by postsurgical chemotherapy. After surgery he was symptom-free until shortly after his fifteenth birthday, when he presented with headaches and nausea and clear evidence of recurrence of his cancer. At that point the only options left open were several experimental chemotherapy protocols. The physicians explained to the parents that K's long-term prognosis was very poor but that these new protocols could probably buy him some time. K is his parents' only child, the family has been close, and the parents have been very involved at all stages of K's care. They definitely wanted the physicians to make every effort to buy some more time for them with K. When all of this was presented to K, however, he was opposed to being enrolled in any further chemotherapy protocols. He said that he was tired of all he had gone through and that he just wanted to be left alone to die in peace. Several conferences involving the physicians, the entire family, and various counselors have been held, but the conflict has not been resolved. There is real tension in this previously close family. What should the treating team do about the conflicting wishes?

## 1.2   The Need for a Theory of Decision Making

The four cases just examined, and the many others presented later in this book, illustrate the difficulty health-care providers face as they make decisions about the appropriate level of care to provide to various patients. We need a proper theory of decision making to deal with such cases.

Such a theory must first address the question of where the burden of decision making falls. In the first illustrative case, should Mrs. A make the decision, should her children make the decision, or should the health-care team make the decision? In the case of Ms. T, should her parents continue to have decisional authority, or should their wishes be overridden in light of their unrealistic hopes? Should the team be allowed to decide not to provide further treatment of Ms. T's infection? In the case of Baby D, should the teenage mother have authority for decision making, should the maternal grandmother have that authority, or should it ultimately rest on the physicians caring for the baby? Should K decide about further chemotherapy, should K's parents make the decision, or does their conflict mean that the physicians will have to decide? These are all procedural questions about the process of decision making and about authority within that process. Any good theory will need to address them.

In recent years discussions of the question of life-and-death decision making have been dominated by consideration of this question of who should decide.[3] Although it is never stated, the impression one often gets from the literature is that this is the only important issue. However, this is not a proper way of looking at these questions. To begin with, those who have the authority to decide still need to confront the question of what to do, and they ought to seek guidance from an adequate moral theory to help them in their own deliberations. If K's parents are to make the decision about further chemotherapy, they will need and/or want some guidance about the right decision given that K so definitely does not want the treatment. If Baby D's mother has the final decisional authority despite the fact that she is a teenager, she may still want to know if there is any way in which one or more of the options open to her is best supported by a proper examination of the moral issues. The same reasoning applies to the cases of Mrs. A and Ms. T. So we need a substantive moral theory as well as a procedural moral theory.

A second consideration is that whatever view we may hold about who should decide, we may also want to impose certain limits on the extent of decisional authority. If we believe, for example, that parents should be entitled to make these difficult decisions even for adolescent children, we might still be prepared to say that when parents go to extremes their wishes should be disregarded. But we will need the guidance of a substantive moral theory to help us identify what constitutes an unacceptable decision, one which requires that the usual rules of procedural authority should be overridden. In short, then, there are two reasons why any adequate moral theory needs to go beyond the question of who should decide and address the question of what is the best decision.

So far we have been considering the sorts of questions raised by the cases that our theory should address. Let's now turn to the question of whether or not the search for an adequate moral theory of decision making is an appropriate search. Some critics claim that a search for an adequate moral theory is unnecessary. Others maintain that the search will not succeed because moral theories cannot do the jobs that I have identified. Each of these claims will be examined separately.

There are many versions of the claim that moral theories are unnecessary for dealing with difficult cases.[4] One version states that we don't need a moral theory; all we need are good human beings. Such people will know what is right in a given case and do not require the aid of a moral theory. A related version admits that more is required than good people. It holds that good people who, in addition, have an adequate clinical exposure to the issues and to ways in which they have been resolved by appropriate role models will be able to make decisions in these cases without any moral theory to aid them.

I believe that examples such as the four cases presented above show that these claims are incorrect. In each of these cases, good people have radically different views about what ought to be done. Both the parents of Ms. T and the members of her treating team are good people. K and his parents are good people. Examples like this illustrate that good people can strongly disagree about what ought to be done in a particular case. This is precisely why the need for a moral theory is so great.

These very same examples also illustrate what is wrong with the claim that all we need is good people who have had adequate role models for dealing with such problems in the course of their clinical training. We need to remember that in cases like these, and in many other cases discussed later in this book, members of the treating team (the physicians, the nurses, and the other allied health professionals) were split over the question of what ought to be done. Yet these were good people with extensive clinical training from some of the finest role models one could want. So that doesn't appear to be sufficient to help deal with difficult cases. Good people, even with ample clinical training under proper role models, can find themselves unsure and can disagree with other such people about what ought to be done. Even experience and training combined with moral goodness are not sufficient. These dilemmas show us why we need help if these cases are to be adequately resolved.

There is, however, a second set of critics whose claims need to be examined.[5] They argue that, while something is needed, moral theory, at least as it has been traditionally understood, cannot provide the relevant guidance. Those who put forward this claim often make the following observations: (1) Moral theories are probably best seen as attempts to explain the rightness or wrongness of various actions when we are already sure about what is right or wrong. As such, the search for them is an interesting theoretical task. But moral theories have never been intended to deal with cases about which we are confused and would be unhelpful in that task. (2) This is so because moral theories are developed at a high level of abstraction and do not generate a clear conclusion about what ought to be done in particular difficult cases. Since this is precisely the type of concrete help that is needed, moral theories can't help.

There is some merit to this set of claims. Some of those who have articulated moral theories have in fact done so at a high level of abstraction, and it is very unclear how they think these moral theories can be applied to particular cases. However, it would be wrong to suppose that this is a necessary or even predominant feature of moral theories. We need to remember that Kant attempted, even in the very abstract *Fundamental Principles of the Metaphysics of Morals,* to illustrate the moral implications of his theory in an examination of four famous cases.[6] He did much more of that in his other, more applied writings, and he drew from his theories many controversial conclusions.[7] Similarly, utilitarian writers such as Bentham and Mill were very keen to insist that their perspectives could help in the formulation of ethical decisions and social policies.[8] So it was certainly no part of the intention of many of the great moral theorists that their theories should only be abstract structures designed to explain what we already know. None of this is to say that it is very easy (or even possible) to ascertain the concrete implications of various moral theories. It is only to say that, from the very beginning, those who put forward these theories intended them to be applied in a way that would lead to nonobvious results. Even if we were to adopt one of the traditional abstract theories of morality, it would be an open question whether or not those theories couldn't do their intended job of helping us to resolve our cases.

There is, however, another point to be made, a point that will become clearer as we proceed. The moral theory advocated in this book is not an abstract moral theory, a theory whose mode of application is unclear. It takes from each of the traditional abstract moral theories a component which needs to be combined with components of other theories in a way that produces a type of model for decision making that can be applied to difficult cases.

In summary, the following response can be made to those who have argued that the development of a moral theory is not what is needed to deal with these cases. The claim that the cases require no theory for their resolution is contradicted by the existence of conflict among good people in these cases. The claim that moral theories can't do the job even if something else is needed is probably wrong but cannot be so easily dismissed. The best way of refuting it is by doing what I shall try to do in this book, that is, by developing a moral theory for medical decision making in life-and-death cases that will help to resolve these cases. If the book is successful, it will show that this viewpoint is wrong.

## 1.3 The Virtues of a Pluralistic Theory

The theory that will be advocated in the following pages is a pluralistic moral theory, one that accepts the legitimacy of a wide variety of very different moral appeals. It differs from traditional monistic theories that emphasize the fundamental legitimacy of only one particular moral appeal. This section is intended to clarify the nature of that difference and the reasons for adopting a pluralistic approach.

The field of moral theory is dominated by the conflicts among a wide variety of competing views. Utilitarianism in its various forms, deontological theories (such as Kant's theory of the categorical imperative), natural rights theories (such as Locke's theory of the rights of individuals), virtue theories (Aristotelian and other-wise), and social contractarian theories (from Hobbes to Rawls) all have their adherents. Various arguments are offered for or against each of these theories, and the conclusion reached by many is that there is no such thing as an acceptable moral theory. There are a great many different moral theories, they are in conflict with each other, each has its strengths and weaknesses, and we don't know which theory should be employed in dealing with concrete practical issues. After all, most of the seemingly plausible ways of dealing with hard cases can be supported by at least one of the conflicting theories. Therefore, lacking any way of resolving the question of which moral theory is correct, we will not be able to get any guidance from moral theory about how to deal with hard cases.

I think we need a new way of looking at the moral theories that have been advocated in the past. We need to recognize that each has emphasized a particular moral appeal whose legitimacy is unquestionable. We also need to recognize that each has failed because it has recognized only one of the many legitimate moral appeals. Rather than seeing the history of moral philosophy as a history of compet-ing theories among which we must choose, we ought to view it as a series of attempts to articulate different moral appeals, all of which will have to be combined to frame an adequate moral theory for helping us deal with difficult cases.

Consider Aristotle's theory of the virtues. This theory, which is about both virtuous persons and the actions they perform, emphasizes a certain type of moral appeal. It says that certain actions are of value because they exemplify such virtues as courage and temperance. An attempt, whether successful or not, is made to define the nature of these virtuous actions. No attention is paid by Aristotle to such moral appeals as the appeal to the consequences of one's actions, the appeal to the rights of individuals, the appeal to moral rules that should govern the behavior of human beings, and so on. Thus, Aristotle's theory emphasizes only one type of moral appeal, the appeal to the virtues. This feature of Aristotle's theory is the source of both its strength and its weakness. Its importance in the history of moral philosophy lies precisely in reminding us of the need to incorporate a consideration of the virtues into moral theory. Its weakness, apart from the question of whether it has adequately defined the virtues, is that it fails to take into account the many other moral appeals which must be incorporated into any adequate moral theory.

The same is true of such classical utilitarian thinkers as Bentham and Mill. They emphasize a very different type of moral appeal, the appeal to the consequences of our actions. The strength of their theory is that it calls our attention to that very important moral appeal, which must be included in any adequate moral theory. Its weakness, apart from the question of whether the theory adequately defines the appeal to utility, is that it fails to take into account other types of legitimate appeals. That is the point of many of the standard objections to utilitarianism, that is, that utilitarianism is insufficiently sensitive to the rights of distinct individuals and that it fails to ascribe enough significance to the moral rules, allowing too many exceptions to them.

Consider, as a third example, natural rights theories, such as Locke's discussion of the rights of individuals to liberty and to property. The strength of these theories is that they remind us of the need to take into account as an extremely important moral appeal the idea that individuals have rights which must be respected. Again, the weakness of these theories, beyond the fact that they haven't fully articulated the content of those rights, is that they fail to take into account other moral appeals such as the appeal to consequences or the appeal to various virtues. Many of the standard objections to rights theories, such as the claim that attending to individual rights may mean that the general well-being is severely diminished, are based precisely upon this observation that rights theorists have failed to take into account other moral appeals in evaluating proposed actions.

In short, moral philosophers over the centuries have put forward many differing moral theories. Each involves a specific type of moral appeal. The strength of each is precisely that the moral appeal it is invoking is a legitimate moral appeal, one that truly needs to be taken into account as we confront real cases. But the difficulty with these theories is twofold. One difficulty is internal, their failure to sufficiently articulate the moral appeals they are invoking. But the other and more important difficulty is that each theory is prone to counterexamples based explicitly on other moral appeals. Utilitarians are challenged by counterexamples that appeal to respect for human rights as an argument against doing what will produce the greatest good. Rights theorists are challenged by counterexamples explicitly based on an appeal to the very bad consequences of respecting the right in question in that case. Virtue theorists are challenged by counterexamples that invoke considerations of consequences or of individual rights. The traditional objections to the traditional theories can be viewed as arguing that the theories are incorrect because they fail to take into account other moral appeals.[9]

There are two options open at this point. One is the traditional approach of attempting to build into these theories, as derivative moral appeals, the moral appeals that a particular theory does not emphasize. Utilitarians are particularly notorious or astute (the adjective you use depends on your attitude toward utilitarianism) in trying to explain why, on good utilitarian grounds, we should attend to moral rules, to the rights of individuals, to virtues, and so on.[10] But they are not unique in adopting the strategy. It would take a whole other book to argue that all of these attempts are failures. But I believe that they are and that this is why we continue to have conflicting moral theories. A second option, which I favor, is to insist that we should not attempt to take one moral appeal from one theory and use it as the basis for all of morality, using other moral appeals derivatively and only to the extent that they can be based on the fundamental moral appeal.[11] Rather, we should regard each of these theories as correct in advocating a moral appeal whose use is certainly legitimate but limited. Thus, we need to incorporate all of these moral appeals, each treated as an independent appeal whose validity is not based on its derivability from some other moral appeal, into a pluralistic moral theory. The model of conflicting appeals, as the name suggests, is an attempt to carry out this second option.

The adoption of such a pluralistic model will help us deal with still another objection to using moral theory to deal with particular choices. If there is a set of conflicting theories, we have to address the question of which theory to use in making any particular choice. If we can synthesize the best ideas from each of the theories into one pluralistic model, that question becomes moot.

Chapter 2 will examine the many moral appeals that have been emphasized in the history of moral philosophy. I will then argue, in Chapter 3, that two models for life-and-death medical decision making are invalid because they fail to incorporate these many different legitimate moral appeals. Chapter 4 attempts to articulate a model for life-and-death medical decision making that does incorporate all of these appeals. The crucial question will be how to put them together into one comprehensive approach, and the answer to that question will dominate the discussion in chapter 4.

## 1.4   The Ontological and Epistemological Basis of a Pluralistic Theory

Before developing the model, there is one other question that must be raised. That is the question of the ontological and epistemological basis of the theory. How do we know which of the appeals that have been advocated in the history of moral philosophy ought to be incorporated into an adequate model for moral decision making? How do we know that we have put them together correctly in our model? Is the resulting theory true? In what does its truth consist?

Are moral judgments true or false, or are they mere expressions of feeling to which the categories of truth and falsity do not apply? And if they are true or false, what is the basis of their truth or falsity? Is it some subjective basis? Are moral claims true only when they report the actual values of a given individual or a given society? Or is there an objective basis for the truth of moral judgments? The answers to these questions form the ontological basis of moral theory. They tell us what is being claimed about the world, if anything of that sort is being claimed, when we make a moral judgment.

Is there any way we can know whether a particular moral judgment is true or false? If so, how? If not, doesn't that mean that we are committed to moral skepticism, to a view that, as far as we know, one moral claim is no better than another? The answers to these questions form the epistemological basis for moral theory. They tell us how, if at all, knowledge is possible in the area of morality.

Any attempt to provide and defend a complete ontological and epistemological basis for moral theory is far beyond the scope of this book. But I will sketch a theory of the ontological and epistemological basis of morality which I have argued for elsewhere and which will serve as background for understanding how this book works.[12]

Let me turn first to the ontological questions. I believe that the traditional meta-

ethical discussions have established that moral properties are supervenient properties, properties whose possession is dependent on the nonmoral properties of individual actions and social arrangements.[13] A moral judgment about a particular
action being right is true if the action in question has the supervenient property of
rightness, a property that depends on the nonmoral properties of the action. Thus,
helping an elderly person cross the street might in some circumstances be the right
thing to do, might be an action that has the supervenient property of rightness,
because it possesses in those circumstances certain other nonmoral characteristics
such as being an act that helps avoid accidents, shows concern for others, and so on.
Moreover, I believe that these same discussions have established that the property
of rightness is not supervenient on sociological properties of how the action is
viewed by individuals or by society. An action is not right just because an individual
agent or his or her society approves of the action. It is other, more objective
properties on which the moral properties depend. In short, then, I am assuming that
the traditional metaethical discussions have established that moral properties super-
vene on objective properties of individuals, actions, and social arrangements.

How do we ascertain which individuals, actions, and social arrangements have
positive moral properties? The view I presuppose is that the intuitionist account is
correct and that we have a fundamental cognitive capacity which enables us to
recognize the moral value of individuals, actions, and social arrangements. But the
intuitionism which I am presupposing is different from the one normally presupposed, and that difference needs to be explained.

Most moral intuitionists have assumed that the fundamental moral intuitions are
indubitable and evident intuitions of the truth or falsity of purported moral rules.[14]
Put another way, they have assumed that our fundamental moral intuitions are
intuitions that particular types of actions have a particular moral quality. This type
of intuitionism is easy to attack. If the rules in question are relatively simple, they
are unlikely to be true because they will fail to take into account the many exceptions that need to be made. If the rules become far more complicated by attempting
to deal with the needed exceptions, it is implausible to suppose that we can directly
intuit their truth. Thus, for example, if one put forward as a fundamental moral
intuition the claim that breaking promises is wrong, one would confront the dilemma that if no exceptions are noted and put into the rule, there is little reason to
believe that the rule is accurate, for there seem to be many cases in which one may
(and even must) break promises in order to obtain far greater moral gains. If, on the
other hand, an attempt is made to modify the principle so that it covers the exceptions, then the new principle is likely to become so complicated that we are unable
to claim with any plausibility that we can intuit its truth. So, if we are to adopt an
intuitionist approach, it will need to be radically different.

The type of intuitionism presupposed in this book holds that the fundamental
moral intuitions are judgments about the rightness or wrongness of particular actions, the justice or injustice of particular social arrangements, the praiseworthiness
of particular individuals, and so on. On this account, we begin by examining the
nonmoral properties of these individuals, actions, and social arrangements. Having
examined them, we often form intuitive moral judgments. These initial judgments
must be tentative, in part because we may not have noticed some of the nonmoral

properties that are relevant or we may have disregarded them. These tentative judgments are the moral intuitions that give us the basis for learning what is right and wrong, just or unjust, good or bad.

The formation of these basic tentative intuitions is not, of course, the whole of the intuitionism I am advocating; it is only the first stage in the process of coming to have moral knowledge. The next stage is that of theory formation.[15] The goal of this stage is to form a theory concerning when actions are right or wrong, agents blameworthy or innocent, and institutions just or unjust. The data about which we theorize are those initial intuitions. The goal is to find a theory that systematizes these intuitions, explains them, and provides help in dealing with cases about which we have no intuitions. In the course of this systematization, it may be necessary to reject some of the initial intuitions on the grounds that they cannot be systematized into the theory. That is another reason for saying that initial moral intuitions are tentative and certainly not evident or indubitable. In short, our theory of intuitionism involves initial tentative judgments, theory formation, and reconciliation between theories and initial judgments. At all stages, the results are tentative and open to revision. The result of this process is a body of particular judgments and theories that (ideally) fit together into a systematic whole.

A number of crucial points must be noted about this intuitionist methodology. (1) Theories are formed at many levels of generality, ranging from simple generalizations covering a small portion of the data to complex theories covering the whole area of inquiry. There are, of course, no rules dictating which level of theory is most appropriate at a given stage of inquiry, but it is not unreasonable to suppose that one will go astray if one jumps from simple data to some high-level theory instead of progressing through intermediate levels of generalization.[16] In fact, I believe the history of moral theory suggests that moral philosophy has been operating in a fundamentally incorrect fashion because full-scale systematizations (such as utilitarianism) have emerged long before we have had successful lower-level moral generalizations. (2) A theory need not account for all the data in its area in order to be successful. Some data can be reassigned to another area, some can be left as anomalies to be dealt with later on, and some can be redescribed and/or totally rejected. As moral systematizations are put forward, they should not be rejected merely because they cannot account for some of the data (some of the moral intuitions). Like the data, these recalcitrant intuitions can be reassigned to another area, left as problems for further inquiry, or even redescribed or totally rejected. The question of when this strategy becomes a dead end requiring that we reject the proposed systematization is a very complex one for moral epistemology. It may be of some consolation to note that the same problem arises in the methodology of the hard sciences.[17] (3) One purpose of developing these moral theories is to have a theory from which we can derive judgments about cases where we have difficulty forming intuitions. To the extent that our theory provides results that seem intuitively acceptable at this later stage, the theory is confirmed. Indeed, this is even more powerful evidence for the theory than is its ability to systematize already-formed intuitions.

What does all of this mean for the arguments put forward in this book to justify the pluralistic model of conflicting values? It means that we shall not be arguing directly for the theoretical structure to be presented in chapters 2 through 4. In those chapters I will certainly note the fundamental features of that structure and will contrast it with other views. But the defense of this theoretical approach will come in chapters 5 through 7, when I apply it to forty difficult cases. To the extent that the theoretical structure described in chapters 2 through 4 helps us deal with these hard cases in what seems at the end an intuitively satisfactory fashion, we will have confirmed the theory. To the extent that it does not, this will count as evidence against the moral theory being developed.

One final methodological point should be noted here. Readers may find one or another of the case resolutions unsatisfactory. They may be willing to accept the theoretical structure and treat those cases as anomalies upon which further work is needed. If not, however, then the methodology suggests that those readers should go back and reexamine the portions of the complex model of conflicting appeals that led to what they take to be an unsatisfactory result. The model, as we shall see, lends itself to a wide variety of modifications. Readers unconvinced by the treatment of some cases may therefore consider how those aspects can be modified to fit more closely with their intuitions about these hard cases. We need to treat the development of complex moral theories, like the development of complex scientific theories, as a tentative process, where there is room for continued comparison of intuitions in particular cases with general moral judgments and room for continued modifications of the theory.

### Notes

1. This is illustrated very clearly in the enthusiasm of the two classical articles introducing cardiopulmonary resuscitation: W. B. Kouwenhoven and J. R. Jude, "Closed Chest Cardiac Massage," *Journal of the American Medical Association (JAMA)* 173, no. 10 (July 9, 1960); and J. R. Jude, W. B. Kouwenhoven, and G. G. Knickerbocker, "Cardiac Arrest," *JAMA* 178, no. 11 (Dec. 16, 1961).

2. Some of the classical articles making this point include "Optimum Care for Hopelessly Ill Patients: A Report of the Clinical Care Committee of the Mass. General Hospital," *New England Journal of Medicine (NEJM)* 295, no. 6 (August 12, 1976); A. Grenvik, D. J. Powner, J. V. Snyder, M. S. Jastremski, R. A. Babcock, and M. G. Loughread, "Cessation of Therapy in Terminal Illness and Brain Death," *Critical Care Medicine* 6, no. 4 (July–August 1978); and "Standards and Guidelines for Cardiopulmonary Resuscitation and Emergency Cardiac Care: A Report of a Consensus Conference," *JAMA* 244, no. 5 (August 1, 1980). The crucial initial court cases were In re *Quinlan*, 355 A. 2d 647; and In re *Dinnerstein*, 380 N.E. 2d 134. This whole approach was summarized and reinforced in the President's Commission for the Study of Ethical Problems in Medicine and Biomedical and Behavioral Research, *Deciding to Forego Life-Sustaining Treatment* (Washington, D.C.: Government Printing Office: 1983).

3. A similar complaint against the dominance of the procedural issue over the substantive issues is voiced in C. D. Clements and R. C. Sider, "Medical Ethics' Assault upon Medical Values," *JAMA* 250, no. 15 (Oct. 21, 1983). While I agree with their complaint, I do not agree with their positive approach, which is a variant of the status model I criticize in chapter 3.

4. I'm not sure where this view has been formally expressed in the literature. However, it is the sort of thing many clinicians say when opposing the formal teaching of medical ethics in the medical-school curriculum.

5. Arthur Caplan, in "Can Applied Ethics Be Effective in Health Care and Should It Strive to Be," *Ethics* 93, no. 2 (January 1983), has usefully dubbed the theory-application model of applied ethics "the engineering model." His own objections to that approach deal more with other issues than the problem of how to apply the theory, although he is somewhat concerned about the deductive structure of that model. See, by way of contrast, a defense of a very deductive structure in A. Donagan, *Theory of Morality* (Chicago: Univ. of Chicago Press, 1977), section 2.5.

6. The case of a man who is contemplating suicide because of despair over a series of misfortunes, the case of a man contemplating borrowing money with a promise to repay even though he knows that he will not be able to do so, the case of a man who is contemplating a life of leisure rather than self-development, and the case of a man refusing to aid others in need. See *Fundamental Principles* (1785), section II.

7. See, for example, Kant's precritical *Lectures on Ethics,* trans. L. Infeld (London: Macmillan, 1930), and the much later *Metaphysics of Morals,* 1st ed. (1797) and 2nd ed. (1798).

8. See the many concrete suggestions in J. Bentham, *Introduction to the Principles of Morals and Legislation* (1789), and J. S. Mill, *Principles of Political Economy.*

9. This is the point, for example, of W. D. Ross's summary of his criticisms of utilitarianism in his *The Right and the Good* (Oxford: Clarendon Press, 1930), pp. 24–28. It is also the point of utilitarian critiques of nonutilitarian theories. See, for example, Jonathan Glover's discussion of the right to life in his *Causing Death and Saving Lives* (New York: Penguin Books, 1977), pp. 83–85.

10. This strategy is nicely illustrated in J. J. C. Smart's classical paper, "Extreme and Restricted Utilitarianism," *Philosophical Quarterly* 6 (1956). A recent, very sophisticated version of this approach is found in L. W. Sumner, "Utilitarian Goals and Kantian Constraints," in B. A. Brody, ed., *Moral Theory and Moral Judgments* (Dordrecht: Reidel, 1988).

11. A similar criticism of this traditional approach, but without a commitment to developing a pluralistic theory, is found in B. Williams, *Ethics and the Limits of Philosophy* (Cambridge: Harvard Univ. Press, 1985), who says: "If there is such a thing as the truth about the subject matter of ethics—the truth, we might say, about the ethical—why is there any expectation that it should be simple? In particular, why should it be conceptually simple, using only one or two ethical concepts, such as *duty* or *good state of affairs,* rather than many? . . . I shall claim that in ethics the reductive enterprise has no justification and should disappear. . . . A good deal of moral philosophy engages unblinkingly in this activity, for no obvious reason except that it has been going on for a long time" (p. 17).

12. B. A. Brody, "Intuitions and Objective Moral Knowledge," *The Monist* 62, no. 4 (October 1979).

13. That traditional metaethical discussion is helpfully anthologized in P. W. Taylor, *The Moral Judgment: Readings in Contemporary Meta-ethics* (Englewood Cliffs, N.J.: Prentice-Hall, 1963).

14. This is true both of such classical intuitionists as William Whewell in his *Elements of Morality* (1846) and of neo-intuitionists such as W. D. Ross in his *The Right and the Good* (Oxford: Clarendon Press, 1930). My criticism is a modification of the one given by H. Sidgwick in *Methods of Ethics* (London: Macmillan, 1907), book III, chaps. 2–10. It only applies to the classical version; we shall return to Ross's theory in chapter 4. On the distinction between the two approaches, see A. Donagan, *The Theory of Morality* (Chicago: Univ. of Chicago Press, 1977), section 1.3.

15. Note that there is no appeal to intuitions about these general principles. This is in contrast to J. Rawls, *A Theory of Justice* (Cambridge, Mass.: Harvard Univ. Press, 1971),

who says on p. 48: "When a person is presented with an intuitively appealing account of his sense of justice (one, say, which embodies various reasonable and natural presumptions), he may well revise his judgments to conform to its principles even though the theory does not fit his existing judgments exactly." It seems that in all those cases in which we have some moral rule that Rawls thinks of as intuitively appealing, we also have many particular intuitions which that rule, in the process of theory formation, might systematize. So we can explain, without postulating any general intuitions, why this theory can be used as the basis for rejecting particular intuitions.

16. J. S. Mill, in chapter 1 of *Utilitarianism,* notes that traditional moral theory differs from scientific theory in that it quickly moves to a high-level theory without first developing intermediate levels of generalization. Apparently, it did not occur to him that this might be a mistake.

17. The writings of authors such as Lakatos testify to the difficulties of this question even in the natural sciences. See, for example, I. Lakatos, *Philosophical Papers: The Methodology of Scientific Research Programs* (Cambridge Univ. Press, Cambridge: 1978), vol. I.

# 2

## Major Ethical Appeals

In this chapter I begin to set out an ethical framework for dealing with the many difficult questions raised by the cases to be presented in chapters 5 through 7. In particular, I introduce the wide variety of legitimate moral appeals mentioned in chapter 1 that must be incorporated into any such framework.

No attempt will be made to set out the fundamental premises of an ethical theory from which one can derive the legitimacy of these moral appeals. As explained in section 1.4, all we will be doing is delineating an ethical framework whose validity is to be established by the intuitively satisfactory consequences derived in chapters 5 through 7. I will try to explain what is involved in each of these appeals and compare my account of them to the account given by other authors. But the validation of my account will only be found in the way it works in resolving specific cases.

### 2.1 The Appeal to the Consequences of Our Actions

The first appeal to consider as we contemplate alternative courses of action is the appeal to the consequences of our actions. This is the appeal emphasized by utilitarian writers in particular and consequentialists in general. However much it may seem that these theories are wrong in reducing all of morality to producing good consequences, it nevertheless is true that an appeal to the consequences of our actions must play an important role in evaluating those actions. All other things being equal, the favorable consequences of an action are good reasons for performing that action, even if not always conclusive reasons, and the bad consequences of an action are good reasons for not performing the action, even if one nevertheless might in some cases have better reasons for doing it anyway.

Sir W. D. Ross, one of the great nonconsequentialist pluralistic thinkers of this century, argued that in building an appeal to consequences into a pluralistic theory one must assign greater significance to nonmaleficence (the avoidance of bad consequences) than to beneficence (the production of good consequences).[1] T. L. Beauchamp and J. Childress continue this tradition, although they distinguish nonmaleficence (avoiding inflicting evil or harm) from three types of beneficence (preventing harm, removing evil, and promoting good).[2] These distinctions, while legitimate, seem to have nothing to do with the appeal to consequences. The usual examples of maleficence include actual infringements of rights (e.g., the right not to be killed) as well as the production of harm, and the greater stringency of nonmaleficence is no doubt due to that fact. From the perspective of the appeal to consequences, there is no difference in significance between nonmaleficence and beneficence, and we can simply speak of performing the actions with the best consequences as beneficial behavior.

In the medical context there are several different bases for appealing to a consideration of the consequences of one's actions. One is the general moral fact, just pointed out, that actions which have good consequences are better to perform than actions that have bad consequences. This general moral fact holds in the medical context. A second basis is the implicit understanding between patients and health-care providers. Patients seek out health-care providers because they believe they will be in a position to help them and those they care about with their problems. Physicians and other health-care providers who accept the care of these patients are therefore in a contractual relationship with those patients and have a contractual obligation to act in ways that benefit them and others they care about. Finally, health-care professionals have committed themselves to be helping and healing agents for individual patients. There is, therefore, a professional obligation to act in ways that are beneficial to patients.

It is important, I believe, to separate these three bases of appealing to consequences when health-care providers are trying to act in ways that are beneficial. In many of the cases with which we will be concerned, one of the crucial questions is, to whom should the health-care provider try to act in a beneficial manner—the patient, the family, or society? Their interests, after all, are not necessarily identical. I think that question, which has often been raised, is badly framed because people have not attended to the distinctions just drawn.[3] To the extent that the health-care provider, all other things being equal, is supposed to do what is beneficial as part of a general moral commitment, the health-care provider needs to consider the consequences of his or her actions for all those affected (in the same way that every person, as part of his or her moral decision making, needs to consider the consequences of his or her actions for all those affected). To the extent that the health-care provider, all other things being equal, is supposed to do what is beneficial as part of a special contractual relationship with the patient, the health-care provider needs to consider the consequences of his or her actions on all those people about whom the patient is concerned and whom the patient wishes the health-care provider to consider. This may be just the patient, or it may be the patient and his or her family and close friends. To the extent that the health-care provider, all other things being equal, is supposed to do what is beneficial as part of the professional ethic of the health-care professions, which addresses itself specifically to the obligations of health-care providers to care for their patients, the health-care provider needs to consider the consequences of his or her actions just for his or her patients.

Much of moral philosophy has debated the question of egoism versus altruism, the question of whose interests need to be considered as we evaluate the consequences of our actions.[4] It is, I suppose, widely believed that altruism has won the day and that we need to consider the consequences of our actions for everyone.[5] I believe that this is both correct in one sense and fundamentally in error in another sense. It is correct in that in deciding which actions are right and which actions are wrong people need to consider, as one moral appeal, the appeal to the consequences of their actions for all those affected. That is, however, perfectly compatible with insisting that some people, including health-care providers, have to take an additional look at the consequences of their actions as part of other moral appeals involving consequences. They may be contractually required to pay special attention to the consequences of their actions only for those people with whom their patient is concerned. They may, as patient helpers, be required to consider the implications of their actions just for the patient. So, for health-care providers, there is no unambiguous answer to the question of whose interests they need to consider. Much debate has been expended on this question, and my point is that it is a pseudo-question. In short, the appeal to consequences in the case of health-care providers and their actions is really three different appeals. Not surprisingly, these appeals may lead to different results in some cases.

Another question that always arises when one talks about the appeal to the consequences of an action is how to evaluate those consequences. It is possible to distinguish three major theories:

*Hedonism.* Consequences should ultimately be evaluated solely in terms of pleasure and pain. All other consequences are good only insofar as they lead to pleasure, and all other consequences are bad only insofar as they lead to pain.

*Preference-satisfaction theory.* Consequences should ultimately be evaluated solely in terms of the satisfaction of preferences. When an action leads to the satisfaction of a preference of someone affected by the action, then that is a good consequence of the action. When an action leads to the frustration of a preference of someone affected by the action, then that is a bad consequence of the action.

*Objective-good theories.* There is a set of consequences whose occurrence is good for those affected whether or not they want those consequences to occur and whether or not they derive pleasure from their occurrence. These objective goods are the basis for the evaluation of consequences. When an action leads to the occurrence of one of these objective goods, then that is a good consequence of the action. When an action leads to its nonoccurrence, then that is a bad consequence of the action.[6]

In this book I adopt the preference-satisfaction theory. Unlike hedonism, the preference-satisfaction theory recognizes that human beings have many preferences besides the preference for pleasure and the absence of pain and that the satisfaction of these preferences is of value independently of any pleasure the satisfaction produces. Hedonists must suppose either that our only preference is for pleasure and the absence of pain or that the satisfaction of these other preferences is of no value. The former supposition is too narrow a view of human nature, and the latter seems arbitrary. Unlike objective-good theories, the preference-satisfaction theory recognizes that human beings vary in their preferences and that the satisfaction of these different preferences are of equal value. Objective-good theorists must suppose either that there is a set of goods that all people "really do desire" or that we can establish what is "really good" for people independently of what they desire. The former view seems implausible, and the latter requires a proof that has not yet been forthcoming.[7] In short, the preference-satisfaction theory's virtue is that it takes seriously the diversity and equal significance of the preferences (values) of distinct human beings. For this reason, it has also come to be called, particularly in the economic literature, the view of consumer sovereignty.

Two types of preferences tempt one to modify the theory of consumer sovereignty: preferences with "immoral content"[8] and preferences formed by "pathologic processes."[9] Consider, for example, the family member who hates the patient and whose preference is that the physician fail in the attempt to cure the patient so that the patient will suffer and then die. Are we required to say that such a failure has as one of its consequences the good result that that malevolent preference is satisfied? Even if the failure is in the end judged to have led overall to bad consequences because of the terrible consequences to the patient, it seems objectionable to say that it has at least some good results because this malevolent family member is satisfied with the outcome. Consider, as a second example, the very disabled patient whose preferences have become so minimal because of his difficult life that they are easily satisfied by what we would view as trivialities. Shall we say that such a patient is not benefited when other things most of us would view as good occur to him, simply because his downtrodden condition has led to a process of desire formation which is so pathologic that he had no hopes that such a thing might occur, had formed no preferences that it would occur, and didn't even enjoy it while it was happening?

Various attempts have been made to construct a modified preference-satisfaction theory which only counts preferences with acceptable contents or preferences formed by appropriate processes.[10] This is not the place to evaluate all of them, but my judgment is that none has succeeded and that, at least for the moment, we need to operate with an unmodified theory of consumer sovereignty. We need to be sensitive, however, to the possibility that this might lead us astray when we consider the cases in chapters 5 through 7.

There remains an additional set of issues raised by the adoption of the theory of consumer sovereignty based on the fact that people's preferences vary over time.[11] Individuals affected by our actions may have one set of preferences before we perform our actions, a second set of preferences at the time when we perform those actions, and a final very different set of preferences at a much later period of time when the effects of our actions are finally felt by them. Which of their preferences should count as we evaluate our actions by appealing to their consequences? My view, which I hope will be supported by its implications for dealing with our cases, is that we should always count the preferences relevant to a particular consequence which were held closest to the time of the occurrence of that consequence.

Consider decisions about the forms of care to be provided to newborn patients currently suffering from many problems. If we succeed in improving their condition, then they may be able to live lives in which they can satisfy many preferences which they will then have but which they don't now have (because they are too young to have such preferences). That means that an appeal to the consequences of our actions supports, at least to some extent, treating them to improve their condition. Or consider the case of elderly patients who recognize the worsening of their mental status and who prefer not to be kept alive aggressively once they become very senile. If they don't change their minds before they become too senile (a state in which, presumably, they have no preferences about the abstract question of continued existence), then that preference is the one that counts.[12] An appeal to the consequences of our actions will then support, to some extent, a nonaggressive approach to their health care, just because keeping them alive aggressively will frustrate their last relevant desires.

This last point introduces a role that the families and friends of patients may play in helping us make decisions about the treatment of patients. We will sometimes be unable to find out directly from individuals what their preferences are. They may be unable to tell us, they may be unwilling to tell us, we may not trust what they tell us, and so on. In such cases, those who know the individuals in question may be able to testify reliably to their preferences, and that testimony will be crucial in deciding what is implied by the appeal to consequences as it relates to those individuals.

In short, then, this book adopts the view of consumer sovereignty, the view that it is those final relevant preferences of individual human beings before consequences occur to them which are the basis of our evaluation as we appeal to the consequences of our actions in determining what is right or wrong. An important confusion often follows adoption of the approach of consumer sovereignty. To say that the evaluation of consequences depends on the preferences of the people affected is not to say that (other things being equal) we are supposed to do what they want us to do. The people affected may want us to act in a certain way because they believe it will lead to the greatest satisfaction of their preferences. We, however, may be in a position to see that, in fact, an alternative course of action will actually lead to the satisfaction of more of their preferences. Contrary to J. S. Mill,[13] people can often be mistaken about which actions lead to what they want. This point may be especially relevant in medical decision-making contexts where, out of ignorance or fear or confusion, patients may often have mistaken views about what course of action will lead to the results they want for themselves. In appealing to the consequences of an action, even if we adopt the consumer sovereignty approach, we are not required to follow these mistaken beliefs. We are only required to determine which courses of action will lead to what the individuals desire, and that may be a very different matter in many cases.

One cautionary remark: many people have a preference that their decisions be respected, even if respecting them leads to other bad results.[14] This preference must also be taken into account, and it sometimes may lead us to decide that, from the perspective of the appeal to the consequences of an action, we ought to do what the person in question wants us to do. Whether it will lead us to that result depends on how strong that preference is in comparison with the other relevant preferences of the person in question.

In any case, none of this by itself determines what health-care providers ought to do in a given case, for appealing to the consequences of our actions is only one of the many things we need to do in deciding what is right.

## 2.2   The Appeal to Rights

The second appeal to be considered is the appeal to the rights of the parties involved in or affected by the actions. This is a very complex appeal, but it is absolutely essential as part of any framework for dealing with difficult ethical issues.

Many have difficulty understanding what it is for someone to have a right.[15] This notion is relatively unproblematic, because, as far as I am concerned, saying that someone has a right can be understood by use of the following matrix:

> X has a right to Y against Z if and only if (just in case) Z has an obligation (not necessarily an overriding obligation) to X not to deprive X of Y or not to withhold Y from X.

Rights are relationships between people which exist as correlatives of obligations. There has been considerable discussion in the history of moral philosophy about whether or not all rights have correlative obligations.[16] Some have challenged that claim and provided putative counterexamples. I believe that there are such correlative obligations even in those putative cases, but I need not defend that thesis here, since all the rights with which we will be concerned can be covered without difficulty by the above matrix.

A failure to understand a number of points about the basic logic of rights is one of the reasons why people misapply the concept of rights to difficult moral problems. The first point is that rights are always waivable. In other words, the obligation that Z has to X is an obligation of which X can relieve Z. When X waives that right, Z no longer has the obligation to X vis-à-vis Y. To use a very simple example, if I have lent you some money which you are supposed to return to me on a given day, then I have a right to that money on that day, which means that you have an obligation not to withhold that money from me on that day. If, however, I waive that right, then you no longer have the obligation to pay me on that day. There are those who have spoken of some rights (e.g., the right to be free) as inalienable.[17] By that, they seem to mean in part that there are some rights that cannot be waived. I cannot accept such a claim; it turns a right into something you are stuck with, and that is not the proper way of understanding rights. I think the point can be better understood in a different way. The people who think of freedom as an inalienable right want to rule out the moral legitimacy of voluntary slavery. One can make that point more effectively by arguing that the slaveholder acts wrongly even if he doesn't violate the rights of the voluntary slave. There are, after all, many other things wrong with slavery. This approach seems superior to the idea that rights are burdens with which we are stuck.

It is important to distinguish individuals who freely waive their rights from other individuals who involuntarily lose their rights because of their behavior. However difficult it may be to develop a full understanding of self-defense, it seems to involve aggressors involuntarily losing some of their rights; it certainly does *not* involve their waiving those rights.

A second point about the logic of rights is that they are not absolute. Suppose I have a right to Y against you. According to the matrix presented above, that means that you have an obligation to me not to deprive me of Y or not to withhold Y from me. There is no reason to suppose that the obligation you have to me is absolute. That obligation which you have to me may be overridden by more pressing moral appeals. In that case, my right is also overridden. To continue the example of my right to be repaid on a given day the money that I lent you, suppose that on that day you have the money but require it for some other morally more pressing purpose (e.g., to buy needed food for your family). Your obligation to feed your family may take precedence over your obligation to repay me.

It is important to note here that when nonabsolute rights are overridden they do not disappear.[18] Suppose once more that my right to have the money repaid is overridden by your more pressing obligations. While you should not then fulfill your obligation to return my money, your failure to do so means that you now have a new obligation, namely to repay me as soon as you can (that is to say, as soon as you have the funds and other more pressing obligations are no longer present). When rights and their correlative obligations are overridden because of more pressing obligations, new obligations are created by way of making up for the failure to carry out the earlier obligations.

The third crucial point about the logic of rights is that some rights are more fundamental than others. Put another way, some rights have greater moral force than others. How shall we give content to the concept of greater moral force? I think our previous point puts us in a position to do this. To say that right A has greater moral force than right B is to say that there are factors that may override B but do not override A, and not vice versa. Thus, the fact that my right to that money on a given day is a less powerful moral right than my right not to be killed on that day means, among other things, that the factors that will justify your withholding the money from me on that day (your family's needs) will not justify your killing me.

It is often said that respecting rights is more important than the pursuit of good consequences.[19] This is understandable, although, put that way, it is an unacceptable view. The utilitarians emphasized the pursuit of good consequences to such a great degree that they seemed to allow us to perform actions that might lead to good consequences even though they result in infringing upon people's rights. It seemed that utilitarianism would justify killing innocent human beings or enslaving them in certain circumstances where the consequences to other people might be very beneficial. Those who noticed this objected to utilitarianism precisely on the grounds that it failed to take into account the significance of human rights.[20] All of this is correct. However, many were misled into drawing the equally extreme conclusion that any right must be respected regardless of the cost to the general well-being, that a consideration of the consequences of our actions can never take precedence over a consideration of rights. We need to reject this extreme alternative to utilitarianism. Some rights may be so strong that it will rarely, if ever, be the case that a consideration of consequences can take precedence over them. However, most rights can be violated if the consequences to other people of respecting them are sufficiently bad. What was wrong with utilitarianism was that it allowed one to violate any right whenever the general well-being was promoted even to the slightest degree by violating that right. This is a mistake; it is equally a mistake to say that we can never violate any rights in the pursuit of very good consequences.[21]

Rights are not mysterious entities. They are the correlatives of the obligations that people have to each other. When you have an obligation to me either to give me Y or, alternatively, not to deprive me of Y, then I have a right against you to Y. My right and your corresponding obligation is waivable, is not necessarily absolute, and may be weaker or stronger than other rights.

These last points are extremely important. The appeal to the consequences of our actions is a crucial part of correct moral decision making. The appeal to rights is a crucial part of correct moral decision making. Other appeals, to be discussed below, are also crucial parts of correct moral decision making. No one factor takes precedence in all cases over the others. The complex web of morality is not structured in such a simple fashion. That is why we must keep in mind that different rights have different moral force and that none of them is absolute.

In a systematic treatise on moral philosophy it would be necessary to say a lot more about the general structure of rights. For our purposes, however, these preliminary observations should be sufficient. I turn, then, to a presentation of a number of rights that will be extremely important in the medical context: the right not to be killed, the right not to have bodily injury or pain inflicted on oneself, the right to be aided against threats to one's life or health, the right to make decisions in cases where the actions decided upon affect oneself, and the right to participate in decision making in cases where the actions decided upon will affect members of one's family.

The right not to be killed is part (but only part) of what is normally referred to as the right to life. When we put this right into the form of the matrix presented above, we get the following:

X has a right not to be killed against everyone since everyone has an obligation to X not to deprive X of X's life (where that means not to cause the loss of X's life).

Notice that on this analysis the crucial point is that one violates X's right not to be killed when one causes the death of X.

Causality is a very difficult concept. A tremendous legal and philosophical literature has been devoted to developing a theory of causality; despite these many attempts, no satisfactory theory has emerged.[22] Some, the American legal realists, have concluded that causality is not a concept that we can fruitfully use in making decisions.[23] It can be used, they say, only to articulate conclusions that have been reached on other grounds. This skepticism about causality is understandable in light of the failure until now to articulate a satisfactory theory of causality. It must nevertheless be rejected; causality is too crucial a notion for every aspect of the theory of rights. As Eric Mack has rightly pointed out, any claim that an action is impermissible because it violates someone's rights involves the presupposition that the action in question causes the loss of that to which the person in question has a right.[24] If we are to appeal to rights in deciding which actions are morally permissible, we must presuppose that we can make causal judgments even if we have no adequately articulated theory of causality.

Some have suggested that causality is less important than intentionality.[25] They are presumably claiming either (1) that we only kill X when we intentionally cause X's death or (2) that we can kill X when we intend X's death even if our action only contributes to, but is not the cause of, X's death. The former claim is shown to be wrong by the existence of unintended killings (e.g., negligent killings). The latter claim is not as easy to dismiss; it has profound implications, moreover, for some of our cases. We shall return to those implications in a moment.

Given the analysis both of killing and of the right not to be killed, that right is not going to be relevant in a large number of cases that raise the question of whether or not to commence or to continue treating a terminal illness. In most of those cases we will not be causing the loss of the patient's life even if we fail to commence or to continue treatment, since the cause of the patient's loss of life will still be his or her underlying disease or disorder. We may or may not be under an obligation to prolong the life of some of those patients in particular cases. That issue will be discussed further as we examine cases in chapters 5 through 7. But one thing we already know is that the right not to be killed cannot be the basis of our obligation to prolong life in most of those cases. It will only be relevant in those cases, if any, in which our failure to act can properly be identified as the cause of the patient's death.[26]

Notice how different things would be if we adopted the view that we can kill someone if we intend that person's death and if our action (or inaction) contributes to that person's death, even if it is not its cause. On that account, we would have killed the patients in all those cases in which we wanted the death and in which we failed to commence or to continue treatment. That would mean either that a great deal of killing is morally permissible or that we are required to treat a very large number of terminally ill patients so as to avoid killing them. It is far more plausible to adopt our strictly causal theory of killing.

The right not to be killed is, like all other rights, waivable. There is an immediate and highly controversial implication of this point: suicide and active voluntary euthanasia (cases in which the patient has requested that his or her life be taken) do not violate this aspect of the patient's right to life.[27] Because the patient can waive the right not to be killed, the patient who commits suicide, or the physician or family member who actively causes the death of a patient who competently requests that his or her life be taken, cannot be violating either the obligation not to kill the patient or the patient's right to life. This is not to say that either suicide or active voluntary euthanasia is always or even sometimes morally permissible. There may be other moral appeals that lead us to conclude otherwise. It is merely to say that the aspect of the right to life which we refer to as the right not to be killed cannot be the moral basis for objecting either to suicide or to active voluntary euthanasia. We must remember our earlier discussion of voluntary slavery. Neither life nor freedom is an inalienable right; if there are moral objections either to voluntary slavery or to voluntary euthanasia, they must be on grounds other than the violation of the rights of the person in question.

The right not to be killed is an extremely strong right. There are few, if any, moral appeals that take precedence over it. The rights to self-defense or to punish are often suggested, even though they rarely arise in the medical context, but self-defense and punishment involve a loss of rights and not the precedence of other appeals. It has sometimes been suggested that another appeal which might take precedence over the right not to be killed is the possibility of saving the lives of many by killing one innocent person.[28] While philosophers have delighted in creating many fascinating stories to raise this point (killing one innocent, for example, to harvest many organs to save many lives), I see few medical contexts in which it has any practical relevance, and I am not convinced by any of those examples. In the context of medical decision making, it is hard to imagine circumstances in which anything takes precedence over this very fundamental right.

One final point: I assume in this book that the right not to be killed is possessed by all living members of our species. Since this point is so crucial for much of the analysis in chapters 5 through 7, let me elaborate and show how it differs from the views of other authors.

At least all of the following views have been held by influential writers:[29]

(a)  Living members of many species, and not just members of our species, have a right not to be killed. To suppose otherwise is to commit a form of speciesism:[30]

(b)  All living members of our species have a right not to be killed. We may not be required to strive to keep all of them alive, but, absent their consent, we would be violating one of their rights by killing them:[31]

(c)  Only some members of our species have a right not to be killed. These are those who fulfill the additional requirements for being a person. There may be various moral reasons against killing nonpersons, but the right not to be killed cannot be one of those reasons.[32]

Naturally, the differences among these views—and there are many variations of each—have profound implications for such diverse issues as animal experimentation, abortion, and the treatment of the terminally ill.

The view I adopt in this book is of type b. Its defense, given our general moral epistemology, rests upon the way it will help us in chapters 5 through 7. Let me say just a little to motivate it, at least against views of type c. First, most will agree that as long as a patient is still alive there are some constraints on what we can do to that patient (we cannot, without the patient's permission, inject the patient with potassium chloride), no matter how bad the patient's condition. These constraints are, moreover, serious ones. The best explanation of this is to suppose that the patient's right not to be killed remains in place, and that claim c in any of its forms is mistaken.[33] Second, as we shall see below, there are crucial ways in which the question of personhood is relevant to the assessment of other moral appeals. To adopt view b is not, therefore, to deny the moral significance of the distinction between persons and living human beings.

The second right with which we shall be concerned is the right not to have bodily injury or pain inflicted on oneself. That right, expressed in our matrix, comes to the following:

> X has a right against everyone not to have bodily injury or pain inflicted on X since everyone is under an obligation not to diminish X's current state of bodily integrity and comfort.

The crucial point is that one violates this right when one causes the diminishment of the current state of bodily integrity or comfort. Therefore, like the right not to be killed, this right will rarely be the basis for an obligation to commence or to continue treating an illness. Usually, if one fails to commence or to continue treatment, the underlying disease or disorder causes the resulting diminishment; one's failure does not. There may be other moral reasons why one is required to commence or to continue treatment, but this particular right cannot be that basis except in those cases in which the failure to treat is the cause of the diminishment.

It is important to note that this right, like all other rights, is waivable. We often for good reasons allow physicians to perform procedures that inflict pain on us, and we sometimes even allow physicians to perform procedures that diminish our bodily integrity (e.g., an amputation to save a life). Why doesn't the action of the physician violate this right of the patient? Presumably, because the patient has agreed. This is why the waivability of this right is an important concept.

It might be suggested that we could justify such actions when the patient does not agree (because the patient is incompetent or unconscious) by appealing to some hypothetical waiving of rights, to the suggestion that the patient would waive those rights if he or she could.[34] This might be so, although one might accept these cases as violations of the patient's rights which are justified on other grounds, such as the positive benefits to the patient. The appeal to hypothetical consent may only reflect an unwillingness to accept the idea that benefits to individuals can take precedence over rights in some cases.

The third right to consider is the right to be aided against threats to one's life or health. The claim that there is such a right is highly controversial; many have argued that this right doesn't exist.[35] They have claimed that while it may be a good thing for people to come to the aid of others in life- or health-threatening situations, there is no obligation to do so. This was the tradition of the common law.[36] It is not, however, the position I adopt. My position is that there is a definite but limited right to be aided against threats to one's life or health. The justification for this will be, of course, that it helps us deal with our cases. In order to spell out the nature of this right, it is helpful to put it into our matrix:

> X has a right to be aided in life- or health-threatening situations against those who are capable of aiding X just because those who are capable of aiding X have an obligation to X not to withhold this aid from X.

Who those people are and how much they are obliged to do are questions that arise to a far greater degree here than in connection with the other rights, and I discuss them more fully in chapter 4.

This right is, of course, significant in the context of emergency decision making; it is one of the foundations of the moral obligation to aid people in such situations. This is not a right that people have only against physicians and other health-care providers; it is a right that they have against everyone, since everyone who is capable of doing so has an obligation to provide the aid in question. This right has special implications for health-care providers only because they are often the people most capable, and sometimes the only people capable, of helping.

This right is also the foundation of many of the obligations of providers to commence and to continue treating patients. This differentiates it from the other two rights. Note, however, that it is only present when the treatment actually aids or has a significant probability of aiding the patient. Moreover, this right, like other rights, can be waived. The provider's obligation to treat is no longer supported by an appeal to this right when the patient waives his or her right to the aid. In other words, an appeal to this right is a possible foundation for the obligation of providers to treat patients, but not when the treatment is no longer an aid to the patient and not when the patient no longer wishes it.

The first three rights are substantive rights, rights that relate to decisions about what should or should not be done to someone. We now turn to a number of procedural rights, rights that concern decisional processes rather than their outcomes.

The first procedural right is the right to make decisions about what health care one will receive. This right has been extensively discussed in recent years, but it has been badly misunderstood by both those who advocate it and those who oppose it.[37] We will need to be very careful in our definition of this right if we are to make any progress in this area.

The most crucial step in clarifying the nature and extent of this right is distinguishing two sorts of cases in which it might be invoked. The first is the case in which a health-care provider wishes to treat a patient in a certain way and the patient does not wish to receive that form of medical treatment. The second is the case in which the health-care provider is opposed to a form of treatment and it is the patient who is requesting that treatment despite the opposition of the health-care provider. These two cases should be analyzed very differently.

In the first case, it seems clear that a competent adult patient (these concepts will be defined in chapter 5) has a right to decide either to accept the recommendation of the health-care provider or to refuse that recommendation and not be treated in that manner. This right to refuse treatment is rooted in the idea that each person is entitled to determine what will be done to his or her body. This right to refuse treatment is distinct from the right not to have bodily injury or pain inflicted on oneself, since it applies even when what will be done involves no pain or bodily injury. It is nevertheless related, since both rights are rooted in this fundamental intuition that we are entitled to control what is done to our bodies.

We can define this right in accordance with our matrix as follows:

> X has a right against everyone to refuse recommended medical treatment, since everyone is under an obligation to X not to take this decisional authority away from X.

This right, like all other rights, can be waived. Not everyone, after all, wants to be a decision maker.[38] This is true in many contexts and may be particularly true in the medical context. Patients may feel emotionally incapable of making difficult decisions at a time of illness, and they may have sufficient trust in their health-care providers to want the providers to assume that authority for them. Patients may feel intellectually incompetent to make some difficult decisions and may wish to leave them in the hands of health-care providers who know better about difficult medical and technical questions. There may be other motives that lead patients to avoid decisional authority. We may positively or negatively evaluate this decision on the part of the patient not to be a decision maker. The crucial point, however, is that the patient, as an autonomous individual, can waive this right to be a decision maker and can put decisional authority in the hands of the health-care provider.

Suppose, however, that the patient does wish to maintain decisional authority. He or she certainly has a right to do so. In order to do so effectively, however, the patient is going to need a wide range of information about the available options, their comparative benefits and costs, and so on. The information the patient is going to need, for the most part, will only be available with the help of the health-care provider. This practical reality (and not the right of the patient to refuse care) has led to the legal requirement of informed consent.[39]

Physicians often claim that the legal requirement of obtaining informed consent is irrelevant and meaningless.[40] They are certainly right in the case of those many patients who do not wish to be decisional authorities; in such cases the providers obtaining informed consent as required by law instead of simply obtaining documentation of the transfer of decisional authority are engaged in a meaningless procedure. If, however, the patient is one of those who wish to retain decisional authority, then that argument is not applicable. Other providers object to the current requirements of informed consent because they find it burdensome.[41] My own view is that providers who find this sufficiently burdensome are certainly free to confine their practices to patients who are willing to transfer decisional authority to them, as long as this is made clear in advance. However, to the extent that providers are willing to take on patients who wish to retain their decisional authority, they cannot object to accepting the accompanying burden of providing relevant information. Finally, some providers object to the current requirement on the grounds that the information to be provided is too complex.[42] This only demonstrates the need to clarify what is essential and what is not.[43]

Finally, this right, like all other rights, may be overridden. One set of circumstances that may justify overriding it is where the patient will suffer irreversible grave losses if the recommended form of treatment is not provided. This is particularly the case when harm will also occur to others, such as the patient's family. Naturally, this exception needs to be invoked sparingly, because the right to be a decision maker is an important right. Still, rights are not absolute, and there will be circumstances in which a consideration of consequences takes precedence over this right, like any other. Exactly what these circumstances are will emerge more fully in chapters 5 through 7. But there is no reason to adopt what seems to be the emerging legal view that the right in question can never be overridden.[44]

In the second set of cases an individual requests a certain form of treatment and the health-care provider believes that this form of treatment is inappropriate. Here the balance of rights shifts radically. Health-care providers also have rights. One of them is the right to decide what they want to do and to act on those decisions as long as their decisions or actions do not infringe on the rights of others. When a health-care provider believes that certain forms of treatment are inappropriate and is firmly committed to not providing those forms of treatment, then he or she has a right to follow that policy, no matter what the patient requests. The patient is naturally free to seek out some other health-care provider who will be willing to provide the disputed form of treatment, but the patient has no right to impose a servitude on the health-care provider. This point raises difficult questions about abandonment. What if the patient cannot find anyone else? What if the patient is a public patient and only private physicians would provide the type of care he or she desires? Can there be cases in which the right of the physician is outweighed by these considerations? We will return to these questions when we consider specific cases.

There are significant differences between the case in which the patient is refusing what the health-care provider wishes to provide and the case in which the patient is demanding what the health-care provider is not willing to provide. In the former case, an appeal to rights favors following the wishes of the competent adult patient; in the latter case, the appeal to rights does not.

The other procedural right is the right of family members to refuse recommended health care on behalf of the patient.

Four cases must be distinguished here. The first involves competent adult patients who are refusing some recommended care. The second involves adult patients who are no longer competent to participate in a decisional process but whose families have some clear understanding that the patients would have refused the recommended care if they could have participated in the process. The third involves adult patients no longer competent to participate in a decisional process and about whom no one has a clear perception of what the patient would have wished if the patient could have participated in the process. And the fourth case involves families of children who are too young to participate in a decisional process and too young to have any serious wishes about what should or should not be done to them.

In many ways, the first case is the easiest to analyze. The patient's right to confidentiality requires that even the flow of information to the family must be guided by the patient's wishes. Health-care providers often assume, without any justification, that patients wish full disclosure of their condition to be made to their families. This is particularly true for hospitalized patients. This assumption should not be made.[45] The relationship between the patient and various family members may differ, and the patient may desire full disclosure to certain family members and none to others. If all this is true even about the flow of information, it is even more true of any role in a decisional process. The role of family members in these cases should be determined by the patient. To the extent that the patient wishes to be guided by the family, the patient may do so, and the family will have a role. To the extent that the patient wishes to maintain the decisional authority alone, that is the right of the patient, and the family has no role. In such cases, the family has no independent right to participate in any decisional process, and a good policy statement would indicate that fact.[46]

Sometimes, when a competent patient is refusing a form of treatment that the health-care provider thinks is appropriate, the health-care provider will turn to members of the family to try to get them to pressure the patient into agreeing to be treated. It would seem, from what I have just said, that this is inappropriate. This, however, is a misunderstanding. What I have said so far does, in fact, entail that when providers do so they are both violating their patient's right to confidentiality and invoking a nonexistent right of the family to be part of the decisional process. However, there may be cases when rights are legitimately overridden out of a concern for the consequences for the patient and/or for others. One extreme way of overriding rights is for the physician to treat without the permission of the patient or the family. Another less extreme way is to violate the rights of confidentiality, let the family know what is going on, and use them to persuade the patient to accept treatment. It is important to keep in mind again that rights are not absolute, and some examples of this type of behavior may be legitimate.

We turn from this relatively simple case to the more complex cases, beginning with the adult patient who is no longer competent to participate in any decisional process but whose family has a clear perception that the patient would have refused the recommended care if the patient could have participated in the process. The family in such a case must be viewed not as people who have a right to make decisions but rather as sources of information about the decisions the patient would have made. In such cases, if the family testimony is credible (the family can be mistaken in their views about what the patient would have done), then we have a reason, based on an appeal to the rights of the patient, for following the refusal of the patient which is being communicated indirectly through the testimony of the family. This helps to explain an important fact about such cases. The advance refusals of patients may deserve greater or lesser respect, depending on such factors as the knowledge the patient had at the time, the extent to which circumstances have changed, and so on.[47] Given that the family's role in such cases is that of informant about the wishes of the patient, the force of the information they convey also depends on these factors.

It is important to distinguish this role of the family from another role they may play, that of testifying about the values of the patient, about how the patient would have valued the consequences of various proposed actions. In both roles the family is testifying about the patient rather than making decisions. But one testimony is relevant to the appeal to consequences while the other is relevant to the appeal to the patient's right to refuse care. The relevance of this distinction will become clear in chapters 6 and 7 when we deal with cases involving incompetent patients.

It is only the third and fourth types of cases that truly involve the right of family members to refuse recommended health care on behalf of a patient. In such cases, and only in such cases, are the family members decision makers.

What is the proper basis for the family's decisions?[48] It is clear from the delineation of these cases that it cannot be the family's judgment of what the patient would have wished, for we are dealing with cases in which that information is unavailable (the adult cases) or perhaps even nonexistent (the pediatric cases). Commentators have suggested that in such cases the family's wishes should be based solely on their perception of what is best for the patient.[49] But it seems to me that in such cases, as in many other nonmedical cases, families need to judge in part upon what is good for the individual directly affected but also in part upon the implications for the rest of the family. When parents decide where a child is to be sent to school, they should certainly consider the implications for the child, but they also may consider the implications for the rest of the family. When children who are responsible for their elderly parents decide in what environment the parents should reside, they certainly should consider the well-being of the elderly parents, but they also may consider the implications for the rest of the family. I see no reason why the medical context should be any different.

The right of family members to refuse health care on behalf of the patient arises, then, only when the patient cannot participate in decision making and only when knowledge of what the patient would have wanted is not available. In such cases families have the right to refuse care, and the refusal should be based in part on their judgment of what is best for the patient and in part on their judgment of what is best for other family members. A difficult question concerns when they lose that right because they show an inability to properly balance a concern for the patient's best interests with other concerns.[50]

Keep in mind that this right, like all other rights, is waivable.[51] The family may decide to leave decisions in the hands of the health-care provider, because they feel either too emotional or too ill-informed to make the decisions, or for any other reason. Moreover, in the case of a family refusing recommended forms of treatment, this right can be overridden if their refusal results in a great loss to the patient. If a patient's right to be a decision maker can be overridden, then the family's right can certainly be overridden. Finally, and crucially, families have no more right to compel health-care providers to administer treatments the providers think are inappropriate than patients do.[52]

## 2.3   The Appeal to Respect for Persons

Immanuel Kant, the great German philosopher, brought the appeal to the respect owed to persons to a central place in moral philosophy.[53] Many of those who consider themselves Kantians have continued that tradition.[54] I believe, however, that this appeal has been misunderstood by many moral philosophers, including Kantians, and has not therefore been properly used, particularly in medical ethics.

The mistaken account of respect for persons might be called the rights account.[55] Its main theses are the following:

1. One shows respect for persons by honoring the rights which they have.
2. There are no cases in which showing respect for persons has moral implications which are independent of respecting the rights of the persons involved.

This account maintains that the appeal to respect for persons really need not be taken into account in evaluating alternative actions because its impact is already covered by the appeal to the rights of the people involved.

I do not see how this account can be accepted.[56] Let me give two examples, one nonmedical and one medical, in which the appeal to respect for persons seems to have a moral significance that cannot be understood along the lines suggested by the rights account:

(a) Someone offers to sell himself into slavery in return for food, housing, etc.
(b) A young person seeks to end his life because he has suffered some severe reverse in his career or in his interpersonal relationships. He shows up in the emergency room overdosed.

Regarding the first example, it is wrong to accept the person's offer to be your slave; part of the reason why it is wrong is that doing so would fail to show respect for his personhood. This is consonant with the earlier point that one can explain what is wrong with voluntary slavery without invoking an inalienable right to freedom. Regarding the second example, it is wrong to let the person die, even if he now wants to die; part of the reason why it is wrong is that allowing him to die in such a case is failing to show respect for his personhood. Again, this is consonant with the earlier point that one can explain what is wrong with at least some cases of allowing suicide without invoking an inalienable right to life. It is clear, however, that no rights account (except one that illegitimately invokes inalienable rights) can explain why it is wrong either to accept the offer or to let the person die. After all, although people have a right not to be enslaved and a right to be aided when their lives are threatened, the potential slave, by making the offer, has waived his right not to be enslaved, and the person who has attempted suicide has, by that act, waived his right to be aided. To be sure, defenders of the rights account can always try to challenge the validity of the waiver, but they may not be successful in all cases. Our account will be. So, if respect for persons is relevant here, it must be something more than just respecting the rights of the persons in question.

This something more involves both a special content and a new type of moral structure. The content of respect for persons seems to be as follows. We think of persons as having the potential to perform a wide variety of actions whose performance we value greatly. These include the potential to make rational (and especially principled) choices, the potential to engage in a variety of interpersonal relations, the potential to appreciate beauty, and the potential to desire to know the truth.[57] We therefore value the person who has those potentials. However, there are conditions that are necessary for (or at least facilitate) a person's ability to fulfill these potentials: the person must be alive, must maintain his or her bodily integrity, must be free to make choices and act upon them, and so on. To show respect for persons is to value them by refraining from eliminating these conditions and by acting to promote their presence. This helps explain the moral opposition both to accepting the offer of the volunteer slave and to letting the suicide victim die. If, for example, we accept the offer of the volunteer slave, we act in a way that limits that person's potential for performing these valued actions, because we are acting in a way that limits his freedom to make choices and act on them. We are not showing respect for that person as a person. If we allow the suicide victim to die, in cases in which the person is otherwise perfectly capable of continuing to perform many of those actions we value so highly, we are failing to show respect for his personhood which consists of his potential to perform those actions.

If respect for persons is to provide the explanation of certain moral facts that infringement of rights cannot, it is because the logical structure of the appeal to respect for persons is very different from that of the appeal to rights. When your action is wrong because it infringes on the rights of others, then it is wrong because you have wrongly interfered in an area that is theirs to control, and that person's consent can eliminate the wrongness of your action. This is why there are no inalienable rights. When, however, your action is wrong because it shows a lack of respect for some person, its wrongness is independent of any infringement on that person's area of control, and that person's consent will not change anything. The obligation to show respect for persons is not an obligation to the person in question. It is just an obligation that may require you to act in certain ways toward that person. Because it is not an obligation to a particular person, even though it is an obligation that has implications for how you should behave toward that person, you are not freed of that obligation by the person's consent.

I would like to suggest the following: to respect people is to value certain actions and to value the people who have the capacity to perform those actions. We show that respect by not lessening the potential of those persons to perform those actions and by aiding them in developing that potential. We have an obligation to show this respect, an obligation which rests on the objective value of the persons in question. This obligation has implications for how we should behave toward individual persons, even though it is not an obligation to those persons. We continue to have this obligation even if the persons in question waive the obligation. This is one of the reasons why it would be wrong for us to accept the offer of the volunteer slave and one of the reasons why it would be wrong to let the suicide victim die.

Because of our analysis of the nature of respect for persons and personhood, we must conclude that the respect which is owed to persons may vary according to the capacities of the individual in question. In this way respect for persons differs considerably from respect for their rights.

Suppose a patient is in a persistent vegetative state. That patient's capacity to perform those human actions which we value is nonexistent. Nevertheless, as I argued in section 2.2 above, this patient is still alive and still has a right not to be killed. Now, in the ordinary case in which someone kills another human being, we criticize the action both on the grounds that it violates the rights of the person in question and on the grounds that it fails to show respect for that person's personhood. In the case of the persistent vegetative patient, however, only the former ground might be applicable. Because of the permanent loss of those potentials for human action, the persistent vegetative patient is not a person whom we have an obligation to respect, although we are obliged to respect his or her rights. This is, of course, an extreme example. We could look at other patients whose conditions are less extreme and who have only a diminished capacity to perform valued human actions. In the case of those patients, we might have, as part of our obligation to respect personhood, a modest obligation to protect and promote their limited capacity to perform valued human actions. However, the respect for personhood in their case is less than the respect for personhood in normal cases. They retain, however, the same rights as the ordinary patient. In short, an important fact about respect for personhood is that it is not owed universally. Moreover, it can be owed to a greater or lesser degree depending on the condition of the person involved. In these ways respect for persons differs from respect for the rights of persons, particularly the right not to be killed. This important difference will obviously have significant implications for the care of patients in the cases in chapters 5 through 7. We shall see then that this is one of the ways in which the quality of the future life of the patient and the extent of his or her personhood is extremely relevant in determining what constitutes appropriate or inappropriate action. Many have suggested that there are patients who, while alive, are no longer fully persons. They have also said that this has significant implications for how such patients should be treated. It is hard to see why this should be so, however, given that we still perceive them as living human beings with their rights intact. Invoking the notion of respect for persons may help clarify this point. Although the patients in question retain their right to life (and cannot, therefore, be killed unless they have waived their right), they are no longer fully deserving of respect for their personhood. In those cases where respect for personhood is central to justifying further intervention, there will not be the normal basis for their receiving that intervention. Some of the examples in chapters 5 through 7 will turn on this point.

## 2.4   The Appeal to the Virtues

Ancient moral philosophy placed great emphasis on the moral virtues. Plato and Aristotle did not discuss such questions as what rights people have or what actions will lead to the best consequences or what actions show the most respect for persons. They discussed what sort of person one ought to be and what sort of actions one ought to perform as part of being the right sort of person. Modern moral philosophy has paid much less attention to these questions, focusing instead on rights, consequences, and respect for persons. In the last few years, however, this shift in focus has come under considerable criticism. There are those who argue that we ought to return to the morality of virtues.[58] I do not see the need for a real conflict here. Looking at the relations of our actions to our character is certainly an important aspect of evaluating actions. Looking at the consequences of the actions, the rights of those affected, and the respect shown are also important aspects. A sound moral philosophy should encompass all of these appeals.

Our interest in the virtues is because of their implications for the moral evaluation of actions. A consideration of the virtues is also relevant to the moral evaluation of individuals, but that is not the concern here, nor is the fundamental theoretical question of the relationship between the virtues as characteristics of actions (e.g., courageous actions) and the virtues as characteristics of people (e.g., courageous individuals). In short, I am not concerned with a full development of a theory of the virtues. I shall simply try to indicate ways in which the appeal to various virtues may affect our evaluation of certain health-care decisions and the actions which carry them out.

Aristotle first suggested the view that an action is virtuous only if it is the right sort of action performed for the right sort of motive.[59] He also saw the possibility of virtuous actions performed for wrong motives. These divergent approaches have continued. Some see a direct connection between virtuous actions and motives. Others do not; for them, a virtuous action is the sort of action that would typically be performed for a certain motive but might still be virtuous when performed for other motives. This is an important dispute;[60] I am neutral about it in my theoretical account, however, for it is not clear that any of our cases will be affected by it.

The first virtue is the virtue of integrity. Many decisions made by health-care providers and/or patients are justified at least in part on the grounds that only by making these decisions can they maintain their integrity. For example, health-care providers will sometimes refuse to provide certain forms of care which patients request on the grounds that doing so is against their values and would therefore violate their sense of integrity. Similarly, patients will sometimes refuse to be treated in certain ways because they believe that being treated in those ways challenges their integrity. In each case, part of the justification for the refusals is just that they display integrity.

Certainly, people who do what they are obliged to do even if they are tempted by personal gains to do otherwise may correctly say that they are performing an act of integrity. But that is not the sort of integrity I am concerned with; that integrity merely reinforces already existing moral obligations and evaluations. Similarly, I am not concerned with at least one type of integrity discussed by Bernard Williams, the integrity of the individual who is concerned not merely with seeing that wrong is not done but particularly with seeing that he or she does not do what is wrong.[61] This is a continuation of the previous notion of integrity, for it too reinforces already existing obligations and evaluations. I am concerned instead with a different type of integrity, one which generates additional moral evaluations.

In order to understand this other type of integrity, we need to keep in mind that not all values are moral values. People frame for themselves conceptions of the goals they wish to pursue, the things they care more about and the things they care less about, and so on. These conceptions form people's personal values. Those who lack such a set of personal values may properly be criticized for lacking a coherent life plan.

These values play a prominent role in the appeal to the virtue of integrity with which I am concerned. A health-care provider, in choosing that career, may have a wide variety of goals in mind. Some are personally oriented (e.g., professional advancement, monetary reward). Others are directed toward the type of medicine they will practice and relate to what they hope to accomplish by the practice of medicine. Some providers, for example, may be particularly excited about the possibility of prolonging conscious human existence. Such providers might find it extremely difficult to participate in decisions that sacrifice that value in order to promote certain other values, such as the relief of pain. They might feel that their participation in such a decision would violate their integrity, just because it calls upon them to abandon their goal and assume the goals of others. Others may have a very different conception of their goal in health care. They may see their primary goal as to be of service to their patients by providing them with what they need to promote their goals. Such providers might very well participate in the same decision without feeling any loss of integrity.

A similar point can be made about health-care recipients. They come to the health-care system with their goals, their life plans, and their personal values. There are decisions that can be made which respect the rights of all, which show respect for personhood, which have beneficial consequences on the whole, and which are still problematic for particular patients because they violate the integrity of those patients. These decisions would not be consonant with their values, and that would be a reason (not necessarily an overriding reason) for their not making those decisions. Consider, for example, a patient who has always placed a high value on being mentally alert, in control of a situation, and capable of making decisions for himself. Such a patient, when confronting the considerable pain of a terminal illness, might find the types of pain relief offered to many patients inappropriate precisely because they would produce a sedated state. Other patients, whose values are very different, might feel otherwise. Decisions which are appropriate when made by one patient might be inappropriate when made by another precisely because they are not consonant with the values of the second patient and because they would therefore challenge his or her integrity.

It is these concerns that the appeal to integrity addresses. It calls upon health-care providers and health-care recipients to stand firm in their values. It evaluates choices at least in part[62] on the extent to which those choices are consonant with the personal values of both the provider and the recipient of the health care.

The second virtue is the virtue of compassion. Many decisions made by health-care providers which are justified at least in part on the grounds that these decisions and the resulting actions show great compassion. For example, a health-care provider who stops to aid an accident victim with whom he or she has no previous professional relationship is certainly to be praised at least in part on the grounds that doing so is a compassionate act of caring for others.

There is an important difference between the virtue of integrity and the virtue of compassion. Compassion is, by its very nature, an other-centered virtue. The compassionate person, after all, is responding to the sufferings and needs of others. The virtue of integrity is not necessarily other-centered. The person of integrity may perform certain actions as a way of pursuing goals that are self-oriented. The person who has adopted as a goal the development of some of his or her capacities (e.g., the capacity to play tennis well) may appropriately be said to show integrity by systematically making certain decisions even if those decisions are of no benefit to others.

To make this distinction between compassion and integrity is not to say that compassion is more important or more valuable than integrity. We ought not to assume that the most important virtues are the other-centered virtues. Such an assumption is one component of the failure to understand that there are many aspects to morality and that the other-centered aspects, however important they may be, are not the whole story.

Is compassion just a way of responding to the suffering of other people? When one responds to the suffering of others by attempting to alleviate that suffering, then one is certainly engaged in a compassionate act. But that is not the only type of compassionate action. Consider, for example, the comatose patient who is not suffering any pain because of his diminished mental status. Such an individual has nevertheless suffered a great loss. To respond to that loss by attempting to care for that patient and attempting to restore his mental functioning is certainly an act of compassion. We need to understand compassion as an attempt to alleviate the losses of others, not merely their suffering.

This brings us to an important question which will have considerable relevance later in this book. How shall we understand this notion of loss which is so essential to the virtue of compassion? In particular, suppose someone feels a great sense of loss because certain of his desires are greatly frustrated. Suppose, moreover, that we judge that he is much better off this way in light of the rest of his own values or in light of our values. Would it be a virtuous act of compassion in such a case to respond to his loss by attempting to help satisfy his desires, or, alternatively, would the compassionate act be to lead him to recognize that he is better off the way he is? As a continuation of our adoption of the preference-satisfaction theory for the evaluation of consequences, we shall define the notion of loss in terms of the individual's values. Therefore, if he is better off in light of his own values, the compassionate action is to lead him to recognize this; but if he is worse off in light of his values, it would be compassionate to help him satisfy the desire in question.

There are clearly going to be some cases of compassionate action where the action performed is one that we have an obligation to perform. Health-care providers with patients who are in pain are certainly under an obligation, absent special circumstances, to help alleviate that pain. That it is an obligatory action in no way prevents it from being compassionate as well. In other cases, however, a compassionate act, although virtuous, is an action that one may have no obligation to perform. Some examples of the Good Samaritan question illustrate this point. I have already suggested in section 2.2 that there will be cases in which we have an obligation to aid strangers who are suffering as a concomitant to their right to that aid. But consider cases in which that obligation is overridden, perhaps because it calls for very large sacrifices. Surely the appropriate thing to say about such a case is that someone (such as a health-care provider) who still aids the stranger has performed a compassionate act, and someone who does not has failed to display this important virtue. The case for helping is sometimes based on our obligation to come to the aid of strangers, but there is a case for helping based on the virtue of compassion whether or not the special obligation to help is present. So appealing to the virtue of compassion may provide an argument for performing actions even when one has no such obligation to the recipient.[63]

I can make one final observation about the virtue of compassion in the health-care context. In the discussion of the virtue of integrity, we saw examples of decisions made by health-care providers and health care-recipients that are valued as acts of integrity or are criticized on the grounds of lack of integrity. So far, in the examination of compassion, all of the examples have involved compassionate or noncompassionate decisions by health-care providers. This is not surprising. In the context of health care, it is the recipient that has suffered the loss, and it is the provider who is in the position to perform the compassionate action. But is this always the case? Are there not at least some possibilities for the display of compassion by health-care recipients toward health-care providers?

Very often health-care recipients are in a position to make requests of health-care providers which impose considerable losses on the providers. It may be nothing more substantial than requesting immediate treatment of a problem that could be deferred for another occasion when it is clear that the health-care provider is tired. Would it not be an act of compassion for the health-care recipient to recognize the needs of the health-care provider and not to impose unnecessary extra burdens on him or her? It may be something more substantial. Some requests that recipients make of health-care providers challenge their integrity. Would it not be an act of compassion to avoid making such requests? When a family puts a physician into a crisis by requesting that he or she heavily sedate a dying patient (where it is understood that this heavy sedation may well result in the death of the patient), this very request may challenge the integrity of certain physicians and yet tempt them because of their own sense of compassion. Isn't the avoidance of making that request a compassionate act, one designed to avoid putting the health-care provider in a very difficult and uncomfortable situation? No doubt these examples constitute an extension of the virtue of compassion in the health-care context, but this extension is neither unnatural nor inappropriate. I am inclined, therefore, to suppose that although in the health-care context compassion is primarily a virtue of health-care providers, health-care recipients also have occasions to behave in a compassionate fashion, their doing so constitutes a display of the virtue of compassion, and an appeal to the virtue of compassion argues for their doing so.

The third virtue I wish to consider is the virtue of courage. There are many decisions made by health-care providers and health-care recipients which are praised at least in part on the grounds that these decisions and the resulting actions show great courage. Any full account of the virtues relevant to health care needs to include this important virtue.

Long ago Aristotle pointed out that courage is not the same thing as foolhardiness.[64] The foolhardy person is totally unconcerned with the possibility that his or her action will lead to pain, bodily injury, or death. The foolhardy person will often perform actions which are inappropriate, involving great risks for very small gains, because the foolhardy person is inappropriately unconcerned with those losses. Foolhardiness, as Aristotle pointed out, is not a virtue. Courage is a virtue precisely because it is not foolhardiness, precisely because it consists of performing appropriate actions as a result of not being swayed by excessive fears.

Courage is the ability to make the appropriate decision without being excessively motivated by such fears as the fear of pain, bodily injury, or death. In the military context, which is the context in which courage is most often discussed, the courageous soldier is the one who does the militarily appropriate action without being excessively motivated by a fear of being killed or injured. Similarly, it is easy to think of many examples of courageous actions performed by health-care recipients. After all, many who are ill confront the possibility of pain, bodily injury, or death and make appropriate decisions despite the fear of those possibilities. The patient who consents to an appropriate surgical procedure, for example, even when there is a real risk of pain, bodily injury, or even death, is properly described as a courageous patient and properly praised for that courage. All too often people have excessive fears of those possibilities, which lead them to reject medically appropriate and necessary courses of action.

But courage is more than the ability to make appropriate decisions without being excessively motivated by fear of pain, injury, or death. Sometimes we make courageous decisions by not being excessively motivated by fear of private guilt or public disapproval. The person who does what he or she believes is the right thing to do, and is not excessively swayed either by a fear of being wrong or by a fear of others disagreeing, is also performing a courageous action. This is why courage can also be a virtue of health-care providers. Health-care providers normally do not face the immediate threat of pain, bodily injury, or death, so they cannot display the same type of courage as that shown by health-care recipients. However, health-care providers are often called upon to make decisions that are problematic, knowing very well that they may later regret the decisions or be criticized by others for them. Courageous health-care providers move forward after careful reflection to make the necessary decisions and are not excessively swayed by such fears.

    This form of courage is also available for those who must be surrogate decision makers for health-care recipients. Family members who have to decide on surgical procedures for their loved ones are one example. If, after weighing the various risks, they make the decision that seems best and move forward with this decision without being excessively swayed by a fear of later guilt feelings or criticism by others, then they too display this form of courage.

    It is important to keep in mind, however, Aristotle's point about foolhardiness. We always need to recognize that we may be wrong. This recognition of our own fallibility should at least motivate us to be extremely careful in important decision making, to consult with others, to consider the various risks several times, and so on. The courageous person is just not excessively swayed by this fear of being wrong. Having gone through a proper decisional process, the courageous health-care provider or surrogate decision maker moves forward with what seems to be the appropriate decision. The cowardly health-care provider or surrogate decision maker harms people by being unable to come to decisions.

    There is one extremely important difference between courage on the one hand and integrity and compassion on the other which has been implicit in our discussion until now. Compassion helps explain why certain actions are praiseworthy which would not otherwise be so. Integrity also helps explain why certain actions are praiseworthy which would not otherwise be so. In this way the virtue of compassion and the virtue of integrity generate values for actions. Courage is not that sort of virtue. After all, the courageous person, by definition, is the person who is performing actions that are otherwise appropriate without being excessively swayed by certain fears. We praise people for being courageous, but their courage is not the basic source of value of the actions they perform. Those actions are independently valuable.[65]

    To say this, however, is not to downplay the significance of the virtue of courage. All too often, especially in the health-care context, appropriate decisions are not made because of a lack of courage on the part of one or more parties. There is this difference between the virtue of courage and these other virtues. This difference does not, however, downplay the significance of courage as a virtue.

    The last virtue is honesty. Many acts of communication between health-care providers and health-care recipients are to be praised at least in part on the grounds that they are honest. Any full account of the virtues relevant to health care must include honesty.

    The first thing to note about honesty and the corresponding vice of dishonesty is that there are at least two different ways in which dishonesty can be displayed. To begin with, there is the making of claims which are known to be false with the deliberate intention of misleading the person receiving the information. The health-care provider who tells a patient that he has a good chance of recovering from a disease if he follows a course of treatment, when the actual chance of recovery is low, is being dishonest. The health-care recipient who insists that he does not drink heavily when he actually does is being dishonest. There is, however, a second way of being dishonest. This is the withholding of information when it is expected and intended that the person from whom the information is withheld will draw wrong inferences. The health-care provider who informs the patient of certain possible side effects of a drug but fails to inform the patient of another serious side effect, and who does so with the expectation that the patient will infer that there are no further side effects, has engaged in a dishonest act of communication. Equally, the health-care recipient who, when asked about abnormal symptoms, reports some but withholds others, with the expectation that the physician will draw the inference that there are no further symptoms, is engaged in a dishonest act of communication.

I am not saying that all withholding of information is automatically dishonest. All I am claiming is that when information is withheld (1) with the expectation that people will draw false inferences and (2) with the intention that they draw these inferences, then the person withholding that information is engaged in a dishonest act of communication.[66] Neither health-care providers nor health-care recipients are dishonest when they simply withhold information; if they were, they would always be engaged in dishonest acts of communication, since they always make choices about how much information to convey.

There is much to be said in favor of honest communication between health-care providers and health-care recipients. To begin with, an appeal to consequences argues for engaging in honest acts of communication. Health-care providers who engage in honest communication with their patients will build trust, will have greater compliance with their recommendations, and so on. Health-care recipients who honestly give information to their health-care providers are likely to get better care, more attention, and so on. Secondly, there are appeals to rights which argue for honest communication between health-care recipients and health-care providers. Each of these parties to the health-care relationship has the right to make certain types of decisions based on information, and when false information is provided or withheld, they are deprived of the opportunity to exercise those rights. So there is much to be said in favor of policies of honesty in the health-care setting even without invoking the virtue of honesty, although an appeal to the virtue of honesty strengthens the case for honest communications.

None of this entails that we ought always to be honest. There may well be occasions on which other moral considerations override the considerations advanced on behalf of a policy of honesty. Compassion, for example, sometimes leads health-care providers to withhold some information from their patients, and that may sometimes be right.[67] Promises of confidentiality may sometimes lead recipients to rightfully withhold information. This should come as no surprise. I have, after all, been arguing throughout this chapter that there are a variety of ethical appeals that need to be considered in making any particular decision, and even the impressive consequentialist, rights, and virtue arguments for honesty may be overridden in certain circumstances.

All of this leads to the conclusion that honesty as a virtue is more like courage than it is like compassion and integrity. In most cases the person who is engaged in an honest act of communication is performing an action that he or she has moral reasons to perform independently of the virtue of honesty. I believe, however, that there are a small number of cases in which honesty may lead one to certain acts of communication that are valuable precisely because of their honest character and not because of any other moral appeal. Imagine cases in which we decide to treat patients against their wishes (perhaps because of a respect for persons). One such case might be providing a blood transfusion to a comatose Jehovah's Witness against the patient's earlier wishes. In such a case, should the health-care provider honesly inform the patient and the family afterwards about what was done? It is hard to see that a consideration of the rights of patients or their families to be decision makers could be the basis for a policy of honesty in such a case since the decision has already been made independently of the wishes of the patient and the family. It is also hard to see that the consequences mentioned above (especially building trust and compliance) are likely to be encouraged by such an act of honest communication. After all, when the patient and the family are told what was done, conflict will certainly be engendered. Nevertheless, it would be appropriate to inform the patient and the family about what was done precisely because it would be the honest thing to do. If that view is correct, then there will be some cases in which the virtue of honesty provides the sole reason for the performance of certain honest acts of communication.

## 2.5   The Appeal to Cost-Effectiveness and Justice

Some health-care decisions should be criticized in part because they are cost-ineffective or because they are unjust, whereas other health-care decisions are justified in part because they are both cost-effective and just. Any attempt to do full justice to these two important moral appeals would require a full theory of distributive justice. In this setting, the most I can do is say a little about the way in which these appeals work and justify their invocation by health-care providers facing particular cases.

It is relatively easy to state the basic concept of cost-effective health care. A health-care decision is said to be cost-effective when the expenditures required to implement the decision are less than the value of the benefits of its implementation. A cost-ineffective health-care decision is one whose cost of implementation is greater than the value of the benefits derived from it.

Judging health-care decisions in terms of their cost-effectiveness is really part of judging them in terms of their consequences. In judging in terms of cost-effectiveness we are simply emphasizing as the negative consequences of the decisions the monetary cost of implementing them. It is nevertheless important to emphasize cost-effectiveness as a separate appeal because people have often paid little attention to this consequence of health-care decisions. They have analyzed the good and bad consequences of decisions in terms of the health benefits to the patient, the family, and the surrounding society. They have not focused on the economic costs. Making cost-effectiveness a separate appeal may help correct this traditional oversight.

There is a well-known difficulty in determining whether or not a particular health-care decision is cost-effective. How are we to weigh the value of all the benefits against the monetary cost? If we would just look at the monetary benefits and the monetary costs, it would at least be conceptually clear how the two are to be compared. But how can we weigh all the gains of the health-care decision (including the psychosocial as well as monetary gains)? It would be nice to say that we could weigh the two by asking whether we would be prepared to pay those economic costs to secure those benefits.[68] This willingness-to-pay approach certainly seems attractive at the individual level, but it runs into trouble when we are trying as a society to decide whether some health care which we are thinking of providing to those who cannot pay for it is cost-effective. How much we are willing to pay for anything depends on how much money we have. If we ask ourselves whether we are willing to pay a certain cost to obtain certain health benefits, then our answer is going to be a function of the number of dollars we have. For example, what we might be willing to pay for as individuals at a certain level of income might not be something we are willing to pay for at a different level of income. In judging on grounds of cost-effectiveness whether we should provide certain types of health care to those who cannot pay for it, we can use their level of wealth to justify saying that certain types of health care are cost-effective for wealthy people and not for poor people, or we can attempt to fix the level of wealth at which the question is raised at some higher level to justify claims of cost-effectiveness, or we can give up the willingness-to-pay approach.[69]

In short, the goal of cost-effectiveness in our health-care decisions is not easy to define in a theoretically satisfactory fashion. The clear-cut cases will be cases of waste, where certain forms of health care are not cost-effective because they involve very substantial costs and no benefits.[70] Other cases, involving substantial costs and some benefits, will be harder to judge. Nevertheless, although we may have a great deal of difficulty in articulating this idea of cost-effectiveness, there is some hope that it will be useful in analyzing clinical cases.

Let's now consider the appeal to the justice of the health-care decision. The intuitive idea of justice is that health-care decisions that provide the health care to which people are entitled are just, whereas health-care decisions that fail to provide that health care are unjust.[71]

There are those who think that such appeals to cost-effectiveness and justice are important for policy makers to take into account as they develop health-care systems but that individual health-care providers should not take them into account.[72] Their view is that individual health-care providers need to do that which produces the best consequences for their patients, respects their rights, and so on; it is not the role of individual health-care providers to worry about cost-effectiveness or justice in health care. I reject this traditional view. It is my claim instead that health-care providers in both the public and the private sector need to attend both to cost-effectiveness and to justice in the provision of health care.

There are three arguments offered on behalf of the traditional claim. The first is an appeal to consequences, an argument that the patient-provider relationship flourishes when patients trust their health-care providers and that that trust is promoted when patients see their providers as their agents. The second is simply the claim that this is essential to the nature of the patient-provider relationship. The third and most important argument is that there is an implicit contractual understanding between patients and their providers that the provider will look out for the interest of the patient. The provider who worries about justice or cost-effectiveness is breaking that understanding and violating the patient's right to have that understanding respected.

The argument that this traditional view is essential to the very nature of the patient-provider relationship begs the question. It just assumes that a social role for the provider, in which the provider considers in individual cases questions of justice and cost-effectiveness, is incompatible with the patient-provider relationship. I see no reason to accept such an essentialist argument. The other two arguments are more serious. They argue against such a social role.

In order to defend my own claim regarding this issue, I need to say something more about the public sector/private sector distinction and about cost-effectiveness and justice in both of those sectors. For the sake of this discussion, we shall understand the public sector/private sector distinction to be based on whether or not the health-care recipient and/or the family are financially responsible for the cost of the health care provided. If they are so responsible (even if they are entitled by virtue of contractual arrangements to pass that cost on to third-party payers), then the health care is being provided in the private sector. If they are not responsible for that cost, then the health care is being provided in the public sector. From this point of view, health care provided to the elderly under Medicare, to the indigent under Medicaid or through local hospital districts, and to veterans in the VA system are all examples of the public provision of health care, even if only some of it is being provided in publicly owned health-care facilities.

There are two types of public programs: programs in which the funding agency (most notably the VA or a local hospital district) provides a budget for the provision of health care, and those eligible receive health care only to the extent of funding provided by the funding agency; and entitlement programs, in which all those eligible will receive the health care, and the funding agency will bear the resulting cost, whatever it may be. The analysis of our issue is somewhat different in these two cases, even if the conclusion I wish to reach is essentially the same.

Those familiar with the first type of program are well aware that the resources allocated to these forms of public health care are rarely sufficient to meet even the most pressing health-care needs of the eligible population, must less all of their needs. As a result, every time some of those resources are used to provide health care to one eligible recipient, other eligible recipients will not receive health care from which they could benefit. In these contexts, every provision of health care is automatically a choice to provide health care to some with the understanding that others will therefore not receive health care from which they could benefit. Suppose, then, that a health-care provider in such a setting insists that his or her responsibility, based on contractual rights and an appeal to consequences, is only to the well-being of his or her patient and that it is inappropriate to consider any appeal to questions of justice and cost-effectiveness. Such a response, in light of the reality of the circumstances, seems inappropriate. To begin with, there is a counterbalancing appeal to consequences which argues that the denial of care to other patients who have greater entitlements or to other patients who could benefit more (and whose care is therefore more cost-effective) produces a decline in trust in the system and in its rationality. Secondly, the rights of those with greater entitlements to the care (those who, according to the appeal to justice, should get that care) may take precedence over the contractual rights of the individual patient. And assuming, as seems reasonable, that recipients have a greater claim to cost-effective health care than to cost-ineffective health care, that may mean that an appeal to cost-effectiveness should take precedence over the appeal to contractual rights.[73]

Let's consider an example.[74] The provision of medical intensive care for a sick patient is an expensive form of health care. Often this expenditure of resources results in a significant improvement in the health and life expectancy of the recipient. There are many cases, however, in which this expensive form of health care is provided with only modest resulting benefits. That seems particularly unjustified in the types of public contexts we are considering. The patient receiving this expensive form of health care is doing so at the expense of other patients who could benefit much more from this very form of health care and yet who are not able to obtain it because the ICU is full. Moreover, the funds used to provide this expensive care could be used in a far more effective fashion to provide different types of health care for others. I do not see how a physician can justifiably say that none of this is his or her concern on the grounds that an appeal to the desirable consequences of trust building and to the contractual rights of patients says that the physician's only obligation is to his or her individual patient. The other patients in the system have rights as well, and the perception that the system is allocating resources ineffectively and unjustly would have terrible consequences. The individual physician needs to keep this in mind and, at least in some cases, to make just (in part because they are cost-effective) decisions, even if this means not doing what is best for the individual patient in front of him or her at the time.

The situation is somewhat more complicated in those cases in which the public program is an entitlement program. One cannot argue that the individual provider is denying the rights of other potential recipients of health care when he or she uses the resources of the program in an ineffective and/or unjust fashion, since those other recipients will receive the health care to which they are entitled anyway. There is nevertheless something wrong with the inefficient allocation of health care resources even in such cases. A recognition of this should lead providers in at least some cases to make cost-effective decisions, even if this means not doing what is best for their individual patients.

Consider once more the health-care provider who is providing health care that is cost-ineffective. This health-care provider is taking the resources of the society and spending those resources for benefits that are not commensurate with the cost (however we define that). It seems unlikely that those who are paying the bill would or should approve of such health-care expenditures.[75] Indeed, there is mounting evidence that they do not.[76] The continued provision of cost-ineffective care may have the terrible consequence of undermining confidence in the system and leading to an unwillingness of those who must pay for the care to do so. Moreover, even in entitlement programs, the health-care facilities may not be available to serve the needs of all people at a given time. In such cases, even if the programs are entitlement programs, the provision of certain health-care services to some automatically excludes others. When health-care providers provide those limited services to those who are less entitled, they do a direct injustice to potential recipients who are more entitled to those services.

In short, whatever the form of the public program, the provision of health-care services that are cost-ineffective and/or unjust will produce bad consequences and will deny the rights of those with greater entitlements. Because of the realities of the situation, health-care providers in the public sector cannot hide behind the familiar claim that their only responsibility is to care for their patients. None of this says that considerations of justice or cost-effectiveness must take priority over all other considerations, including the appeals invoked by the defenders of the traditional view. As I have said so many times in this chapter, I am merely indicating the appeals that need to be examined as we decide what to do in difficult cases. All I am claiming is that providers must be sensitive to the fact that their decisions need to be evaluated at least in part based on their cost-effectiveness and justice and that such evaluations may lead them in at least some cases to deny care to those who could benefit from it.

We turn now to the private sector. There is a powerful argument to suggest that health-care providers should not withhold private health care on grounds of cost-effectiveness. Suppose a provider is considering a costly form of treatment whose benefits to the patient seem, at least to the provider, modest in light of the costs. If the patient agrees with the provider's assessment of the benefits as compared with the costs, then clearly the health care in question should not be provided, but that is the patient's decision and involves no withholding of care by the provider. If, however, the patient disagrees and feels that the benefits are worth the cost, then why shouldn't the health-care provider provide those services? After all, if the party paying for it (the health-care recipient) judges that the benefits are worth the cost, then it is an appropriate expenditure for that person. The provider's role is to give the patient some proper understanding of the costs of the health-care procedures and the possible benefits that might result from them. Having done that, the provider has fulfilled his or her responsibility in the area of cost-effectiveness. It is the patient's judgment of how much the benefits are worth that will ultimately determine whether the health care will be provided and whether it is cost-effective.

Note that this argument can be used only in the private context and not in the public context. We can certainly use willingness to pay as a measure of cost-effectiveness in the private sector; it is the health-care recipient who is incurring the financial costs of the health care provided. We can therefore use willingness to pay as a measure of cost-effectiveness in the private sector. In the public sector, however, where society in general is bearing the cost, this argument will not hold. The patient may be quite willing to see the heavy costs incurred in order to receive the benefits in question, but that is only because the patient pays none of the costs. It is in the public sector, of course, where problems of defining cost-effectiveness are most critical. It cannot be defined by reference to the recipient's judgment when the recipient bears none of the costs.

Some would say that the introduction of insurance and third-party payers radically changes the validity of this argument. They would say that since the vast majority of the costs incurred in the private sector are paid by third parties rather than by the recipients, the willingness of the recipients to have the procedure performed does not indicate that it is truly a cost-effective procedure. Those who raise this objection say that with the advent of insurance the distinction between the private sector and the public sector breaks down, and providers in the private sector need to do more than simply inform prospective patients about the relevant costs and benefits.

I am not convinced by this point. I would agree that insurance policies with small co-payments lead to strange decisions about which health care is provided, since the recipients find most of the care cost-effective in light of their minimal payments for it. And that may be a good reason for society's encouraging the creation of insurance policies with higher co-payments or insurance policies with other vehicles for introducing cost considerations. But the purchaser of a health insurance policy with a low co-payment has purchased the right to receive the care that he or she judges cost-effective in light of that low payment.[77] There seems to be no moral basis for the physician to take that authority from them.

I conclude, therefore, that the role of the appeal to cost-effectiveness during medical decision making is radically different in the private sector and in the public sector. In the public sector the fact that a certain form of health care is not cost-effective may offer the health-care provider a strong, although not necessarily conclusive, reason for not providing that form of health care, because its provision may produce bad consequences and/or because its provision may be unjust to other recipients. In the private sector the role of the appeal to cost-effectiveness is much more limited. The costs and benefits of a proposed form of health care are something that the provider needs to let the recipient know about, but the provider has no reason on grounds of cost-effectiveness for withholding that form of treatment if the patient requests it. Cost-ineffectiveness is not like medical inappropriateness. Medically inappropriate health care is something that providers in any sector may in some cases not provide as part of their professional integrity. Putatively cost-ineffective health care is a very different matter. If the recipient wishes it and is willing to pay for it, then, from the perspective of the person who has to pay, it is cost-effective and ought to be provided.

It would seem that very similar things have to be said about the appeal to justice in the provision of health care in the private sector. After all, if a patient requests and is willing to pay for some form of health care, and if the provider is willing to provide it, then the patient is entitled to it. If that is the case, then, given our definition of justice in the provision of health care, it would seem to follow that providing that health care cannot involve engaging in an unjust act. This is radically different from the public sector. There, in the nonentitlement segment, there is a real possibility of doing injustice if one gives the care to the person who is less entitled to it.

One complication must be kept in mind. There are cases in which the form of health care to be provided involves the use of certain health-care facilities that can serve only a limited number of patients at a given time. On some occasions there will be more patients who will be in need of or who desire that particular form of health care than the facilities can handle. In such cases there remains a real possibility that the entitlement of some other patients to those health-care facilities may be greater than an entitlement simply based on some patient's or some entitlement program's willingness to pay. In such cases the health-care provider will need to recognize the injustice of assenting to the wishes of his or her own patient and should take that into account in deciding whether or not the patient ought to be treated at that time. For the most part, this sort of case is less pressing in the private sector than in the public sector. A continuing fact about American health care is that these problems of limited facilities seem far more acute in the nonentitlement public sector than in the entitlement public sector and the private sector, and the possibilities of this form of injustice are therefore greatest in the nonentitlement public sector.

## 2.6   Conclusions

I have set out in this chapter a wide variety of ethical appeals that health-care providers and recipients need to take into account as they decide on the appropriate actions in a given case. To do this, however, is not to set out a full framework for dealing with difficult cases but only to indicate the sort of appeals that need to be considered as such a framework is developed. In the next chapter we will look at two models of health-care decision making and see whether or not they are successful in bringing all of these relevant appeals into an appropriate framework for decision making.

### Notes

1. W. D. Ross, *The Right and the Good* (Oxford: Clarendon Press, 1930) pp. 21–22.

2. T. L. Beauchamp and J. Childress, *Principles of Biomedical Ethics,* 2nd edition (New York: Oxford Univ. Press, 1983) pp. 107–8.

3. The question has come up most recently in debates over the role of physicians in cost-containment efforts. See, for example, the very good summary of that issue in M. Angell, "Cost-Containment and the Physician," *JAMA* 254, no. 9 (Sept. 6, 1985).

4. That discussion is summarized in R. Brandt, *Ethical Theory* (Englewood Cliffs, N.J.: Prentice-Hall, 1959).

5. This is so true that some important authors feel entitled to assume that an egoistic evaluation is simply an amoral evaluation, not just an incorrect moral evaluation, and to use that assumption as the basis for important theoretical arguments. See, for example, section 3 of J. C. Harsanyi's "Morality and the Theory of Rational Behavior," in A. Sen and B. Williams, eds., *Utilitarianism and Beyond* (Cambridge: Cambridge Univ. Press, 1982).

6. Forms of hedonism have been held by a wide variety of figures in the history of moral theory (going back to the Greeks), including many of the classical utilitarians such as Benthan and Mill. Its most vigorous recent defense may be in R. Brandt's "Two Concepts of Utility," in H. Miller and W. Williams, eds., *The Limits of Utilitarianism* (Minneapolis: Univ. of Minnesota Press, 1982). Forms of the preference-satisfaction theory have been held by such diverse philosophers as R. B. Perry and J. Harsanyi as well as by most economists. Its history before this century is not well known and is deserving of study. A form of the objective-good theory was suggested by G. E. Moore in *Ethics* (London: Oxford Univ. Press, 1912) chap. 7.

7. The importance for moral philosophy of the failure to establish an objective theory of the good has been stressed by such diverse authors as A. McIntyre, *After Virtue* (Notre Dame: Univ. of Notre Dame Press, 1981); and H. T. Engelhardt, Jr., *The Foundations of Bioethics* (New York: Oxford Univ. Press, 1986).

8. This type of objection is forceably advocated by R. Dworkin in his discussion of discriminatory preferences in *Taking Rights Seriously* (Cambridge, Mass.: Harvard Univ. Press, 1977), pp. 234–37. His attempt to deal with it by rejecting all external preferences, including all altruistic and caring preferences, is a tribute to the difficulty of dealing with this problem.

9. I. L. Peretz, in his classic "Bontsha the Silent," reprinted in I. Howe and E. Greenberg, eds., *A Treasury of Yiddish Stories* (New York: Meredian Books, 1954) pp. 223–31, presents a marvelous story of how God himself is embarrassed by this consequence of the consumer-sovereignty theory. Our more prosaic example is indebted to A. Sen in "Well-Being, Agency and Freedom: The Dewey Lectures 1984," *Journal of Philosophy* 82, no. 4 (April 1985), pp. 196–97.

10. The idea seems to date back to the German neo-Kantian philosopher Leonard Nelson. A brief summary of some of the options (with an appeal to the need for such a theory) is found in sections 7 and 8 of Harsanyi's "Morality and the Theory of Rational Behavior."

11. Brandt, most notably in "Two Concepts of Utility," has stressed the significance of this problem.

12. Of course, they may have other preferences whose satisfaction requires their continued existence, and that will complicate the consideration of our appeal. Also, we need to remember that other appeals will be relevant to both of these cases.

13. This is the crux of Mill's argument in chapter 4 of *On Liberty* (1859) that the individual is far more likely to get these judgments right than is society.

14. This point is made with great vigor by J. Glover in *Causing Death and Saving Lives* (New York: Penguin Books, 1977), pp. 80–82.

15. This is particularly true of authors in the utilitarian tradition. Bentham began this type of critique. For a discussion of Bentham's conceptual doubts about the meaningfulness of rights, see H. L. A. Hart, *Essays on Bentham* (Oxford: Clarendon Press, 1980), chap. 3. An argument in that spirit, but stated more carefully, is presented in L. W. Sumner, "Rights Denaturalized," in R. G. Frey, ed., *Utility and Rights* (Minneapolis: Univ. of Minnesota Press, 1984).

16. A useful introduction to this debate and to many other points about the logic of rights is R. Martin and J. W. Nichel, "Recent Work on the Concept of Rights," *American Philosophical Quarterly* 17, no. 3 (July 1980).

17. Such a view was presumably held by the Founding Fathers of the United States when they described the existence of such inalienable rights as self-evident.

18. This point has recently attracted much attention. A classic statement of it is found in R. Keeton, "Conditional Fault in the Law of Torts," *Harvard Law Review* 72, no. 3 (January 1959).

19. A good example of this is C. Fried's insistence in *Right and Wrong* (Cambridge, Mass.: Harvard Univ. Press, 1978), p. 9, that the right is "prior to the good." Fried comes very close to holding the extreme conclusion, although he draws back from it at the end by his theory that norms are categorical rather than absolute and hold only within a domain that does not include extreme circumstances.

20. This is the thrust of such diverse critics of utilitarianism as Nozick, Fried, and Dworkin. It is interesting to note how this theme of rights, which is so predominant in such recent critics, was not as prominent in earlier critics of utilitarianism such as Ross.

21. I suggested that this was equally mistaken years ago in a review of Nozick's *Anarchy State and Utopia,* published in *Philosophia* in 1976. The suggestion has not been picked up. I hope it will be this time.

22. These legal and philosophical literatures have been joined ever since the publication of the classic treatiste by H. L. A. Hart and A. M. Honore, *Causation in the Law* (Oxford: Oxford Univ. Press, 1959). There is a great need for a careful summary of the immense literature on this topic published since then.

23. A marvelous expression of this view is found in the dissent of J. Andrews in *Palsgraf* v. *Long Island Railroad Company,* 248 N.Y. 339, 162 N.E. 99 (1928), who said: "Each cause brings about future events. Without each the future would not be the same. Each is

proximate in the sense it is essential. But that is not what we mean by the word. Nor on the other hand do we mean sole cause. There is no such thing. . . . The words we used were simply indicative of our notions of public policy. . . . It is all a question of expediency. There are no fixed rules to govern our judgment."

24. E. Mack, "Moral Rights and Causal Casuistry," in B. A. Brody, ed., *Moral Theory and Moral Judgment* (Dordrecht: Reidel, 1988).

25. This general thesis about intentions is defended in Fried, *Right and Wrong*, pp. 20–29. It is applied to draw a distinction between killing and death-causing behavior in G. Grisez and J. M. Boyle, Jr., *Life and Death with Liberty and Justice* (Notre Dame: Univ. of Notre Dame Press, 1979), pp. 392–401. They certainly hold point 1 and almost certainly hold point 2 as well.

26. This emphasis on causality making a difference has been challenged by J. Rachel's *The End of Life* (Oxford: Oxford Univ. Press, 1986), pp. 111–14. His argument is as follows: "The reason we think it is bad to be the cause of someone's death is that we think death is a great evil—and so it is. However, if we have decided that euthanasia, even passive euthanasia, is desirable in a given case, then we have decided that in this instance death is no greater an evil than the patient's continued existence. And if this is true, then the usual reason for not wanting to be the cause of someone's death simply does not apply" (p. 115). The opening sentence, of course, begs the question against the more appropriate view, the one adopted here, that being the cause of someone's death is bad in part because death is a bad consequence and in part because it violates the person's right to life. The violation of the right remains even if the bad consequence disappears; the violation requires that the patient waive the right before it disappears as well.

27. The right not to be killed, therefore, cannot be the basis for objection to the recent Dutch protocol for active voluntary euthanasia. Also, this means that in many cases active euthanasia will be as justified as passive euthanasia. To say this, however, is not to accept Rachel's equivalence thesis.

28. This suggestion is not new. It was raised by the defendants in the classic lifeboat case of *Regina* v. *Dudley and Stephens*.

29. These are views on the question of who has the right not to be killed. This is a different question from the question of whether we need to consider consequences for members of many species, for members of our species only, or for persons only when we evaluate the consequences of our actions. Carl Cohen, in his very important article "The Case for the Use of Animals in Biomedical Research," *NEJM* 315, no. 14 (Oct. 2, 1986), sees, as many have not, that these are separate questions but seems to think that a type b answer to our question also dictates a type b answer to the question of the consequences-for-whom question.

30. The most influential recent proponent of this view is T. Regan, *The Case for Animal Rights* (Berkeley and Los Angeles: Univ. of California Press, 1983).

31. See, for example, Cohen, "The Case for the Use of Animals."

32. The most complicated (and most plausible, but still, I believe, fundamentally wrong) version of of this view is to be found in chapter 4 of H. T. Engelhardt, Jr., *The Foundations of Bioethics* (New York: Oxford Univ. Press, 1986).

33. Alternative accounts, such as the one that speaks of the merely symbolic significance of not injecting potassium chloride, fail to sufficiently explain the seriousness of those constraints.

34. This suggestion is not found in the classic case of *Canterbury* v. *Spence*, 464 F. 2d 772 (1972), which simply announces the emergency exception without articulating any reasons for it. R. Faden and T. L. Beauchamp, *A History and Theory of Informed Consent* (New York: Oxford Univ. Press, 1986), say quite appropriately that "Consent to treatment is often said to be 'implied' in an emergency, but this 'implication' is based on a standard of the

reasonable person, not the particular individual. This language and strategy are evasive, because the implicit claim is that consent has been obtained when in fact no authorization has occurred" (p. 36). They only need to add the point I try to make here, that we could justify the intervention on the grounds that it is so beneficial.

35. The whole debate about the Good Samaritan problem is about the question of whether you have a right against strangers that they aid you when you are threatened. The classical summation of this debate is found in J. M. Ratcliffe, ed., *The Good Samaritan and the Law* (Garden City, N.Y.: Anchor Books, 1966). A very important recent discussion, with extensive references to the literature, is chapter 4 of J. Feinberg, *Harm to Others* (New York: Oxford Univ. Press, 1984).

36. A good statement of this position is the following: "With purely moral obligations the law does not deal. For example, the priest and the Levite who passed by on the other side were not, it is supposed, liable at law for the continued suffering of the man who fell among thieves, which they might and morally ought to have prevented or relieved." *Buck v. Amaroy Mfg. Co.,* 69 N.H. 257, 44A. 809 (1898).

37. It is probably the most discussed issue in recent medical ethics. The standard consensus is expressed in the President's Commission for the Study of Ethical Problems in Medicine, *Making Health Care Decisions,* Vol. I (Washington, D.C.: Government Printing Office, 1982).

38. In this context, it is important to distinguish between patients wanting to understand decisions and patients wanting to help make them. There is some evidence that, in at least some clinical contexts, patients are more interested in the former than in the latter. See, for example, W. Strull, B. Lo, and G. Charles, "Do Patients Wish to Participate in Medical Decision-Making," *JAMA* 252, no. 21 (Dec. 7, 1984).

39. One could, after all, imagine a world in which patients have the right to refuse care but are obliged to get the information on their own, perhaps from independent consumer-information groups. There may even be some merit in such a scheme. It is not, however, the scheme we have adopted. Our scheme, in which physicians are required to provide the information, is based on a separate policy choice and is not just part of the patient's right to refuse care.

40. This is presumably a major part of the basis for the divergence between what patients say they want to know and what physicians say patients want to know. See, for example, Ruth Faden et al., "Disclosure Standards and Informed Consent," *Journal of Health Politics Policy and Law* 6, no. 2 (Summer 1981).

41. My own impression is that physicians see informed consent as more burdensome paperwork; they think that hospital consent forms (especially presurgery forms) are the heart of informed consent. When they are reminded that the heart of informed consent is effective communication, physicians express a very different attitude.

42. A very thoughtful example of this type of argument is found in A. F. Patenaude, J. M. Rappeport, and B. R. Smith, "The Physician's Influence on Informed Consent for Bone Marrow Transplantation," *Theoretical Medicine* 7, no. 2 (June 1986). They claim that "for bone marrow transplantation, at least, the vast amount of relevant technical information, the many uncertainties, and the high level of patient anxiety, make it impossible for the potential bone marrow transplant patient to digest all of the relevant data to make a truly autonomous decision without editing and selective emphasis from the physician" (p. 169). I have no doubt that many other specialists would make similar claims for their procedures.

43. To continue the bone-marrow transplant example, consider the adolescent patient with acute lymphoblastic leukemia who has relapsed after the first remission, who has a compatible donor, and in whom a second remission has been induced. The crucial points are presumably just these: (1) the chemotherapy regimen which has been tried until now (and

others like it) has a low probability of long-term success from now on; (2) there is an alternative approach which has emerged recently and has a much better success rate but which produces quicker and more painful deaths in many of the cases in which it fails; (3) it involves totally destroying the patient's current bone marrow and transplanting new marrow from the donor; (4) the great risks are infections when the old bone marrow is destroyed before transplantation and the grafted marrow producing substances that attack portions of the patient's body after transplantation. One can then offer to provide further details as requested. It may be even more important to provide this information in light of new data which suggest an alternative to bone-marrow transplantation in such cases. These data are presented in G. K. Rivera et al., "Intensive Retreatment of Childhood Acute Lymphoblastic Leukemia in First Bone Marrow Relapse," *NEJM* 315, no. 5 (July 31, 1986). Patients now need to be told that (5) much more intensive chemotherapy has recently been reported to work just as well, so there is a choice here with no clear indications of which alternative is more likely to result in survival.

44. Such a view was strongly argued by the Legal Advisors, Committee of Concern for Dying in "The Right to Refuse Treatment: A Model Act," *American Journal of Public Health* 73, no. 8 (August 1983). To quote their own abstract: "Although the right to refuse medical treatment is universally recognized as a fundamental principle of liberty, this right is not always honored. A refusal can be thwarted either because a patient is unable to competently communicate or because providers insist on continuing treatment. To help enhance the patient's right to refuse treatment, many states have enacted so-called 'living will' or 'natural death' statutes. We believe the time has come to move beyond these current legislative models, and we therefore propose a Model Act that clearly enunciates an individual's right to refuse treatment, does not limit its exercise to the terminally ill or to heroic measures, and provides a mechanism by which individuals can set forth their wishes in advance and designate another person to enforce them" (p. 918). The act allows for no exceptions to this right to refuse care.

45. Many clinicians with whom I have discussed this question agree, however, that it is usually made.

46. An excellent example of a good policy statement on this point is the following: "Patients should be encouraged to discuss forgoing life-sustaining treatment with family members and (where appropriate) close friends. However, a patient's privacy and confidentiality require that his order not to enter into such a decision or not to divulge to family members the patient's decision to forgo life-sustaining treatment must be respected." This quotation comes from A. Meisel et al., "Hospital Guidelines for Deciding about Life-Sustaining Treatment: Dealing with Health 'Limbo,'" *Critical Care Medicine* 14, no. 3 (March 1986): 245.

47. Unfortunately, statutes such as the Natural Death Acts make no allowance for any of these factors except for language like the following: "The attending physician shall comply with the directive unless the physician believes that the directive does not reflect the present desire of the patient" (section 4A of the Texas Natural Death Act).

48. Two bases are normally put forward: "substituted judgment" and "best interest." A tremendous literature surrounding many crucial court cases has grown up around these concepts. The point is, of course, that the bases in question deal with different sorts of cases and are not really competing with each other. Failure to see this can have disastrous consequences. The Texas Natural Death Act (as amended in 1985) attempted to deal with the problem of patients who had not expressed any wishes about life-sustaining procedures by allowing family members to make decisions together with the physician. Their decision "may, based on knowledge of what the patient would desire, if known, include a decision to withhold or withdraw life-sustaining procedures from the patient" (section 4C[a]). The Texas

legislature clearly wanted to adopt a substituted judgment approach, presumably viewing it as a competitor to the best-interest approach. The legislature has failed to deal with the question of what to do in the case in which this knowledge of the patient's wishes is not available.

49. That is, of course, the usual meaning of the best-interest standard. The President's Commission suggests, in *Making Health Care Decisions,* pp. 180–81, that this can be extended to a consideration of the interest of the family only when there is convincing evidence of the patient's interest in the family's well-being. Both sides are wrong, because they haven't attended to how families are normally entitled to make decisions for family members.

50. This question is equivalent to that of when family decisions result in sufficient neglect to a dependent family member that they constitute abuse by neglect. That question is notoriously difficult to answer.

51. The family's right to waive their right to be decision makers and to refuse care must be distinguished from the family's right to waive any of the patient's rights. For example, can the family waive the patient's right not to be killed, thereby eliminating one of the major obstacles to justifying active euthanasia? We shall return to this question at several points in chapters 6 and 7.

52. Since I first wrote this section, I have had the pleasure of consulting Allen Buchanan's very important *Surrogate Decisionmaking for Elderly Individuals Who Are Incompetent or of Questionable Competence,* a report prepared for the Office of Technology Assessment and dated November 1985. Many of Buchanan's conclusions parallel mine, but I want to note several points of disagreement. First, Buchanan believes that if we must fall back on judgments about the patient's best interests, the determination should focus solely on the individual's self-regarding interests and not on alleged interests in the good of others. This leaves out the possibility that family members as decision makers are entitled, independently of any alleged interest on the part of the patient, to consider the interests of others. Second, Buchanan thinks that permanently unconscious patients are beyond the scope of the best-interest principle since they cannot benefit because they are unaware of what is occurring. This view presupposes that we can only benefit from consequences if we are aware of their occurrence. That presupposition is not necessarily true on the preference-satisfaction theory, since one may have last relevant preferences (e.g., to continue one's biological life as long as possible) which can be satisfied even if one is not aware of their satisfaction.

53. As is well known, Kant, in both *The Fundamental Principles of the Metaphysics of Morals* (1785) and *The Critique of Practical Reason* (1788), emphasized three fundamental themes: universalizability, treating humanity as an end, and autonomous choice. The second theme, that of rational beings as entities whose existence is an end in itself, is the intellectual origin of the theory of respect for persons that I am advocating here. I first introduced it in "Toward a Theory of Respect for Persons," in O. H. Green, ed., *Respect for Persons: Tulane Studies in Philosophy,* Vol. XXXI (New Orleans: Tulane Univ., 1982).

54. Two notable recent examples in the theoretic literature are A. Donagan, *Theory of Morality* (Chicago: Univ. of Chicago Press, 1977), and Fried, *Right and Wrong.*

55. Many writers in bioethics suggest these ideas. The following quotation is representative: "In evaluating the autonomous actions of others we ought to respect them as persons with the same right to their choices and actions as we have to our own." T. Beauchamp and J. Childress, *Principles of Biomedical Ethics,* 2nd edition (New York: Oxford Univ. Press, 1983), p. 63. Note how respect for persons is seen in honoring a procedural right of the individual.

56. To say this is not to deny that we fail at least sometimes to show respect for persons when we violate their rights. It is only to say that there are failures to show respect which have nothing to do with violating rights.

57. Notice that our list is not very Kantian. I include his emphasis on rational deliberation and choice, but I include other things as well, such as capacities to engage in interpersonal relations, to appreciate things of beauty, and so on. The severely demented patient who can make few rational choices but who still smiles when he sees a loved one or when he is taken out to a pretty garden on a warm spring day is still entitled to some respect as a person, and the strict Kantian way of understanding respect for persons fails to see this.

58. This suggestion, particularly as it applies to an Aristotelian theory of the virtues, has been argued for by A. McIntyre in *After Virtue* (Notre Dame: Univ. of Notre Dame Press, 1981). He writes: "My own conclusion is very clear. It is that on the one hand we still, in spite of the efforts of three centuries of moral philosophy and one of sociology, lack any coherent rationally defensible statement of a liberal individualist point of view; and that, on the other hand, the Aristotelean tradition can be restated in a way that restores intelligibility and rationality to our moral and social attitudes and commitments" (p. 241).

59. See, for example, his definition of the courageous man: "The man, then, who faces and who fears the right things and *from the right motive,* in the right way and at the right time, and who feels confidence under the corresponding conditions, is brave" (1115b, 18–20).

60. It becomes an important dispute in cases of potentially virtuous actions performed for dubious motives. I discuss in this book few examples of such actions where the virtues are relevant. There are many real cases not discussed in this book in which the dispute does become very relevant.

61. Williams, in J. J. C. Smart and B. Williams, *Utilitarianism: For and Against* (Cambridge: Cambridge Univ. Press, 1973), pp. 98–99, raises the case of Jim, who is faced with a choice of killing one innocent individual or of allowing the evil Pedro to kill twenty. Williams has much to say about the case, including: "A feature of utilitarianism is that it cuts out a kind of consideration which for some others makes a difference to what they feel about such cases: a consideration involving the idea, as we might first and very simply put it, that each of us is specially responsible for what he does, rather than for what other people do. This is an idea closely connected with the value of integrity" (p. 99). Later in that same essay Williams talks about integrity in a way that is closer to what I have in mind, although his emphasis seems more on projects and less on personal values.

62. I emphasize "in part" to remind us that, like any moral appeal, the appeal to the virtue of integrity can be overridden by other considerations.

63. This is one way in which the idea of supererogatory actions (actions which have moral value, even if they are not obligatory) can be built into a moral theory. See J. O. Urmson, "Saints and Heroes," in A. I. Melden, ed., *Essays in Moral Philosophy* (Seattle: Univ. of Washington Press, 1958); R. Chisholm, "Supererogation and Offense," *Ratio* 5 (1963); and J. Feinberg, "Supererogation and Rules," *International Journal of Ethics* 71 (1961). Despite the important initial work on this topic, the ways in which supererogatory actions relate to the various moral appeals require considerable additional investigation.

64. *Nicomachean Ethics,* book III, chap. 7.

65. This is to say that the thief cannot be courageous in his acts of theft. That seems somewhat counterintuitive, but perhaps I could make it seem less so by explaining that this just means that there is nothing virtuous about the thief's behavior.

66. The law has struggled with these questions for a long time. See, for example, the discussion of nondisclosure in W. L. Prosser, *Handbook of the Law of Torts,* 4th ed. (St. Paul: West Publishing, 1971), section 106.

67. It is this type of appeal to compassion which lies behind the therapeutic privilege much discussed in the context of informed consent. That privilege is the right to withhold information in those cases in which it is thought that disclosure might harm the patient. The

therapeutic privilege is discussed in Faden and Beauchamp, *A History and Theory of Informed Consent,* pp. 37–39, and in the literature cited there.

68. A very good introduction to the economic literature surrounding this suggestion and alternative suggestions is found in S. Rhoads, "How Much Should We Spend to Save a Life," *Public Interest* 51 (Spring 1978).

69. See, in particular, the discussion in chapters 2 and 3 of P. Menzel, *Medical Costs, Moral Choices* (New Haven: Yale Univ. Press, 1983).

70. Exactly what is a case of waste is not always easy to ascertain. See, on this issue, B. Brody, "The Ethics of Cost-Benefit Analysis in OB/GYN Practice," *The Female Physician* 11 (August 1986). On the political significance of this concept, see M. A. Baily, "Rationing and American Health Policy," *Journal of Health Politics Policy and Law* 9 (Fall 1984).

71. I am using the word *entitled* here just to mean "what's due to them." I do not want it to carry all of the theoretical associations it has come to have in its use in the libertarian literature.

72. The classic recent statement is C. Fried, "Rights and Health: Beyond Equity and Efficiency," *NEJM* 293 (1975).

73. A major reason for making this assumption may just be that no one has a claim against the public to provide health care which is not cost-effective.

74. This example is motivated by two very important recent discussions: H. T. Engelhardt, Jr., and M. Rie, "Intensive Care Units, Scarce Resources, and Conflicting Principles of Justice," *JAMA* 255 (March 7, 1986); and R. Strauss et al., "Rationing of Intensive Care Unit Resources: An Everyday Occurrence," *JAMA* 255 (March 7, 1986).

75. The claim that they should not and would not approve is connected with the claim above that we are not a society obliged to offer to those who cannot pay for it themselves forms of health care that are not cost-effective. Any attempt to justify this claim would require a full theory of justice in health care. Short of that, the reader might consult A. Gibbard, "The Prospective Pareto Principle and Equity of Access to Health Care," *MMFQ* 60 (1982), for an argument that could support this conclusion.

76. The evidence is all of the attempts to control health-care expenditures, particularly those (e.g., those which raise co-payments and deductibles) which are designed to give patients an incentive to reject forms of care which provide little benefit at considerable cost.

77. The exception to this would be policies which build into their explicit terms the right of the insurer to refuse to pay for forms of health care which are not cost-effective.

# 3

## The Contractual and Status Models: Strengths and Weaknesses

The last chapter outlined a variety of ethical appeals that should be incorporated into any model of decision making which will enable us to deal with the cases to be discussed in chapters 5 through 7. In this chapter we will examine two standard models of the patient-physician relationship and health-care decision making within that relationship to see whether or not they are successful in incorporating all of the ethical appeals.

Each of these models draws its strength from the fact that it does incorporate some important ethical appeals. The weakness of each lies precisely in the fact that it only incorporates some of these appeals while others are left out.

By the end of the chapter, we will be in a position to see how difficult it is to develop an appropriate model for the patient-physician relationship and for medical decision making within that relationship. It is easy to incorporate some of the appeals we have discussed, but it is very difficult to develop a model that incorporates all of the important ethical appeals. In chapter 4, I hope to show that it is nevertheless possible to develop a model that does appropriately incorporate all of them.

### 3.1  The Contractual Model

I call the first model of decision making the contractual model, since it presents a contractual approach to the patient-physician relationship.[1] It makes five basic claims:

1.  Neither party in the patient-physician relationship is under an obligation to enter into that relationship.
2.  Each party enters into the relationship only on the basis of the terms to which each freely

agrees, and these terms will dictate (among other things) the type of decision making that will legitimately take place in that particular patient-physician relationship.

3.  The relationship legitimately exists only when the terms set in advance by each party are the same.
4.  Society's main role in connection with the patient-physician relationship is to protect both parties against nonperformance or malperformance and against fraud or coercion, and society has no special role in seeing that certain decisional processes or outcomes come about.
5.  Society has no special obligation resulting from the patient-physician agreement to pay for the health care that results from the decisions made in the relationship.

Even this brief statement makes it clear why this model is properly called the contractual model. After all, according to this model, the patient-physician relationship and the decisions made in it are analogous to normal commercial relationships created by normal contractual processes. However, the aptness of this name will be even clearer after we look more carefully at each of the five claims.

The first claim is that neither party in the patient-physician relationship is under any moral obligation to enter into it. This, of course, means two things. First, no physician is under an obligation to provide services to any particular patient, even when there is an emergency situation in which help is needed immediately. Second, no potential patient is under a moral obligation to consult a physician about his or her medical problems, even if the potential patient is in serious need of medical treatment. A physician who fails to offer services, even in an emergency situation, has not, according to this model, failed to fulfill his or her obligations as a physician. A patient who fails to seek medical help, even when it is seriously needed, has not, according to this model, failed to fulfill an obligation to seek that help.

The second claim is that each party enters into the relationship only on the basis of the terms to which he or she has freely agreed, and these terms will include the way in which decisions will be made in that particular relationship. For the physician, this means that he or she is free to provide services at some set time, in some set place, for some set fee, in some set manner, according to some set decisional process. To be more precise, the physician is free to provide these services in accordance with the terms acceptable to him or her, providing that he or she can find someone who desires the services subject to those terms. For the patient, it means that he or she is free to accept such medical services as are offered in accordance with such terms regarding time, location, manner, price, and form of decision making that are acceptable to him or her. More precisely, it means that the patient is free to accept such services according to terms acceptable to him or her providing he or she can find someone who wishes to provide those services in accordance with those terms.

The third claim is really a summation of the first two, and it expresses the heart of the contractual model of the patient-physician relationship and decision making within it. It says that the patient-physician relationship legitimately exists only when both parties have agreed to the same terms governing the provision of medical services. In particular, the relationship legitimately exists only when, among other things, both parties have agreed to the same approach to decision making. One caveat about this third claim. Even in a commercial case, a relationship can, in extraordinary circumstances, be created unilaterally.[2] If, for example, your property is threatened by destruction and I can save it but you are unavailable to consent, then if I do save it I can obtain certain payments from you. In such a case, we may allow the relationship to come into effect on the basis of your hypothetical consent, the consent you would have given had you been able to consider the offer of my services. Similarly, in a medical context proponents of this model say that a legitimate physician-patient relationship may exist when a physician provides services in an emergency situation in which the patient's consent cannot be obtained. The legitimacy of the relationship is based on the physician's actual agreement and the patient's hypothetical agreement.[3]

The fourth claim is that society's main role in connection with the physician-patient relationship is to protect both parties against nonperformance or malperformance and against fraud or coercion. This is the classical liberal conception of the social role in connection with any commercial transaction.[4] To begin with, society must protect people against the use of fraud or force to obtain consent to relationship-creating agreements. In recent years these requirements have deepened as we have come to understand more about subtle fraud and subtle coercion.[5] Secondly, society must protect both parties against nonperformance or malperformance. Malperformance gives rise to a tort suit and nonperformance to a suit for damages or for specific performance. The crucial point this model wants to make is that there is no place for society to do anything beyond these limited tasks. In particular, the decisional processes that will be utilized in a patient-physician relationship and the decisions that will be made are something for the parties to agree on. This model is saying that there are no clearly appropriate decisional processes and decisional outcomes society should enforce independent of the agreed-upon wishes of patients and physicians.

The fifth and final claim of the contractual model is that society is under no special obligation resulting from the patient-physician agreement to pay for the services rendered by the physician. This important aspect of the model grows out of its insistence that the patient-physician relationship should be created by agreements between those parties into which they are under no obligation to enter. The patient's agreement to create a certain patient-physician relationship can oblige him or her to pay certain fees; it is unclear how it can create a social obligation to pay those fees, and the contractual model insists that there is no such obligation. All this is perfectly compatible with the idea that some third party (e.g., an insurance company) can have an obligation, created by some agreement in advance between the patient and the third party, to reimburse the patient for the fees paid. More crucially, all of this is compatible with many different versions of the idea that society may have a special obligation to provide health care to the indigent, ranging all the way from the idea that society should directly provide that care it judges appropriate (socialized medicine), to the idea that society should pay the fees it finds appropriate for forms of care it judges appropriate (national health insurance), to the idea that society should provide funds out of which the indigent can purchase the health care they desire (voucher scheme).[6] All that is being claimed here is that the purchase of medical care creates no special obligation for social payments.

## 3.2  Strengths and Weaknesses of the Contractual Model

There are obvious strengths of the contractual model of the patient-physician relationship and of decision making within it. It certainly incorporates some of the crucial ethical appeals.

We will begin with the procedural rights outlined in section 2.2. The first of those rights was the right to make decisions affecting oneself. This right was had by both patients and physicians. It included the right of the patient to refuse forms of treatment that a physician wished to perform and the right of the physician to refuse to perform procedures and treatments that a patient might desire. The contractual model is obviously sensitive to both important aspects of this decisional right. In this respect it is a significant advance over the popular view that simply emphasizes the patient's right to decide what will happen to his or her body.[7]

There is an additional way in which the contractual model correctly understands this procedural right. We saw in section 2.2 that the patient may waive the right to be a decision maker and may give the appropriate decisional authority to a provider that he or she trusts. The contractual model certainly captures this right of a patient. As it says in its second claim, each party must freely agree to the type of decision making that will take place in that particular physician-patient relationship. This means, among other things, that patients may agree to give total decisional authority to their physicians, who then have that authority providing that they are willing to take it.

The contractual model is less helpful when considering the other crucial procedural right, that of the family to participate in decision making when the patient is no longer competent. The model, as presented, makes no reference to any form of collaborative decision making between the physician and the family. It is possible, however, to modify the model to incorporate this additional element. One way to do this would be to suppose that there is an implicit understanding in the contract between the patient and the physician that the patient's family will act in place of the patient when the patient is no longer competent to do so. One advantage of thinking of it this way is that it enables us to deal with a certain class of cases in which the family has no right to participate in decision making. These are the cases in which the patient, while competent, has made it clear that he or she does not wish the family to participate in decision making for him or her. Sometimes, for example, a patient may say to a doctor that he or she mistrusts family and does not want them to be involved in any decision making about his or her care. In other cases, the patient may wish to spare the family the agony of decision making and may indicate this to the physician. If we suppose, as our modification of the contractual model suggests, that the right of the family to participate in decision making when the patient is no longer competent is an implicit term of the contract between the physician and the patient, then this implicit understanding will, of course, be overruled by any explicit statements to the contrary by the patient.[8] In short, then, it is possible to extend the contractual model so as to encompass in helpful ways the right of the family to participate in decision making.

Turning from the procedural rights to the substantive rights discussed in section

2.2, the contractual model does not explicitly refer either to the right not to be killed or to the right not to have bodily harm inflicted on oneself. However, both of these rights (and even the stronger right simply not to have one's body touched by anyone else) are presupposed by the contractual model. According to the contractual model, there is a legitimate physician-patient relationship in which the physician can treat the patient only when the two parties have come to some agreement. Absent such agreement, it would be wrong for the physician to treat the patient, and the basis for that is that the patient has a right not to be touched by anyone, much less harmed or killed, without his or her consent.

There is one further substantive right, the right to be aided in times of need. This right is obviously not incorporated in the contractual model, which gives the physician the right to refuse to come to the aid of the patient unless the appropriate agreement has been reached, and this is an obvious weakness of the model, one to which we shall return.

We turn now to the virtues, beginning with the virtue of integrity, which, as we saw in section 2.4, essentially refers to decision makers being true to their values. The contractual model has the advantage that it does leave room for the display of integrity because it allows both health-care providers and health-care recipients to refuse to enter into relationships. They are not required to enter into any relationship unless they can obtain terms which are acceptable to them. This at least allows them to be true to their values and to maintain a sense of integrity by refusing to participate in health-care relationships that are destructive of that integrity. In this respect the model incorporates the virtue of integrity. There is, however, another way in which this model does not make sufficient allowance for integrity. It does not require the health-care provider and the health-care recipient to remain true to their values in coming to their agreements with each other. The model does not mandate integrity; it merely allows for it. In allowing for it, there is a certain strength to the model. In merely allowing for it and not demanding it, the model falls short of an ideal moral model.[9]

Very similar remarks can be made about the virtues of compassion and courage. The contractual model allows both parties to insist that the relationship be structured so as to allow them to exhibit their courage and compassion. It does not, however, criticize a health-care relationship in which both parties have agreed to behavior that is cowardly or incompassionate. In not doing that, this model suffers from a serious weakness.

The virtue of honesty is treated somewhat differently by this model. Honesty in the process of creating a health-care relationship is mandated by the model. An agreement between a provider and a recipient that is not arrived at honestly is not a valid agreement and does not create a legitimate patient-physician relationship. The virtue of honesty, at least in the creation of health-care relationships, is mandated by the contractual model. It says nothing, however, about the honesty that should obtain in such a relationship after it has come into existence. Once more, the model certainly allows for a patient-physician relationship based on honesty if that is what both parties desire. If, however, both prefer a relationship in which a certain amount of dishonesty is present, then, as far as the contractual model is concerned, this is a legitimate health-care relationship. After the creation of the physician-patient relationship, honesty is treated by this model no differently from any of the other virtues.

The contractual model explicitly incorporates certain procedural rights of both health-care recipients and health-care providers, it implicitly presupposes certain substantive rights of those recipients, it mandates a certain honesty in the creation of the health-care relationship, and it allows for the exhibition of a variety of important virtues of both providers and recipients. These are all important strengths of the model. Unfortunately, there are also significant weaknesses.

The first weakness of the contractual model is one to which we have already alluded in our discussion of its strengths. While the contractual model allows for the exhibiting of a variety of important virtues, it does not insist that these virtues be incorporated into a proper health-care relationship.

A few examples will illustrate this point. Consider the virtue of integrity. In section 2.4, I pointed out that different health-care providers may have different goals in their practice of medicine. Consider, for example, a provider whose personal goal is to find ways to extend the possibility of prolonging conscious human existence. According to this model, a legitimate health-care relationship might exist between such a provider and a recipient who has very different goals, such as the relief of pain. Such a provider may, according to the contractual model, create a legitimate health-care relationship if the provider agrees to adopt the goals of the recipient, even if this means relieving pain by methods that shorten the patient's life. The contractual model finds this agreement acceptable, even if it is based on the physician's desire to increase his or her income by increasing patient load. Many would find it objectionable, however, not because of what has been agreed to but because of the dissonance between the terms agreed upon and the values of the person who has agreed to them. This failure of provider integrity would strike many as a fundamental flaw in this particular health-care relationship. By not demanding that health-care providers and recipients display integrity, the contractual model fails. The same point can be made in connection with the important virtue of compassion. The contractual model, at best, allows for the structuring of health-care relationships that are compassionate, but it does not mandate that compassion. This is one of the reasons why the contractual model is forced to fall back on the hypothetical consent of the patient in order to allow the health-care provider to come to the aid of a stranger. All of this seems in error. And the same is true for the compassion that should be shown by a health-care recipient. A recipient who requests immediate treatment of a problem that could be deferred for another occasion when it is clear that the health-care provider is tired has failed to show the proper compassion. If, however, the provider agrees to this immediate provision of health care, perhaps out of a felt need to keep up patient load, the contractual model can find nothing faulty. This is a further indication of the poverty of the contractual model in the health-care context.

It might be thought that these difficulties with the contractual model could easily be remedied. After all, could we not simply expand the model to build into it the idea that health-care relationships should incorporate these virtues? This suggestion, while initially attractive, misses the crucial point. The basic idea behind the contractual model is that the only values that are required in health-care relationships are the mutually agreed-upon values of the health-care provider and the health-care recipient. As long as the two parties agree through a process that is procedurally acceptable, then there are no further moral demands on the health-care relationship. To impose the additional values that the virtues in question call for, and to impose them independently of the agreement of the two parties, is not to add to the contractual model. It is instead to challenge the fundamental presupposition of that model. I am not arguing that it would be inappropriate to mandate the display of the appropriate virtues in the health-care relationship; on the contrary, I am insisting that it would be appropriate to mandate this but that doing so is contradicting the fundamental spirit of the contractual model.

A very similar point must be made about the question of respect for persons in the health-care relationship. If respect for persons was simply a respect for their rights, then the contractual model would have no difficulty with it. As we have seen, the model certainly makes provision for respecting the procedural and substantive rights of recipients and providers. However, as we saw in section 2.3, there is an additional content to respect for persons. Respecting persons is, in part, valuing their potential to perform certain types of actions. We show that respect by not lessening these potentials, and our obligation to show this respect is independent of the wishes of the persons in question. It is this aspect of respect for personhood which the contractual model cannot take into account. The reason for this is straightforward. The logical structure of the appeal to respect for persons leads us to have certain obligations to people independently of their insisting on our fulfilling these obligations. This respect for persons will lead health-care providers to promote the life and bodily integrity of their patients, even in some cases where this goes beyond the wishes of the patients in question. Respect for persons is like respect for the virtues in that it introduces values into the health-care relationship that may be independent of the wishes of a particular recipient and a particular provider at a particular time. Such values cannot be accommodated in the contractual model without challenging its fundamental claim that the health-care relationship is legitimate when and only when the terms set in advance by each party are the same. That fundamental claim mandates that the values to be exhibited in a health-care relationship are simply those set by the parties in question. Respect for persons, like respect for the virtues, introduces further values, and this undercuts the fundamental point of the contractual model.

It might be thought that this is also true in connection with the appeal to the consequences of our actions, which might be thought to mandate a value which is independent of the wishes of the parties. A further weakness of the contractual model could be that it cannot properly handle the moral legitimacy of the appeal to consequences in evaluating health-care decisions. This is not completely accurate. As we saw in section 2.1, there are really several appeals to consequences in the health-care context. It is relevant to consider the impact of health-care decisions on society in general, on the patient alone, and on those with whom the patient is concerned. These are three different appeals, the moral root of each of them is different, and the implications of them for the contractual model are different.

The consideration of the impact of the health-care decision on those with whom the patient is concerned is perfectly compatible with the contractual model. If the patient wishes the physician to be primarily concerned with the implications of health-care decisions for the patient's family, and if the physician agrees to do so, then both the contractual model and this aspect of the appeal to consequences agree that the morally appropriate thing to do is to focus attention on the implications of decisions for the family. This aspect of the appeal to consequences is therefore compatible with the contractual model. In the classical example of the dying patient who refuses further treatment because of the economic disaster it will impose on his or her family, the contractual model would agree that the physician should judge possible health-care decisions for this patient in light of the impact on the patient's family.

There are, however, other aspects of the appeal to consequences which the contractual model cannot handle because they do introduce values which are mandated for the health-care relationship and which do not grow out of agreements between recipients and providers. To begin with, there is the appeal to the general consequences of our actions. As we saw in section 2.1, the denial of utilitarianism is not equivalent to the claim that such an appeal to the consequences of our actions for people in general is totally wrong. We certainly need to take those consequences into account. Even if the provider and the recipient are perfectly prepared to come to an agreement that health-care decisions will be made without taking into account any of the implications for people in general, there is good reason to believe that such an agreement sometimes leads to morally inappropriate actions. In short, the value that utilitarians have always talked about certainly needs to be built into the evaluation of health-care decisions. As an imposed external value, it cannot be accommodated in the contractual model.

In a similar fashion the contractual model cannot do justice to the professional value of attending simply to the implications of one's health-care decisions for one's patients. The oldest of the traditional values of the medical profession is that one should do no harm to one's patient.[10] One does not need to agree with the traditional claim that this is a rule to which there is no exception to agree that it represents a fundamental value to be incorporated into any moral evaluation of particular health-care relationships. The contractual model certainly allows for that traditional value, but it does so only if both parties agree to it. The contractual model fails because it only allows for its incorporation without mandating it.

We turn finally to the question of whether or not the contractual model can properly handle questions of justice and cost-effectiveness in its evaluation of health-care relationships. The contractual model finds nothing wrong with the provision of very expensive health care with minimum benefits in the private sector providing that both recipient and provider understand and agree to the cost and benefits of the health care being provided. We saw in section 2.6 no reason to disagree with this aspect of the contractual model. However, there remains the possibility of the need to justly allocate limited health-care resources even in the private sector, and here the contractual model is in trouble. It presupposes that the health-care relationship is entirely structured by the terms of the agreements between the providers and the recipients, and it cannot address the moral question of what to do when not all providers can possibly provide what they are willing to provide and recipients are willing to receive. The model, of course, is even less able to incorporate the demands of justice and cost-effectiveness in the public sector. These are appropriate demands, independent of any particular agreement between physicians and patients. The imposition of such moral values is not consonant with the whole approach of the contractual model.

In short, there are two major weaknesses with the contractual model. The first is that it cannot accommodate any external imposition of values on the health-care relationship. For this reason it cannot do justice to the appeal to the virtues, the appeal to respect for personhood, the appeal to the right to be aided, and the appeal to certain types of consequences in the evaluation of health-care relationships and decisions. Second, it cannot do justice to the social dimension of the evaluation of health-care decisions, whether in the public provision of health care or in the private provision of health care. The model's strength is that it incorporates some of the ethical appeals discussed in chapter 2. The model's weakness is that it fails to incorporate the rest of them.

## 3.3   The Status Model

I call the second model of decision making the status model.[11] It is based on a fundamentally different approach to the patient-physician relationship, and it makes five basic claims about the patient-physician relationship and decision making in it:

1.   Both parties in the patient-physician relationship are under an obligation in certain conditions to enter into that relationship.
2.   Some of the appropriate terms of the relationship, including some of the terms that dictate the type of decision making that will legitimately take place, are independent of and may conflict with the wishes of one or both of the parties. Other terms should be set by their joint agreement.
3.   The patient-physician relationship legitimately exists only when (a) these independent terms are met and (b) the other terms are set by mutual agreement of both parties.
4.   Society's main roles are to ensure that the two parties enter into this relationship when they are obliged to do so and to ensure that the relationship is governed by the appropriate independent terms. In addition, society has the role of protecting both parties against nonperformance or malperformance in connection with any of the terms and against fraud or coercion in the agreement on those terms which are properly settled by the agreement of the two parties. As a result, society has a special role in seeing that certain decisional processes and certain decisional outcomes come about.
5.   Society may have a special obligation to pay for required health care if the recipient is not in a position to do so.

The contrast with the contractual model is clear even from this brief statement of the status model. Before elaborating, I want to say something about the name of this model. Henry Maine, in his classic work *Ancient Law* (1861), drew the contrast between societies in which relationships are governed by terms freely agreed upon by the parties, which he called contractual relationships, and societies in which relationships among individuals are governed by terms that are in part determined by independent external norms, which he called status relationships. Since it is crucial to this model that some of the terms are set by independent norms, it seems appropriate to call this model the status model of the patient-physician relationship.

Two sources of these independent norms are usually mentioned.[12] One is a set of norms grounded in a professionally shared understanding of what is medically appropriate for the patient. Given the patient's physical and mental condition, medical standards dictate that certain treatments be applied, and any legitimate patient-physician relationship must involve the physician providing those services and the patient accepting them. This consensus of medical judgment about what is the appropriate form of treatment for some conditions generates, according to this version of the status model, the conclusion that certain decisions may well be inappropriate even if both parties agree to them, just because they violate the established professional consensus. The second source addresses itself to other questions (questions concerning fees, availability, types of decisional processes) as well as questions of forms of treatment. This involves the ethical factors of the type discussed in chapter 2. There are many different versions of the status model which differ in their emphasis on these two sources and in their understanding of the norms arising out of them. But they all share an acceptance of the idea that there are independent external norms governing the health-care relationship.

The first claim of the status model is that both parties in the patient-physician relationship are under an obligation in some circumstances to enter into that relationship. This claim means different things when it is applied to the patient and to the physician. The potential patient is under an obligation to seek out a physician's help when he or she has a serious medical problem, and the obligation becomes greater as the problem becomes more serious. A patient who fails to seek medical help for a serious medical problem is not merely a stupid patient; on this model, the patient has also failed to fulfill his or her obligations, which are rooted in an appeal to consequences and/or an appeal to respect for his or her own personhood. The physician is under an obligation to provide services to people in need, particularly in emergency situations. A physician who fails to offer services, especially in an emergency situation, may, on this model, be accused of a failure to respect the patient's right to aid, a lack of compassion, and a failure to attend to the consequences of his or her action.

The second claim is that each party to the patient-physician relationship enters into that relationship under terms which are at least in part independent of their wishes, and these terms will include, among other things, how decisions will be made in the relationship. Again, this claim means different things for the patient and for the physician. For the physician, there are constraints on the forms of treatment that he or she may legitimately provide, and there are limits on the conditions (including fees, availability, etc.) under which these services are to be provided.[13] For the patient, there are constraints on the types of treatments that he or she may legitimately request and constraints on the conditions for receiving treatment. None of this is to say that all of the terms of the patient-physician relationship, including the terms of decision making, are independent of the wishes of both parties. What is being claimed is that there are certain crucial terms that are independent of the wishes of the two parties; the remaining terms are determined by their wishes.

The third claim is really a summation of the first two, and it summarizes the heart of the status model. It says that the mere agreement of patient and physician to terms for the provision of health care does not guarantee that the resulting relationship (and the provision of health care in it) is a legitimate patient-physician relationship. Legitimacy, according to this model, is based on more than simply the consent of both parties. It requires that the basic independent norms governing the physician-patient relationship be observed. It also requires an agreement from both parties on the remaining terms governing their particular relationship.

The fourth claim is that society's main role is to ensure that the parties enter into the relationship when they are obliged to do so and to ensure that the relationship is governed by the appropriate terms. This is not surprising. After all, the main role of society in both the contractual and the status model is to ensure the legitimacy of the patient-physician relationship. In the case of the contractual model this puts the major emphasis on supervising the process by which the relationship is formed. In the case of the status model it emphasizes the legitimacy of the terms.

The fifth and final claim of the status model is that society's role may extend to having a special obligation to pay for required medical treatment if the patient is incapable of doing so. It is easy to see how this final claim arises out of the earlier claims. Suppose we have a case in which society has insisted that a patient who cannot afford medical treatment obtain that medical treatment on the grounds that it is needed and has insisted that a physician provide that treatment. Suppose, moreover, that society's insistence is legitimate according to this model. Who is to bear the cost of the physician's care? It cannot be the patient, because the patient doesn't have the ability to pay. We might impose the cost on the physician, but it is unclear why it should be the physician's burden alone, and in any case he or she is likely to pass it on to the rest of us through his or her fees.[14] Realism, combined with a sense of fairness, seems to lead to the conclusion that society must sometimes bear the cost. This obligation will exist independently of any other theory of justice in health care. In this final way, then, the status model differs from the contractual model.

## 3.4   Strengths and Weaknesses of the Status Model

The obvious strength of the status model of the patient-physician relationship and of decision making within it is that it incorporates some of the crucial ethical appeals which were outlined in chapter 2.

The model is sensitive to important aspects of the appeal to the consequences of actions. As we saw in section 2.1, the commitment of the health-care profession is to be a helping and healing profession. This means that the health-care provider should be trying to do what is beneficial for his or her particular patient. To some extent, health-care providers need to focus on the implications of their actions just for their patients and not for society in general or for others with whom the patients are concerned. This aspect of the appeal to consequences is directly captured by the status model. After all, the model derives some of its most important norms which are mandatory for any legitimate health-care relationship from a medical consideration of what is best for the individual patient being treated. In addition, the status model can incorporate without any difficulty the appeal to the general consequences of one's actions. A second source of the external norms which are mandatory for any legitimate health-care relationship involves moral appeals which are independent of any professional ethic. The appeal to the general consequences of one's actions is one of those independent moral appeals which becomes an external norm for legitimate patient-physician relationships.

We turn then to a consideration of the rights of the parties involved. Like the contractual model, the status model has little difficulty incorporating the right not to be killed and the right not to have bodily injury or pain inflicted on oneself. Absent most unusual circumstances, actions that result in the killing of a patient or the infliction of bodily injury or pain on the patient are not in accord with professional norms and with appropriate independent values and are not therefore morally permissible in a legitimate patient-physician relationship. More crucially, the status model has little difficulty incorporating the right of the patient to be aided in life- or health-threatening situations. After all, according to the first claim of the status model, the patient is under an obligation in those circumstances to seek medical help, and the physician is under an obligation as part of his or her professional responsibilities to provide that help.

The status model finds it easy to incorporate the appeal to respect for persons into its general approach. As we saw in section 2.3, respecting people is shown by behaving toward them in ways that will not lessen their potential for acting in valued ways. It is an obligation that has implications concerning how we should behave toward persons, even if it is not an obligation we have to those persons. This fits very well with the picture of independent norms which are compulsory in the patient-physician relationship, providing that we assume, as seems quite reasonable, that those independent norms mandate that members of the health-care profession provide treatments which will promote the abilities of patients to act in those valued ways. It also fits very well with the first claim of the status model, which mandates that patients receive the care required to maintain their abilities and that physicians provide that care. The status model, with its emphasis on the correctness of certain types of decisions independent of the wishes of the parties involved, has no difficulty incorporating the appeal to respect for persons.

Some of the virtues discussed in section 2.4 are clearly mandated by the status model. Consider, for example, the virtue of courage, which is the ability to move forward resolutely to implement appropriate decisions despite the fear of pain or error. This virtue ·of both health-care recipients and health-care providers is not merely allowed for but is mandated by the status model. According to the status model, when a medical decision is the appropriate decision in light of independent professional and moral standards, it is a decision which must be made and implemented, despite fears that both parties might have, if the patient-physician relationship is to be legitimate. In this way the virtue of courage is mandated by the status model.

There is also an important aspect of the virtue of compassion which is mandated by the status model. The status model dictates that health-care providers are professionally obliged to provide health care for those in need of that care. This, of course, is the mandating of a certain form of compassion. And there is no reason why the virtue of compassion, as a source of independent values, cannot mandate other forms of compassion, much as other virtues such as honesty and integrity can, as a source of independent values, mandate other actions.

Finally, the status model is in a position to address those questions of justice and cost-effectiveness that were raised in section 2.5. One of the crucial claims of the status model is that society may be obliged to pay for some of the health care in legitimate patient-physician relationships when the recipient is not in a position to do so. The health-care provider, who is society's agent in providing this health care, can without any difficulty be perceived as being under an obligation to justly provide the health care in a cost-effective fashion so that people can get the health care they are required to obtain and are entitled to even though resources are limited. In this way the status model, even if it does not explicitly make reference to questions of justice and cost-effectiveness, is in a position to incorporate these important ethical considerations.[15]

Therefore, the status model definitely incorporates some of the important moral appeals discussed in chapter 2. It explicitly incorporates aspects of the appeal to consequences, the substantive rights both of health-care recipients and health-care providers, respect for persons, and some of the virtues. While it does not explicitly incorporate considerations of justice and cost-effectiveness, it has the potential of being expanded to incorporate them. That it does all of this is the major strength of the model. There are also, however, significant weaknesses.

The first major weakness of the status model is that it fails to incorporate at least one aspect of the appeal to the consequences of actions. With its emphasis on professional norms grounded in a professional understanding of what will lead to the best consequences for the patient, the status model emphasizes the appeal to consequences as they affect the patient. With its emphasis on other value norms, it can take into account the ways in which medical decisions affect society in general. But it has great difficulty incorporating that aspect of the appeal to consequences which focuses just on those with whom the patient is concerned. This is part of its general failure to emphasize sufficiently what the patient wants. Because of this failure, the status model is in no position to ascribe particular importance to considering the consequences of medical decisions just for those people with whom the patient is concerned.

This last point deserves emphasis. As we saw above, the contractual model, because of its emphasis on the authority of the individuals creating the health-care relationship, is able to emphasize properly the consequences of proposed actions just for those with whom the patient is concerned. The status model, because of its roots in standard professional norms, is able to emphasize properly the consequences for the patient. It can also use independent value norms as a basis for emphasizing consideration of the consequences for society as a whole. But these independent norms, professional and value, leave only a residual place for terms agreed upon by both parties, and this makes it difficult for the status model to allow for anything more than a residual role for a consideration of the consequences just for those whom the patient wants to be considered.[16]

The status model incorporates the substantive rights of the parties involved, but the second problem with the model is that it is much weaker in dealing with the procedural rights. To be sure, the status model can allow some significance to the rights of the parties involved to make decisions concerning which health care will or will not be provided. They may make the decisions in all those cases in which professional and independent value norms do not dictate a particular decision.

However, when these norms dictate a particular decision, then the status model insists that the norms take precedence over the wishes of both the health care-provider and the health-care recipient. There is no doubt that this claim is sometimes true. But we need to allow for the cases where these norms can be overridden by the desires of both the provider and the recipient. There are cases in which patient and physician wishes should take precedence over independent norms, much as there are cases in which independent norms should take precedence over patient and physician wishes. The status model, which assumes that independent norms must always take precedence over the wishes of those involved in the health-care relationship, fails precisely because it does not allow enough room for that autonomy.

Finally, another major weakness of at least some versions of the status model is their limited picture of the role of some of the virtues in the provision of health care. The model certainly insists on courage and compassion on the part of both parties in the health-care relationship. It also allows for honesty as a source of independent value. However, honesty seems to play little role in many versions of the status model. It is interesting to note that classical statements or codes of medical ethics, such as the Hippocratic oath, mandate no requirement of telling the truth in the patient-physician relationship.[17] While the traditional medical codes did not explicitly call for deception, they certainly made no appeal for full revelation, and it was widely believed that the withholding of much information might well be justified. Those versions of the status model which rest on traditional codes of medical ethics suffer, then, from a failure to give honesty a significant place in their model. The problem is even more fundamental with regard to the virtue of integrity. If we identify integrity simply with the performance of that which is independently mandated, then, of course, the status model mandates integrity. But if we go on to identify integrity as the virtue of acting in accordance with one's personal values, then we will encounter a problem. Integrity emphasizes decisions which are in keeping with the decision maker's personal values, personal life plans, and personal conceptions of the good. This emphasis on personal conceptions and on making decisions in accordance with them has only a modest role in the status model, where so many of the terms are set by independent norms, so the status model is not in a position to properly emphasize integrity.

In short, while the status model definitely incorporates many of the important moral appeals discussed in chapter 2, it also fails to incorporate other crucial appeals. There is at least one aspect of the appeal to consequences that it neglects, it pays insufficient attention to the procedural rights of health-care recipients and health-care providers, and it does not do sufficient justice to some of the virtues. In each of these cases the source of the problem is that the status model calls for the independent professional and value norms to take complete precedence over the desires and choices of those in the provider-recipient relationship.

## 3.5  Conclusions

The main moral to be drawn from our analysis of the two standard models is very straightforward. Each model draws its strength from the fact that it incorporates some of the important ethical appeals. Each model suffers from the fact that it fails to adequately incorporate the rest of the appeals.

Obviously, what is required is the rejection of these two models and the development of a third which provides a proper emphasis on all of the moral appeals that were outlined in chapter 2. Developing such a model is, as might be expected, a very complex matter, and it will be taken up in the next chapter.

## Notes

1. I first introduced this account in "Legal Models of the Patient-Physician Relation," in E. Shelp, ed., *The Clinical Encounter* (Dordrecht: Reidel, 1983). I argued there that this model is presupposed by classical common law. For reasons that I explained in my "Response to Franck and White" later in that same volume, I still believe that it is the model presupposed by that body of law. Robert Veatch, in "Models for Ethical Medicine in a Revolutionary Age," *Hastings Center Report* 26 (1972), and more fully in *A Theory of Medical Ethics* (New York: Basic Books, 1981), distinguished four models (the engineering model, the priestly model, the collegial model, and the contractual model) and argued for the merits of the contractual model. Veatch's contractual model, however, involves an additional basic social contract which articulates a social morality and an additional second contract between society and the medical profession which spells out the role-specific duties regarding interactions between laypeople and professionals.

2. On the many issues arising out of such cases, see Wade, "Restitution for Benefits Conferred without Request," *Vanderbilt Law Review* 19 (1966).

3. A classic case which analyzes this issue, particularly the implications of the idea of an implied contract for the appropriate physician fee, is *Cotnam v. Wisdom,* 104 S.W. 164 (1907). Note, of course, that other models may not need to apply this idea of implied contract at all. This, in light of the argument in chapter 2 about the Good Samaritan issue, is a virtue of those models.

4. For an elegant contemporary defense of this position, see C. Fried, *Contract as Promise* (Cambridge, Mass.: Harvard Univ. Press, 1981).

5. The issues are discussed in ibid., chaps. 6 and 7.

6. These ideas are the views of the British National Health Service, the Canadian National Health Insurance scheme, and A. Enthoven's proposal for American health care in his *Health Plan* (Reading, Mass.: Addison Wesley, 1980). America's actual scheme for providing health care to the indigent is a mixture of all three. It should also be noted that claim five is certainly compatible with the idea that society has no obligation to provide any health care to the indigent.

7. That language seems to have become popular in the abortion debate.

8. These remarks refer to the case of adult patients who are no longer competent. I argue in chapter 4 that the situation is very different in the case of children or never-competent adults, because the right of the family to be decision makers in such cases is based on very different considerations.

9. It must be remembered that this is a model for a moral understanding of the physician-patient relationship. All too often, because of the interaction of law and morality in this area, people have left out moral considerations which they think the law cannot accommodate. A separate question, by the way, is whether the law can accommodate questions of virtues. Some preliminary remarks on that issue are found in my "The Role of Private Philanthropy in a Free and Democratic Society," *Social Philosophy and Policy* 4, no. 2 (Spring 1987).

10. "Primum non nocere" is so often used (and badly mispronounced) by physicians as a way of avoiding serious ethical questions. A fine discussion of this principle, questioning its antiquity, is found in R. Veatch, *A Theory of Medical Ethics* (New York: Basic Books, 1981), pp. 159–62. Of particular interest is footnote 8.

11. I first introduced this account in "Legal Models of the Patient-Physician Relation." I argued there that the status model is presupposed by rabbinic law. For reasons that I explained in my "Response to Franck and White" later in that same volume, I still believe that it is the model presupposed by that body of law. A contemporary presentation of that approach is D. M. Feldman and F. Rosner, eds., *Compendium on Medical Ethics*, 6th ed. (New York: Federation of Jewish Philanthropies, 1984).

12. The shared professional understanding approach is emphasized in C. D. Clements and R. C. Sider, "Medical Ethics' Assault upon Medical Values," *JAMA* 250, no. 15 (Oct. 21, 1983). The rabbinic material mentioned above, while also talking about professional understandings, emphasizes the independent ethical norms.

13. A splendid example of such a constraint is found in the following: "As far as fees are concerned, the Tur writes in the name of Nachmanides that one can be compensated for the time and effort expended but not for the study one has first undergone. . . . As God says about doing good deeds, much as I act without a fee, so should you act without a fee." Y. Epstein, *Aruch Hashulchan, Yoreh Deah* 336: 2–3. In fact, however, it appears to have been Nachmanides's view that the patient can be obligated to pay a higher fee if he or she agrees to do so.

14. This point can be generalized to other situations. If, for example, we insist that physicians and hospitals must provide emergency care to indigent patients who lack any insurance, we need to consider carefully why they should bear that burden rather than being reimbursed by society. Moreover, we need to be realistic about the inevitable cost shifting and its moral dilemmas. On these issues, see G. Graham, "The Doctor, the Rich, and the Indigent," *Journal of Medicine and Philosophy* 12, no. 1 (February 1987).

15. Unfortunately, many of its traditional adherents failed to do so.

16. The residual role of this appeal, plus the appeals mentioned in the next two objections, results precisely from the fact that the status model incorporates a lexical ordering of appeals, where the independent norms always take precedence over patient-physician decisions.

17. The finest (and at the same time most irritating) statement of that classical approach is quoted by S. Bok, *Lying* (New York: Vintage Books, 1978), from the essays of Oliver Wendell Holmes: "The face of a physician, like that of a diplomatist, should be impenetrable. Nature is a benevolent old hypocrite; she treats the sick and the dying with illusions better than any anodynes. . . . Some shrewd old doctors have a few phrases always on hand for patients that will insist on knowing the pathology of their complaints without the slightest capacity of understanding the scientific explanation. . . . I think nothing on the whole has covered so much ground, and meant so little, and given such profound satisfaction to all parties, as the magnificent phrase 'congestion of the portal system' " (p. 232).

# 4

## A New Model for the Patient-Physician Relationship

In chapters 2 and 3 we explored the many moral appeals that need to be taken into account in the development of an adequate model of the patient-physician relationship. We also saw that two standard models for that relationship fail precisely because they take into account only some of these moral appeals. This chapter presents a new model for the patient-physician relationship which properly incorporates all of these many different appeals.

I call this the model of conflicting appeals because the name captures the fundamental moral claim that there are many different moral appeals that may conflict with each other and to which both parties in the patient-physician relationship need to respond. A proper model for that relationship must be sensitive to all of these different moral appeals and the ways they must be meshed together.

This chapter has three major sections. In the first I set out in a schematic fashion the basic claims of this new model, comparing them with the analogous claims of the contractual model and the status model. The basic claims will make reference to the concept of conflicting moral appeals but will say nothing about how these conflicts ought to be resolved. The second section discusses techniques for dealing with conflicting moral appeals and shows how they are to be applied in the articulation and further development of our model. The third section of the chapter consists of an elaborate development of the model.

## 4.1 The Model of Conflicting Appeals

The model of conflicting appeals makes five basic claims about the patient-physician relationship and about decision making in it:

1.  Both parties in the patient-physician relationship are under an obligation in some circum-
    stances to enter into that relationship. However, this obligation can in some cases be
    overridden, no matter how serious the medical problem, because the patient's and/or the
    physician's autonomous choices or some other value considerations override this
    obligation.
2.  Some of the terms governing the relationship, including some of those that dictate the
    type of decision making that will legitimately take place, are independent of and may
    override the wishes of one or both of the parties. Wishes of one or both parties may,
    however, sometimes override these independent terms. In any case the remaining terms
    are to be set by the joint agreement of the two parties.
3.  The patient-physician relationship legitimately exists only when (a) these independent
    terms are met in those cases in which they take precedence over the wishes of the parties
    and (b) the remaining terms of the relationship are set by mutual agreement of both
    parties.
4.  Society's main roles are to ensure that each party enters into this relationship when he or
    she is obligated to do so and to ensure that the relationship is governed by the appropriate
    independent terms in those cases where they should govern the relationship. In addition,
    society has the role of protecting both parties against nonperformance or malperformance
    in connection with any of the terms and against fraud or coercion in the agreement on
    those terms which are properly settled by the agreement of the two parties. As a result
    society has a special role in seeing that certain decisional processes and certain decisional
    outcomes come about.
5.  Society may have a special obligation to pay for health care when it is required if the
    recipient is not in a position to pay for it.

The contrast between this model and the contractual and status models is clear
even from this brief statement of the new model. On the one hand, it challenges the
contractual model and agrees with the status model in introducing the notion of
independent terms for the legitimacy of the patient-physician relationship. On the
other hand, it agrees with the contractual model in contrast to the status model in
allowing that there are circumstances in which autonomous wishes take precedence
over these independent terms. Finally, it contrasts with both of the earlier models in
recognizing that the terms that need to be incorporated into a legitimate patient-
physician relationship derive from many different moral appeals and that neither the
autonomous wishes stressed by the contractual model nor the medical and other
value factors stressed by the status model are always subordinate to the other.
Legitimate patient-physician relationships in this new model are going to be far
more complex than in the earlier models.

The first claim of the new model seems closer to the position of the status model
than to the contractual model since it recognizes that both parties in the patient-
physician relationship may in some circumstances be under an obligation to enter
into that relationship. It agrees with the status model in claiming that a patient who
faces a serious medical problem may be morally required to seek help and that a
physician may be required to provide that help when other help is not available.
However, unlike the status model, it does not see these obligations as always
overriding. In deference to some of the considerations raised by the contractual
model, the model of conflicting appeals recognizes that these obligations may
sometimes be overridden either by autonomous choices or by other value considera-

tions. In this way the model of conflicting appeals puts forward claims that are in between the claims of the status model and the contractual model.

A similar middle-of-the-road position emerges as we compare the second claim of the model of conflicting appeals with the analogous claims of the status model and the contractual model. Once more, in agreement with the status model, the model of conflicting appeals says that some of the terms governing the patient-physician relationship are independent of and may override the wishes of one or both of the parties. The status model, however, makes a stronger claim about these independent terms, namely that these terms always take precedence over the autonomous wishes of the two parties. The model of conflicting appeals, while accepting the existence of these independent terms, agrees with the contractual model that they can be overridden in at least some cases by the autonomous wishes of one or both parties.

The third claim of this model, like the third claims of the other two models, is really a summation of the first two and expresses the heart of the model's view of the patient-physician relationship and of decision making within it. Legitimacy is based on the meeting of the terms that have the consent of both parties, the meeting of the basic independent terms growing out of medical understandings, and the meeting of other basic ethical norms. Legitimacy requires the proper balancing of these different appeals, recognizing that they are often in conflict with one another. In short, for the model of conflicting appeals the patient-physician relationship legitimately exists when the proper balance is drawn among various conflicting moral appeals.

Like all other models, the model of conflicting appeals says that society's main role is to ensure that patient-physician relationships are legitimate.[1] Within the contractual model, where legitimacy rests only on the ways in which the relationship was formed and the ways in which the agreed-upon terms were carried out, society's only roles were to protect the process of relationship formation and to ensure that the terms agreed upon were carried out. Within the status model, where legitimacy rests primarily on the relationship's being in accord with the appropriate independent terms, society's main role was to ensure that individual patient-physician relationships satisfied those terms. For the model of conflicting appeals, where legitimacy rests on the proper balancing of the conflicting appeals that should govern the patient-physician relationship, the primary role of society is to ensure that these conflicting appeals are properly balanced. This is, in effect, what the fourth claim says.

The model of conflicting appeals comes closer to the status model and is farther from the contractual model in its fifth and final claim that society's role may extend to having a special obligation to pay for medical treatment if the patient is unable to do so. It is easy to see how this final claim arises from the earlier claims. Suppose we have a case in which society has properly insisted that a patient who cannot afford medical treatment get that medical treatment because it is something that he or she is obliged to receive and has properly insisted that a physician provide that treatment. Who is to bear the cost of the physician's treating the patient? It cannot be the patient, because he or she doesn't have the capacity to pay. We might impose the cost on the physician, but it's unclear why it should be the physician's burden alone, and in any case the physician is likely to pass it on to the rest of us through his or her fees. These arguments, which were used by the proponents of the status model, can be used equally well by proponents of the model of conflicting appeals to conclude that in those circumstances society has a special obligation to pay for the health care. The only difference between the status model and the model of conflicting appeals on this point is that the model of conflicting appeals claims that patients are obliged to receive health care in fewer cases, and it will therefore conclude that society has a special obligation to pay for that health care in fewer cases.

## 4.2   Dealing with Conflicting Appeals

The fundamental claim of the model of conflicting appeals is that both parties in the patient-physician relationship are subject to a wide variety of moral appeals which they need to satisfy. This model says that the legitimacy of the patient-physician relationship depends on the proper balancing of these conflicting moral appeals. But how are they to be properly balanced? That is the question that will occupy us for the rest of this chapter. In this section we will look in an abstract way at the general question of the possible ways in which conflicting moral appeals can be properly balanced.

One approach, the hierarchical or lexical ordering approach, is to rank particular moral appeals by saying that some are the most important and always take precedence over all others, a second group takes precedence over all others except those in the first group, and so on. In effect, this way of thinking about conflicting moral appeals perceives the world of morality as hierarchically ordered and says that in any given case we do not need to think about any lower-ranked moral appeals until we are sure that none of the higher-ranked appeals makes any claims on us in that case.

This idea of a lexical ordering or a hierarchy of appeals became very popular as a result of the influence of John Rawls. In his writings on the theory of justice Rawls emphasized the idea that one of his principles of justice (the equal distribution of liberty principle) should always take precedence over the second (the principle justifying some social and economic inequalities).[2] This idea has been adopted in general moral theory by Charles Fried in his claim that the right has priority over the good[3] and in medical ethics by Robert Veatch in his claim that nonconsequentialist principles (such as promise keeping, autonomy, honesty, avoiding killing, and justice) have lexical priority over the consequentialist principle of beneficence.[4]

This is a comfortable way of thinking about the world of morality, but it is also highly implausible. First, it is hard to think of any moral appeal that always takes precedence over all others. It seems as though there are always circumstances in which one takes precedence over a second while the second takes precedence over the first in other circumstances. In fact, our two rejected models provide us with good examples. The contractual model sees the appeal to provider and recipient autonomy as always taking precedence over all other appeals, including appeals to what is best for the patient, appeals to the integrity of the parties involved, and appeals to respect for persons. The status model, on the other hand, sees the physician's following certain imposed terms as always taking precedence over such appeals as the appeal to autonomy. Each embodies the hierarchical approach, and each fails precisely because it does so.

It is of some value to remember that one of the major bases for the appeal of the hierarchical approach is the feeling that it is needed to avoid utilitarianism. To quote Veatch:

> In fact, if the nonconsequentialist principles are to have any power in a medical ethical system, it may be that they together have to be given a lexical priority over the principle of beneficence. Otherwise a consideration of consequences can always swamp the other moral considerations.[5]

But this argument is, of course, a non sequitur. All that is needed to avoid the "swamping" is that the nonconsequentialist principles should sometimes take precedence over beneficence, and this is compatible with beneficence sometimes taking precedence.[6]

There is a second difficulty with this hierarchical approach to the world of morality. Even if I were able to think of a moral appeal that always took precedence over any other appeal taken by itself, I would still have trouble with the view that it should take precedence over other appeals taken jointly. We have to consider the possibility that A might always take precedence over B, might always take precedence over C, and might always take precedence over D, but would not take precedence over B, C, and D when those three jointly favored one action while A favored another.

These two considerations should move us from this simple hierarchical approach to a more complex approach. One possible picture is the following. In different circumstances, each of the moral appeals has a different weight. For any given circumstance we can assign a weight which the appeal has in that circumstance. We can then add up the weights of all the appeals favoring one action and all of the appeals favoring another action and come to a conclusion about which set of appeals takes precedence over the other set in the given case. In this fashion we can deal with conflicting moral appeals. I call this approach the scale approach to conflict.[7]

Consider the common example of the adult Jehovah's Witness who refuses blood transfusions because it is against religious principles and the physicians who wish to transfuse the patient because it would save his or her life. On the one side are the right of patients to control what happens to them and to their bodies and the virtue of integrity which calls on patients to live by their moral/religious principles. On the other side are the physicians' obligations to produce the consequences that are best for their patients, physicians' integrity which calls upon them to save salvageable lives, and a respect for persons which calls for saving lives. The scale approach suggests that we assign weights to the significance of each of these appeals in this case, then add up the weights, see which side has the greater sum weight, and perform that action. We have no way of doing this at the present moment, but the proponents of this approach hope that we could at least go through this exercise in an informal fashion and reach some conclusion.

The scale approach has the virtue of dealing with the two objections posed to the hierarchical approach. The hierarchical approach presupposed that we could identify one moral appeal that always took precedence over all others, another that took precedence over every one except the first, and so on. This seemed unlikely because moral appeals would have different strengths in different contexts. The scale approach captures this insight. It insists that the very same moral appeal can have different strengths in different contexts and that we need to take into account its strength in a particular context when deciding what to do. Furthermore, the scale approach to moral conflict can deal with the other objection to the hierarchical approach, that several weaker moral appeals can combine together to take precedence over an opposing appeal that is stronger than each of them individually. While the right of the Jehovah's Witness to control what happens to his or her body might have the greatest strength in a particular case and might take precedence over any one of the appeals listed on the other side, the scale approach could allow for the possibility that all the other appeals taken jointly might take precedence over the right of the Jehovah's Witness. I do not say that it would or should. All I am pointing out is that the scale approach has the virtue of at least allowing for such a possibility.

There is one major difficulty with the scale approach. We have absolutely no reason to believe that it is possible to do the things it requires us to do. Its first task, indicating when a given moral appeal has greater or lesser significance in a particular case, is perhaps possible. The second task, constructing a common scale so that we can add the strengths of the various appeals on each side, is a different matter. We may be able to develop an account of when the right to autonomy is more significant or less significant. We may be able to develop an account of when the virtue of personal integrity is more significant or less significant. We may be able to develop an account of when considering the consequences for the patient is more significant or less significant. I see no reason to believe, however, that we will be able to construct a common metric for all of these so that we can add up the strengths of the appeals favoring each proposed action and come to a conclusion about which set of appeals takes precedence in a given case. I know of no attempt to do so, and I see no reason to believe that such an attempt will be successful.

We seem forced to adopt a third and in some ways very disturbing approach to facing conflicting moral appeals. I shall call this the judgment approach.[8] It agrees with the claim of the scale approach that we can and must develop a theory of when a given moral appeal has greater or lesser significance in a particular case. In approaching a particular case of moral conflict we must, according to this third approach, identify all of the moral appeals relevant to that case and then use the theory to ascribe a significance to each. According to the judgment approach, however, this is as far as moral theory can take us. Having identified the various moral appeals that back the various proposed actions and having ascribed to them a significance in light of the theory we have developed, we are not in a position to use a common metric to derive a conclusion of what is the appropriate action. This final process, rather than being a weighing process, is a process of judgment. We look at the various appeals and their significance, and then we judge what we ought to do.

A theory of the significance of a given appeal for a given case compares that appeal's use in different cases *against one another* and ranks the uses of the appeal in terms of likelihood to override other appeals *all other things being equal*.

I described this third approach as disturbing. There are three reasons for this.

(1) There will be many cases in which an individual decision maker, seeing the significance of the various appeals supporting the different courses of action, will feel very unsure about what judgment to make. In such cases the individual decision maker may well want some further guidance from moral theory. It is not enough, he or she might say, that moral theory enables one to identify the relevant appeals and ascribe to them their significance in a particular case. One wants the moral theory to provide an answer. The judgment approach is not comforting in dealing with moral conflict precisely because it insists that moral theory cannot do this. (2) In many cases the several people involved in making the decision, although agreeing upon the relevant appeals and their significance, disagree about which set of appeals should take precedence. At this point they may wish that moral theory would give them a way of deciding whose judgment is correct so that the dispute among them can be resolved. When they are told, as the judgment approach tells them, that moral theory has done all it can do and that this is a conflict in judgment which moral theory cannot resolve, they may find this approach less than comforting. (3) A judgment approach is always open to abuse by those who are interested in justifying a prechosen alternative.[9] They can always say that their judgment is that the appeals arguing for their alternative take precedence in the case in question. Their opponents will not be able to mount a theoretical argument against them, and this will lead them to frustration. No doubt, any moral theory can be abused, but this observation, however accurate, is still less than comforting.

Despite these reasons for being uncomfortable with the judgment approach, there are two reasons for accepting it. The first is the negative reason that the hierarchical approach and the scale approach seem implausible. However much we would prefer it to be the case that one of those two approaches were correct, we have seen that there are good reasons for being dubious. Therefore, by default, we may have to accept the judgment approach.

There is, however, another, more positive reason for accepting the judgment approach. It seems to do justice to the reality of moral ambiguity. We experience in our own lives the varieties of moral ambiguity alluded to above. We often find ourselves in situations in which, even after we have identified all of the relevant appeals and assessed their significance, we are unable to decide what we should do. This is a type of personal moral ambiguity that we have all experienced and whose reality needs to be accounted for by any moral theory. Moreover, we have all experienced the interpersonal form of moral ambiguity, cases in which good people, after carefully examining and assessing the significance of the relevant appeals, still disagree about what should be done. The reality of this type of interpersonal disagreement needs to be explained by any moral theory. The other approaches to conflicting moral appeals, the hierarchical approach and the scale approach, do not properly explain the reality of these types of moral ambiguity. For them these moral ambiguities must be the result of a failure to take into account certain appeals and/or a failure to properly weigh them. For them, if one has taken into account the relevant appeals and has properly identified the weights that ought to be ascribed to them in a given case, then one will be led by moral theory to a determinate conclusion. Only the judgment approach recognizes that it is possible, even after one has identified all of the relevant moral appeals and properly assessed their significance, to be unsure about which set of appeals dominates and therefore unsure about what to do. A positive reason for accepting the judgment approach is, therefore, that it can account for these deep moral ambiguities.

It might be thought that the adoption of a judgment approach to conflicting moral appeals leads to a certain form of relativism. Since moral theory, even after we have provided it with all of the relevant moral facts, may lead to no determinate conclusion, there is no such thing as right and wrong but only the particular and often differing judgments people make. This confusion needs to be avoided. The adoption of the judgment approach does lead to the conclusion that it is possible for people to identify all of the relevant moral appeals and their significance in a given case and yet be unsure about what to do because all that information does not entail a conclusion about the appropriate thing to do. But none of this entails that there is no such thing as the right thing or the wrong thing to do. The judgment approach is compatible with moral objectivism, with the view that there is a right thing and a wrong thing to do; its claim is about the extent to which moral theory determines what is the right thing and the wrong thing. The judgment approach is a picture of the epistemology of morality, of how we can come to know what is right and wrong. It is totally neutral on the question of the ontological status of morality, on whether moral judgments are or are not objectively true.[10]

What does the adoption of the judgment approach mean for our model of conflicting appeals for the patient-physician relationship? For each of the moral appeals we have identified as relevant to the patient-physician relationship, we need to develop a theory of their respective significance in particular cases, an account of when they have greater or lesser significance. This account is the most a moral theory can provide.

In the following section I complete this account of the model of conflicting appeals by reviewing the relevant moral appeals and indicating when they have greater or lesser significance for a particular decision. That will be as much as can be done by way of articulating a proper theoretical basis for morally legitimate patient-physician relationships. That account and my best judgments will be used in the last three chapters to analyze difficult cases.

## 4.3   Assessing Conflicting Appeals

### Assessing the Appeal to the Consequences of Our Actions

Health-care providers, as part of their professional ethic, are required to evaluate their actions in terms of the consequences for their patients. Health-care providers, as a consequence of the contractual element of their relationship with their patients, are required to evaluate their actions in light of the consequences for all those with whom their patients are concerned. Health-care providers, as moral agents, are required to consider the consequences of their actions for all those affected by those actions. In taking into account all of these consequences they should judge consequences as good only if they satisfy the final relevant preferences of those affected. This does not mean, however, that health-care providers should simply do what those affected wish them to do, for those affected may have very mistaken beliefs about which actions will lead to the consequences they desire. The appeal to consequences merely offers health-care providers a reason for performing those actions which will, in their professional judgment, lead to the consequences that the affected people desire.

What factors lead this appeal to have a greater or lesser significance in a given case? The following seem to be the major considerations. (1) The first factor is the likelihood of the consequences occurring. We live in a world of uncertainty in which we rarely can predict with complete certainty what will be the consequences of our actions. If this is true about the world in general, it is even more true about the world of medicine. When a physician believes that a certain action is right because it will lead to the best consequences for those affected, he or she must consider how likely it is that those consequences will result. The more likely it is that those consequences will result, the stronger the physician's reason for performing the action. The less likely it is that those consequences will result, the weaker the reason for performing the action. Economists often say that what we take into account in evaluating our actions is not their consequences but their expected consequences.[11] I prefer to put this first point simply by saying that the appeal to consequences has greater or lesser significance according to the likelihood of those consequences occurring. (2) Next comes the value of the consequence for a particular person. The appeal to consequences is an argument for performing certain actions because they lead to good consequences and for not performing other actions because they lead to bad consequences. In a given case, however, there may be several actions open to us that lead to good consequences for a particular affected person, or it may be that all the actions open to us lead to bad consequences for that person. In each of those circumstances we still need to choose one of the alternatives open to us. In the former case we should choose the action which leads to the best consequences. In the latter case we should choose the action which leads to the least bad consequences. In both cases the appeal to consequences provides a greater reason for performing (or not performing) some action according to the degree of positive or negative value of the consequences for the person affected. More generally, the extent to which the appeal to consequences provides us with a reason for performing an action is a function of how much the person affected wishes those consequences will occur, and the extent to which it provides us with a reason for not performing an action is a function of the extent to which the person affected wishes that those consequences will not occur. (3) The third factor is the extent of the impact of the action. Decisions and actions of health-care providers often have implications for many desires of their patients. Parts of the appeal to consequences call on us to take that into account. Moreover, these decisions and actions can have positive implications for some people and negative implications for others. Obviously, all other things being equal, we should perform the action which most benefits more people and least harms fewer people. Consider a situation in which one person was greatly benefited by an action while many were harmed in a very limited way and in which intuitively the gains to the one person vastly outweigh the losses to the others. Our formula means that we should perform the action which benefits one even though it harms many. So it is not just a question of counting how many gain and how many lose. But there is a problem here. We have at present no theoretical foundation for comparing the benefits to some and the losses to others. This technical problem is referred to as the problem of the interpersonal comparison of utility. While we can meaningfully talk about the number of people who benefit and suffer, the probability that they will benefit or suffer, and how much each prefers to suffer or not to suffer the consequences, can we meaningfully talk about how much the gains to some outweigh the losses to others? I believe we can, even if we have no adequate theory of how to do this. It seems to be connected with our ability to put ourselves in the shoes of these many others and to suppose that the gains and/or losses to them are comparable to the gains and/or losses to us in their shoes.[12]

It might be suggested that we need to take into account the proximity of the consequences. The sooner the good consequences of the action result, according to this suggestion, the greater the significance of those consequences. The less proximate they are, the less their significance. There seems to be some truth in this suggestion, but the truth in it can be accounted for by the factors mentioned above. One reason why we treat consequences that occur relatively soon after the action as more significant is that the probability of these proximate consequences occurring is much higher. Another factor that may be involved is based on the fact that preferences change over time. It is judged unlikely that the preferences of the people affected will change in the relatively near future. Therefore, in looking at the consequences of our actions for them, we feel reasonably confident that performing the action that will lead in the relatively near future to the consequences that they *now* desire will be performing the action that leads to good consequences for them *then* because they will still desire those consequences. However, when we are considering long-range consequences we also have to take into account the possibility that the preferences of the people in question may change, so that by the time the consequences occur they will no longer be desired consequences, and we will have performed an action that leads to bad consequences for those affected.[13] In short, we can explain why we should be more concerned with the proximate consequences of our actions than with their long-range consequences without postulating that as an additional factor in assessing the significance of the appeal to consequences.

It might also be suggested that the death of a patient is a consequence that has an extra significance in some radically different way from any other possible consequence. I believe this suggestion needs to be firmly repudiated. Obviously, the death of a patient is usually a very negative outcome of an action. But this can be understood in light of the factors mentioned above, particularly the second factor. The death of a patient is usually something the patient strongly wishes to avoid, and it will moreover lead to the frustration of many of his or her other desires. As a result, we need postulate no special significance to death to understand why it should normally (but not always) be treated as a very bad consequence. Moreover, to accord it some special significance beyond the significance dictated by the preferences of the patient is to challenge the fundamental doctrine of consumer sovereignty. This is perfectly compatible with recognizing that there are other moral factors that may lead us to treat the death of a patient in a very special way. All I am claiming now is that the assumption of consumer sovereignty does not allow for a consequence to have a special negative value beyond that resulting from the fact that it is something the patient very much wishes to avoid. And if, because of the patient's condition, death is not something he or she wants to avoid (and if, more-over, there are not, because of the patient's condition, a large number of preferences which would be satisfied if the patient remains alive but which will be frustrated if the patient dies), then the appeal to consequences will *not* argue for keeping the patient alive.

### Assessing the Appeal to Rights

Health-care recipients have certain rights which need to be taken into account by health-care providers as they evaluate proposed actions. Some of these rights are substantive rights, including the right not to be killed, the right not to have bodily injury or pain inflicted on oneself, and the right to be aided in life- or health-threatening situations. Others are procedural rights, rights about roles in decisional processes. The most crucial of these is the right of the patient to refuse medical treatment despite the recommendation of the health-care provider. The other impor-tant procedural right is the right of family members to participate in decisions concerning the treatment of a patient and to refuse care on behalf of the patient when the patient is for some reason incapable of participating in decision making. These rights, whether substantive or procedural, are waivable, are not absolute, can be overridden by a variety of factors, and are therefore of varying degrees of moral force (measured by what factors can override them).

What factors lead the appeal to rights to have a greater or lesser significance in a given case? We can only answer this question by examining the rights separately.

There are at least three factors we take into account when we assess the signifi-cance in a given case of the right of the patient to refuse treatment and to have that refusal respected by health-care providers.[14] The first is the competency of the patient who is refusing the treatment. The second is the nature of the refusal. The third is the basis for it.

An analysis of competency will be presented in chapters 5 and 7. All I want to note for now is that it will show competency to be a matter of degree. This point is particularly crucial in assessing the significance of the patient's right to refuse to be treated in a given case. The more we judge the patient to be competent, the more significance we must assign to the patient's refusal of treatment. This is not to say that a patient whose competency is assessed as high is necessarily one whose refusal must be respected or that a patient whose competency is assessed as low is one whose refusal can be disregarded. All I am saying is that there are various factors that influence the significance of the patient's refusal, and the greater the competen-cy of the patient, all other things being equal, the more reason we have to respect the right of the patient to refuse treatment. Other factors, however, may not be equal, and they may support a less significant right to refuse treatment while overriding a more significant right to refuse treatment.

The nature of the refusal refers to two aspects that we take into account when we assess the significance of the patient's right to refuse treatment in any given case.

The first is the force with which the patient refuses treatment. Sometimes people refuse treatment in a way that makes one suspect that they are not refusing, just resisting. At the other extreme are refusals of treatment that are clearly very strongly held. The greater the force of the patient's refusal of treatment, the more significance we must accord to that refusal. The other relevant aspect is the duration of the refusal. Sometimes patients have made it clear for a long time that there are certain treatments they do not desire. These long-term repeated refusals have greater significance than first-expressed or very recent refusals. When we understand the refusal of treatment to be not just an immediate reaction to bad circumstances but a deep-seated and continuing judgment, then we find it deserving of greater respect.

Regarding the basis for the refusal, there are cases in which the patient's refusal of treatment is based on some fundamental beliefs or values of the patient. If we treat the patient despite that refusal, then we are attacking the patient's fundamental beliefs and values. In such cases the right to refuse treatment is of great significance and must be accorded great respect. There are other cases, however, in which the basis of the refusal of treatment is much less central to the value system and/or belief system of the patient. Failing to respect that refusal of treatment would still be failing to respect the wishes of the patient, but it would not be as serious a violation of the patient's rights. In such cases the right to refuse treatment would be of lesser significance. Centrality of belief and value is, of course. a matter of degree, and that is why this third factor provides us with varying degrees of significance for the right to refuse treatment in particular cases.

It might be suggested that there is a fourth factor: the consequences of accepting the refusal of treatment.[15] If the consequences of accepting that refusal are very grave, then that refusal has less significance than if the consequences are more modest. If a patient's refusal to accept treatment results in death, for example, then the right to have that refusal respected is of lesser significance (although it still may be of considerable significance) than if the consequences of the patient's refusal of treatment are less drastic. I don't accept this suggestion, although I think there is a point to it. From the perspective of the model of conflicting appeals, this factor is not relevant to assessing the significance of the right to refuse treatment in a given case. It is instead relevant to assessing the significance of the appeal to the consequences in deciding when the appeal to consequences overrides the right to refuse treatment.[16]

The second of the procedural rights is the right of family members to participate in decisions concerning the treatment of the patient when the patient is incompetent to participate in that decision making and when there is no evidence for what the patient would have wished. Before we look at the significance of family refusals in particular cases, we need to consider the preliminary question of whether a particular family member has acquired the right to participate in decision making and to refuse suggested treatments. Two factors seem relevant: the competency of the patient and the degree of closeness of the family member.

Since the right of the family members to be surrogate decision makers presupposes the incompetency of the patient and since competency is a matter of degree, it seems that the right of family members to be surrogate decision makers is going to be a function of the degree of incompetency of the patient. The more incompetent the patient, the more family members acquire the right to be surrogate decision makers. Those who view competency as an all-or-nothing matter deal with the patient as long as they view him or her as competent and deal with the family when they feel the patient is no longer competent. This practice, I believe, is undercut by the insight that competency is a matter of degree. The more appropriate approach is to substitute family wishes for patient wishes to an increasing degree as the patient becomes less and less competent.

There is often more than one family member present when an incompetent patient presents with a medical problem. Which of these family members acquires the decisional authority? This would not be such a difficult problem if all the family members were in concurrence about their wishes. In the real world, however, this is often not the case. One possibility would be to take into account the varying wishes of each, giving their wishes greater or lesser significance depending on their relationship to the patient. The difficulty of doing that in practice has led to a standard answer which seems acceptable but conceals a fundamental ambiguity: the closest family member acquires the right to be the surrogate decision maker for the incompetent patient.[17]

The ambiguity that undercuts the helpfulness of this standard answer is in the word *closeness*. There is, on the one hand, the closeness of a formal relationship: meaning spouses are closest, parents and children next, then siblings, and so on. This is the closeness to which the law often refers.[18] There is, however, a second meaning to *closeness*. This refers to the actual quality of the relationship which exists between family members. There is no reason to assume that this closeness always corresponds to the formally defined closeness. Sometimes your closest family member may be a distant cousin. Sometimes, in fact, the closest person to you may not even be a family member. Which of these meanings of *closeness* should clinicians employ as they accept the right of the closest family member to be the surrogate decision maker for the incompetent patient? Who actually has the moral right to be a surrogate decision maker? We need to distinguish two cases. The first is the pediatric case where the incompetency of the patient is because of age. In that case, where the patient has never yet acquired any decisional authority, such authority should rest in the family member with the closest formal relationship. The situation is very different in the case of the formerly competent adult patient who is no longer competent to make decisions. Here we should rely on the actual quality of the relationship. The reason for this difference is relatively easy to see. In the latter case, where the patient had already acquired decisional authority, that authority should be transferred to the person to whom it is most likely that the patient would have wished it to be transferred. In the case of the formerly competent adult patient, the surrogate decision maker who steps in should be the person the patient would most have wanted to step in if he or she had had a chance to decide. Usually that is the person who has the deepest real relationship with the patient, and that is often not the formally closest family member.[19] In the pediatric case, however, the family members making the decision are exercising authority on behalf of someone who has not yet had any decisional capacity, and it makes no sense to have the surrogate decision maker be the person that person would have chosen.[20]

So far we have examined the question of when surrogate decision makers come to have their right to be decision makers. We turn now to the factors that need to be taken into account when we assess the significance of the right of the surrogate decision maker to participate in decision making, including the right to refuse care for the patient. It goes without saying that we need to consider at least the three factors mentioned above in connection with the significance of the right of the patient to refuse treatment. If a surrogate decision maker refuses treatment for a patient, thereby exercising the right to be a surrogate decision maker, then the strength of the surrogate's right to have the refusal respected is certainly going to be greater in those cases in which the surrogate decision maker is very competent, is expressing a long-standing decision to refuse that treatment for the patient, and is basing the refusal on fundamental beliefs and values either of the patient or of the surrogate. It will have lesser significance in those cases in which the surrogate decision maker refusing treatment for the patient is less competent, is expressing a sudden decision against the treatment, and is basing that refusal on less fundamental beliefs and values.

There is an additional factor to be considered here. Imagine a case in which the surrogate decision maker is not properly considering the best interests of the patient. How should that be taken into account as we attempt to assess the significance of this right to be a surrogate decision maker? Some think that surrogate decision makers should always decide solely in terms of what is in the best interest of the patient. I have argued in chapter 2 that this view is incorrect and that surrogate decision makers may consider the interests of larger groups. This is true in the case of parents serving as surrogate decision makers for children as well as of surrogate decision makers acting on behalf of no longer competent adult patients. However, there are upper limits to this. Sometimes surrogate decision makers come close to exceeding those limits. The closer they come, the less significance their decision has. In the extreme case, when those limits are exceeded, society should take away the right by transferring custody of the patient to a specially appointed guardian. Whether or not that legal mechanism is employed, it certainly remains true that this is an additional factor relevant to the significance of the right of family members to serve as surrogate decision makers for incompetent patients.

Turning from the procedural rights of health-care recipients to their substantive rights, these substantive rights include two negative rights—the right not to be killed and the right not to have bodily injury or pain afflicted on oneself—and one positive right—the right to be aided in life- or health-threatening situations. Like all other rights, these rights are always waivable, are not absolute, and can be overridden by a variety of factors.

Let us begin with the right not to be killed. Little needs to be said about the factors that give this right greater or lesser significance. To be sure, this is a waivable right, and the importance of that fact has been noted. However, in all cases where it is not waived it seems to have an equally great significance. Moreover, as noted in chapter 2, it is a right held by all living members of our species.

The situation is slightly more complicated when we consider the other negative right, the right not to have bodily injury or pain inflicted on oneself. Like the right not to be killed, this right is waivable, and its being waived by the patient is essential for allowing physicians to act in ways that would otherwise constitute battery. But what about cases where this right is not waived? Again, the right in question always seems to possess a significant degree of strength. Still, it has greater or lesser significance in particular cases depending on the bodily injury or pain being inflicted. The greater the injury or bodily pain an action inflicts on an unwilling victim, the more serious the violation of the right of the victim.

In many ways, these two negative rights are among the most fundamental rights. Organized societies, from the very beginning, have had as one of their main functions the enforcement of these rights. Health-care professionals have always recognized that they have a corresponding obligation neither to kill their patients nor to inflict bodily injury or pain on them. The only major exception traditionally recognized is the inflicting of bodily injury or pain on the patient when necessary to avoid a greater evil (particularly when performed with the consent of the patient). In that special case it is easy to see why this right is overridden by other moral considerations.

The account of the significance of substantive rights becomes far more complicated with the last of them, the right to be aided in life- or health-threatening situations and the corresponding obligation to provide that aid. As we saw in chapter 2, the very existence of this right has been challenged by many, although I am assuming that it does exist. It is, again, a waivable and nonabsolute right. But what gives this right greater or lesser significance in particular cases?

There seem to be at least four factors to consider in assessing the significance of the right of the person faced by a life- or health-threatening danger to receive aid.[21] (1) First is the probability and gravity of the threat. Not all threats to the life or health of people are the same. Some raise greater probabilities of loss of life or health, while others involve a less likely risk. Naturally, the more likely the loss of life or health, the more significant the obligation to come to the aid of the person. Similarly, some threats are of greater losses than other threats. The graver the threatened loss of health, the more significant the person's right to aid. (2) Second is the burden of providing that aid. Sometimes, when a person is facing a threat to his or her life or health, we are in a position to help without accepting any great burden. In other cases, however, the burden of providing the aid becomes quite great. Sometimes, for example, we can only provide that aid by risking our own lives or health. In other cases we can only provide aid by incurring tremendous financial losses. Whatever the nature of the burden, it seems correct to say that the right of the threatened person to be aided (and our corresponding obligation to provide that aid) has a greater significance when the burden of providing the aid is low, and its significance decreases as the burden of providing that aid increases. (3) The third factor is the existence of a special relationship. In some cases the person facing a threat to life or health stands in a special relationship to the party who is in a position to provide that aid. The two people may be members of the same family; they may be friends, neighbors, or fellow citizens. There may be an earlier professional relationship existing between them. A prominent example of this is when the person needing aid is a patient of the person who is in a position to provide the aid. As these special relationships between parties become more significant, the obligation to provide the aid against life- or health-threatening situations becomes greater. The obligation is weakest in the case of the absolute stranger, where the person in need

87

of help bears no special relationship to the person who is capable of providing that help. (4) The fourth and final factor is the fault of the person in need. In some cases the person whose life or health is threatened is in that situation without being at fault. The person struck down by a disease whose causes are in no way related to that person's earlier behavior is a prime example. In other cases the person who is in need of help is in that situation precisely because of earlier behavior for which he or she can properly be blamed. The patient who has cirrhosis because despite ample medical warning he insisted on drinking two six-packs a day for many years is a classic example. Perhaps even more common is the person suffering from lung cancer or chronic obstructive pulmonary disease who has a long history of smoking one or more packs of cigarettes a day. It is not that these people have no right to be aided. Their right to be aided has a lesser significance, however, precisely because they are responsible (causally and morally) for being in the situation which requires that they be aided. The unfortunate and innocent victim has a greater right to our aid in times of need.

It might be suggested that there is a fifth factor: the number of previous occasions on which the person who is in need of aid has made his claim to aid and the number of previous occasions on which the person who is in a position to aid has provided that aid to that person. I think that is not a relevant factor. To be sure, the person who has often provided aid may now be under a lesser obligation to provide further aid, but this is true, when it is true, because the provision of additional aid is often a greater burden than the provision of the initial aid. If the provision of the additional aid continues to be no additional burden, I see no reason why there isn't a continuing obligation of equal significance to provide that aid. The other purported factor, how often the person who is to receive aid has previously received the aid, seems totally irrelevant. A failure to recognize this irrelevance would lead to the unacceptable conclusion that people with chronic medical problems have only modest rights to be helped just because their problems are chronic.

## Assessing the Appeal to Respect for Persons

The appeal to respect for persons is an appeal to behave in ways that will promote the capacity of people to live lives full of the human actions we value so much. Helping them maintain their lives, their bodily integrity, and their capacity to choose and act is an important element of this respect for personhood. It is a respect that is owed whether or not the party in question wishes to be respected in this way, for it is an obligation that we have concerning them, not an obligation to them.

How important is the appeal to respect for persons going to be in dealing with particular cases? What are the factors that lead this appeal to have a greater or lesser significance in a given case? We need to contrast the appeal to respect for persons with two other appeals: the appeal to the rights to life and bodily integrity (which I accept) and the appeal to the sanctity of life (which I reject). The appeal to the rights to life and bodily integrity is different from the appeal to respect for persons because the former has no significance when the person in question waives those rights, while the latter continues to have significance even in such cases. That is the point of saying that the appeal to respect generates obligations we have concerning people, not obligations we have to them. This might lead one to suppose that the appeal to respect for persons is a sanctity-of-life appeal. It is true that the appeal to the sanctity of life, like the appeal to respect for persons, obligates us to respect the life and the bodily integrity of people whether they wish us to do so or not. Where these appeals differ is on the question of whether this obligation is always present with equal significance. The appeal to the sanctity of life is an appeal present with an equal degree of significance in all cases.[22] It mandates with equal significance life- and health-respecting actions in all cases. The appeal to respect for persons does not. It mandates, to be sure, life- and health-respecting actions regardless of the wishes of the person in question. It does not do so with equal significance in all cases, however, and in this it is radically different from the appeal to the sanctity of life.

Several factors must be taken into account in deciding on the significance of the appeal to respect for persons in a given case. The most significant is the capacity of the person in question to perform, after our help, those actions whose performance we value. The more those capacities will be present (and I take this to be what we should properly mean when we speak of an objective notion of the quality of life of the person in question), the more we are under an obligation to respect that person by promoting his or her life and bodily integrity.[23] The less those capacities will be present, the less we have an obligation to respect that person in that way.

What are those valuable actions the capacity for which determines the significance of our obligation to respect the person in question? I think they include at least the following:

1. *Capacities for rational choice.* The capacity to recognize the facts of a situation for what they are, to deliberate about options for actions in those cases, to choose (especially on principled grounds) one out of a series of alternative actions for that case, and to act upon that choice.
2. *Interpersonal capacities.* The capacity to feel a variety of emotions, such as love and friendship, relating to other people, and the capacity to act on the basis of those emotions.
3. *Other emotional capacities.* The capacity to appreciate things of beauty, the capacity to desire to know the truth, the capacity to enjoy what is pleasant or humorous, and so on.

This list is meant to be illustrative rather than exhaustive. The crucial point it brings out is that there are a wide variety of actions that persons typically have the capacity to do whose performance we judge to be of great value. A person who has those capacities is an object worthy of respect. That respect provides us with an independent reason for not taking the life or interfering with the bodily integrity of such a person, whatever that person's wishes, and for aiding and promoting his or her life and bodily integrity when they are threatened.

The complexity of this appeal to respect helps explain the complex feelings we have about medical care for severely demented patients. The more demented they are, the less their capacity for performing these valued actions, and the less the significance of the appeal to respect for persons. All of this leads us to suppose that we are not obligated to provide vigorous medical care to keep them going. Still, there are other moral considerations to keep in mind. Even in those cases where the person's capacities to perform the valued actions are very low, we may still be under a significant obligation not to impair life or bodily integrity and even under an obligation to promote it, but the source of that obligation will have to be found elsewhere. We may also have other reasons (e.g., limiting pain and indignities) for not promoting life and bodily integrity. All I am providing at this point is an account of the significance of the obligation to respect persons in a particular case. That obligation is not the only moral factor we have to take into account, however, so what we are actually obliged to do in a given case of a severely demented patient will be determined by many other factors.

I said above that the objective quality of life of the person after our action is the most important factor determining the significance of respect for persons in a given case. What other factors also help determine the significance of that appeal in a given case? To begin with, the more likely it is that one's actions will enhance the person's resulting capacities, the more significant is the appeal to respect for persons. Also, the greater the burden of one's action on oneself, the less significant is this appeal.[24]

## Assessing the Appeal to the Virtues

We have analyzed four virtues: integrity (standing firmly by one's values and choosing in accordance with them), compassion (caring attempts to alleviate the losses of others), courage (acting on appropriate decisions without being excessively motivated by various fears), and honesty (not intentionally misleading people by providing false information and/or withholding other information). These virtues can be displayed by both providers and recipients. Some of these virtues provide a basis for a positive or negative evaluation of actions that would not otherwise have moral signifiance. Others simply provide an additional basis for a positive or negative evaluation of an action. A failure to take the virtues into account results in an incomplete moral evaluation of various health care decisions. The consideration of these virtues is then very important, but the appeal to virtues is of greater or lesser significance in particular cases.

The first virtue is integrity. People involved in a particular decision, providers and recipients alike, have framed for themselves conceptions of the things they care more about and the things they care less about, and in this way they have developed a set of personal values. Some of the decisions they can make will be in accord with these values; others will be in conflict with them. Displaying the virtue of integrity is making decisions that are in accord with one's own values; failing to display integrity is making decisions that are in conflict with one's values. This suggests that there are at least two factors relevant to assessing the significance of the appeal to integrity in the evaluation of health-care decisions. One is the centrality of the values with which a particular decision is in accord or in conflict, and the other is the relationship between the values and the life circumstances of the person.

Not all of the values and goals that a person has adopted are of equal importance in the life of that particular individual. Some values and goals are central to our lives because we have made a great commitment of time, energy, and resources to them. Others are far less central because we have made far less of a commitment to them. A particular decision's integrity is of great significance if it consists of a consonance between that decision and a value that is central in the life of the decision maker. A particular decision's integrity is of lesser significance if it consists of a consonance between the decision and a value that is less central to the life of the decision maker. Thus, for example, the integrity displayed by the Jehovah's Witness who refuses blood transfusions in life-threatening situations makes the refusal very significant precisely because that decision grows out of one of the central values of the patient. Conversely, if that Jehovah's Witness agrees to the blood transfusion, then the agreement is open to serious criticism precisely because the lack of integrity shown involves a conflict between the patient's decision and one of his or her central values. None of this is to say that the health-care provider should accept the first decision and challenge the second decision. That is a separate issue which involves the evaluation of many other moral factors besides the question of integrity. It is only to say that the centrality to one's life of the value one is deciding in accordance with is one of the major factors that gives the appeal to integrity a greater or lesser significance in a particular case.

Regarding the second factor, consider the patient who is contemplating risky surgery in the hope of restoring his or her health so that he or she can engage in various strenuous physical activities. Suppose, moreover, that engaging in those strenuous activities has been important in the life of that patient until now. The decision for surgery would then be a display of integrity. But how important is that? To begin with, being able to engage in these strenuous activities may not have been as central to the life of this person as the beliefs and values that led the Jehovah's Witness to refuse a transfusion. But even if they have been, if the person's physical health changes engaging in these strenuous physical activities may retreat in centrality, and engaging in other activities may take their place without any change of mind about the value of the activities. These values may be more changeable because of changes in circumstances. We need to take this into account before we assess the significance of the integrity of a decision.

These are examples of assessing the significance of health-care recipients displaying or failing to display integrity in the decisions they make. Similar examples could be given for assessing the significance of the display of integrity on the part of the health-care provider. In short, a health-care decision that displays integrity is a better decision, all other things being equal, than one that is marked by a failure of integrity. But the importance of this fact in deciding which decision to make is not a simple matter. It relates to the centrality of the values in question in the lives of the decision maker and the permanence of those values in the changing circumstances in which people find themselves.

One final remark about integrity. It is easy to see why individuals should be concerned about maintaining their own integrity, but why should we be concerned that others maintain their integrity? In particular, why should we evaluate choices as better or worse because they are consonant or dissonant with the values of the chooser, not our values? The answer is just that this type of consonance is seen as something of objective value, a reflection of the way people should relate to their values. We see the formulation of values and goals as a valuable activity but one which would be undercut by a lack of integrity, and we therefore see integrity as something objectively good.

Compassion is the virtue displayed when we attempt to alleviate the losses suffered by others. Obviously, all other things being equal, the compassionate decision is morally superior to the noncompassionate decision. But that fact has a greater or lesser significance in particular cases. At least two factors are involved. (1) First is the seriousness of the loss suffered. Some compassionate acts are responses to grave losses suffered by other people. Other compassionate acts may be responses to much less significant losses. The latter are nevertheless compassionate acts worthy of praise. That they are compassionate acts, however, is of less significance in the decision about what to do than the fact that an act is a compassionate response to a major loss suffered by someone. (2) The second factor is the amount one is able to do by way of alleviating the loss. In some cases there is little we can do to alleviate the losses of others, while in other cases we are in a position to alleviate most of the losses suffered. Displays of compassion are always admirable, but the fact that a response is compassionate is of greater significance in deciding what to do when the alleviation we can offer is greater.

Some might suggest that we need to add such factors as the nature of the relationship between the two parties (the closer the relationship, the greater the significance of the compassion), the burden of providing that aid (the greater the burden, the less the significance of the compassion), and the degree of fault of the party suffering the loss (the more they are at fault for having suffered the loss, the less the significance of the compassion). These are, after all, factors we used in evaluating the significance of the appeal to the right to be aided, and there seems to be some resemblance between the appeal to the right to be aided and the appeal to the virtue of compassion.

I think this suggestion is a mistake which displays a failure to understand the differences between the appeal to a right and the appeal to a virtue. People who are closer to me have a greater claim on me to be aided; that is why their right to be aided is of greater significance than the right of strangers. People whose aid would impose a lesser burden on me have a greater claim on me to be aided; that is why they have a more significant right to be aided. The crucial point is that the right to be aided is connected with the claims that people can make on me and the resulting obligations I have to them. The virtue of compassion is a different type of moral consideration. It has less to do with the claims of others on me and my obligations to them and more to do with the moral value of my being willing to help others who have suffered losses. Showing compassion should not be done indiscriminately, and we have seen that there are reasons why the appeal to compassion has a greater or lesser significance in particular cases. But showing compassion for others is different from recognizing their claims on us, and the moral factors that need to be considered in assessing claims do not seem to be relevant in assessing a virtue's significance. We may therefore have strong reasons based on an appeal to compassion for alleviating the losses of strangers, even if we are under only a very weak obligation to do so.

We turn now to the virtue of courage, of acting on appropriate decisions without being excessively motivated by various fears. Courage is radically different from other virtues in that there are no actions we could be led to do just because they are the courageous thing to do. Courage is the virtue of doing what is appropriate (even if more than what we are obliged to do) without being swayed by our fears. The appropriateness of the action is settled independently of the fact that its being performed in a fear-invoking situation makes it a courageous action. That being the case, we do not need to provide a theory of the significance of the appeal to courage in deciding what to do in particular cases. The courageous recipients and providers are those who, having assessed the relevant factors, make a decision about what is appropriate to do and then display their courage by doing it despite the fears that would prevent others from carrying out that decision. Still, we can at least say that the greater the fears, the more likely it is that others would be dissuaded, the more courageous the action, and the more deserving it is of praise.

Finally, there is the virtue of honesty. Being honest is in many cases mandated by many moral factors. There are, however, a special set of cases in which it is only the appeal to the virtue of honesty which would lead us to act in a certain way. One such case involves being honest to patients and their families about what we are doing when we have decided, on independent grounds, to do what they don't want. In such cases there may be moral factors that call on us to mislead these people. An appeal to compassion or to the disastrous consequences of knowing the truth might suggest that we misleadingly withhold information or even provide false information. Moreover, as I pointed out above, many of the usual arguments for honesty (such as the right to make informed decisions) will not apply in such cases. We therefore need to have a theory of how we should assess the significance of the appeal to honesty in particular cases.[25]

It seems that there is only one factor that we need to take into account here, and that is the extent to which the people with whom we are communicating want to receive honest and complete information. The more they want to have that information, the greater the significance of the appeal to honesty.

There may be many reasons why people want to have accurate information. They may want to act on it, but they may just want to know what is going on. Whatever their reasons, people often want accurate information. But the extent to which they want it varies from person to person and from case to case, and the significance of the appeal to the virtue of honesty varies in a directly proportional fashion

One of the implications of saying this is that there will be cases in which the appeal to the virtue of honesty has absolutely no force at all. There will be cases in which the people with whom one is communicating will indicate in one way or another that they do not wish to have certain information. In such cases the appeal to the virtue of honesty provides no reason for honestly conveying that information or even for avoiding lying. But we need to be careful about this point. After all, health-care providers are often tempted not to convey honest information of an unfortunate or tragic nature to health-care recipients because of the extreme unpleasantness of having to provide that information. In such cases it is easy and natural for them to mistakenly assert that the recipients really don't want to know the truth. So they lie or avoid telling the truth. This temptation and this self-deception must, of course, be resisted. However, its existence does not undercut the theoretical point that the appeal to honesty as a reason for providing information has a significance proportionate to the wishes of the people with whom one is communicating to have that information.

## *Assessing the Appeal to Cost-Effectiveness and Justice*

I distinguished the role of the appeal to cost-effectiveness and justice in evaluating health-care decisions in three settings. The first is the setting in which public funds are used to create an agency which directly provides health care to some eligible population, but the funding is a set amount which will not be augmented no matter what the needs of the population. In such settings health-care providers are required to justly allocate the health-care dollars available, and this requires them to consider among other questions the question of cost-effectiveness. There are also consequentialist reasons for considering that question. The second setting is where all those who are eligible receive health care, and the public pays the bill. In such cases, in order to avoid undercutting the very existence of the program, health-care providers are required to ensure that the health care they are providing is cost-effective. In the third setting, that of privately financed care provided in the private sector, health-care providers are at least required to make sure that the recipient understands the costs and possible benefits of a procedure so that the recipient can make an informed judgment about whether he is prepared to bear the cost in order to obtain the benefits. In all of these settings, if there are circumstances in which special technologies are being used and there is an inadequate supply, the health-care providers are required to allocate them in a just fashion.

In each of these settings the appeal to cost-effectiveness is relevant in some way. In different ways, depending on the setting, it is going to play a role in determining whether or not the health care in question will be provided. We need to ask ourselves how we shall assess the significance of the appeal to cost-effectiveness. In particular, when does a claim that a particular form of care is not cost-effective have a greater or lesser significance?

It seems that the only relevant factor is the extent of the cost-ineffectiveness. Some provisions of health care are extremely cost-ineffective. Those are the cases in which the excess of costs over benefits is very high. In such cases the fact that the health care in question is not cost-effective will be a very significant reason for not providing it. In other cases the costs may exceed the benefits but only modestly. In these cases the fact that the health care is not cost-effective will be less of a reason for not providing it.

It is not surprising that this is the only factor that needs to be taken into account as we assess the significance of the appeal to cost-effectiveness in determining whether a particular form of health care should be provided. Cost-effectiveness is, after all, desirable just because we want to get the most impact for the dollars we have. We want to do the most good with the resources available to us. The greater the excess of costs over benefits, the less we achieve that goal, and the more the costs in question should lead us to not provide that form of health care.

It might be suggested that there is another important factor, namely the amount of money being spent. The suggestion is that the more money required to provide a particular form of health care, the less we have a reason for providing it. This suggestion is based on a confusion. If the cost of providing the health care in question is high, then the benefits will have to be even higher in order for that provision of health care to be cost-effective. Suppose they are; suppose the relevant benefits outweigh these costs. Then why should that higher cost lessen the significance of providing that health care?

Let us turn finally to the question of justice. We are contemplating cases in which there are a group of people who would benefit from the provision of some health care and are entitled to it but in which the health care in question will not be provided to all of them, either because sufficient funds have not been allocated (the first type of public-sector case) or because it involves technologies available in an insufficient amount (all settings). In such cases we need to consider claims of justice. At least some of those putting forward their claim to receive the care will be claiming that justice demands that they get it.

The following factors are relevant to assessing the significance of the appeal to justice. (1) First is the loss suffered by the person if he or she does not receive the health care. In our lives we all suffer injustices. Some produce great losses. Others bother us but do not result in such great losses. Clearly, the appeal to injustice is going to have a greater force when the person who is making that appeal can show that he or she is suffering a great deal because of the injustice. (2) Second is the number of people suffering the injustice. In some cases a decision to allocate health-care resources in a certain manner will result in an injustice to only a few. In other cases (particularly when limited resources are allocated to expensive health-care technology provided only to a few while a large number are denied the ordinary health care to which they are entitled) the injustice in question is an injustice to a great many people. The larger the number of people who are unjustly denied health care, the greater the significance of the appeal to the injustice of the decision. (3) The third factor is the extent of previous injustices. Suppose those who may be denied the care have previously been unjustly denied health care to which they were entitled. It seems that their appeal will have greater significance. This is partly caused by the probability that the previous denials have made their needs greater and would make their losses greater if they were denied care again. But that does not exhaust the entire extra significance of their claim. The previous injustices seem to give their appeal to injustice a greater significance. So we seem to have here an additional factor that is relevant to the significance of the appeal to justice in a particular case.

## 4.4   Conclusions

We are now in a position to clarify the claims of the model of conflicting appeals because we have identified the various appeals which need to be considered in determining the morality of a health-care decision and the factors that give each of these appeals greater or lesser significance in a particular case.

The first claim of the model is that both parties in the patient-physician relationship are in some circumstances under an obligation to enter into that relationship. The circumstances are presumably ones in which the life or health of the patient is threatened. The patient's obligation to seek out health care may be based on at least the following appeals: consequentialist considerations which indicate that the patient and/or family and/or others affected by the decision will be better off if the patient is treated; considerations of respect for the patient's own personhood which obligate him or her to maintain life and bodily integrity; and considerations of integrity which may entail that the patient should get better so that he or she can attain goals. The physician's obligation to provide that health care, if that physician recognizes that he or she is the one who can best provide that care, may be based on at least the following appeals: the above-mentioned consequentialist considerations and considerations of respect for personhood; the patient's right to be aided, if he or she does not waive it; a sense of compassion for the patient in need; and considerations of integrity based on his or her own values as a physician.

There is, however, another part to the first claim of our model. Even in the above-described circumstances, this obligation to enter into a patient-physician relationship can be overridden, in some cases by the patient's exercising the right to refuse care or the physician's exercising the right not to provide care, in other cases by the existence of special consequences which mandate another course of action, and in still other cases by the fact that the provision of the required health care may violate the integrity of one or another party.

Which will be the cases in which the obligation to enter into the patient-physician relationship exists, and which will be the cases in which it does not? There is no quick answer, and we will be looking at it more closely as we examine our case examples. But we can at least say that for each of the appeals indicated above there are factors that lead to their having a greater or lesser significance in a given case. When we confront the cases we will be able to check for the presence of these factors, and that will help resolve the issue of the significance of these appeals as arguments for the existence of an obligation to enter into the relationship.

A very similar analysis applies to the second claim of our model about the terms that must govern the patient-physician relationship. Once more, the model identifies many moral appeals relevant to setting the terms of that relationship. The following appeals generate terms independent of the wishes of the participants: consequentialist considerations which indicate that health care of a certain sort is most likely to produce good results; considerations of respect for personhood and of substantive rights; considerations of cost-effectiveness and/or justice which may rule out certain forms of health care that the recipients desire and the providers are willing to provide; and considerations of integrity, compassion, and honesty which may lead to an argument for certain types of health care being provided in certain ways, even if both parties are willing to adopt a different approach. On the other hand, many terms cannot be settled by these appeals, and those will be set by the mutual desires of both parties. Moreover, in at least some cases the procedural rights of both parties to make decisions may take precedence over the above-listed appeals and lead to different terms, the ones desired by both parties. When this will happen will depend on the significance of the various appeals, and I have provided an account of that.

The third claim of the model is a summation claim. The legitimate patient-physician relationship is structured in an appropriate fashion by a proper assessment of the significance of all of these appeals. Some of the resulting terms will be based on the desires of the parties, while others will be based on considerations of consequences, substantive rights, respect for personhood, the virtues, or cost-effectiveness and justice. The fourth and fifth claims, extending this point, conclude that society's roles are to ensure that patient-physician relationships are legitimately structured and to pay for some of the resulting health care.

This model of conflicting appeals, as I have already indicated, is very complex. But that may be just what is required for complex cases.

One final remark before we turn to the cases. The reader may find a particular resolution I offer satisfactory. That should confirm the model, the theory of the assessment of the significance of the various appeals, and the final judgment. The reader may, however, disagree with some of my resolutions. That disagreement is certainly not an argument against the model itself. It will probably be the result of a different final judgment and/or a feeling that the theory for the assessment of significance needs modifying. I accept those possibilities with equanimity. Moral casuistry of the type called for by this model has been neglected in recent centuries. A first attempt, like that in the next three chapters, is likely to need modification. With that invitation to disagreement and joint exploration in mind, let us turn to the cases themselves.

## Notes

1. How society should carry out this role is a question for political philosophy and the philosophy of law. The methods may range all the way from the use of the criminal law to educational efforts. Moreover, society may choose different methods for different aspects of ensuring legitimacy. I shall not consider these questions further in this book.

2. Most notably, J. Rawls, *A Theory of Justice* (Cambridge, Mass.: Harvard Univ. Press, 1971).

3. C. Fried, *Right and Wrong* (Cambridge, Mass.: Harvard Univ. Press, 1978), pp. 7–9.

4. R. Veatch, *A Theory of Medical Ethics* (New York: Basic Books, 1981), pp. 298–303.

5. Ibid., pp. 299–300.

6. Fried, *Right and Wrong,* pp. 10–13, recognizes this point by allowing for the catastrophic and the trivial as areas in which the nonconsequentialist considerations of the right are overridden by consequentialist considerations. In this he follows the famous footnote of R. Nozick, *Anarchy State and Utopia* (New York: Basic Books, 1974), p. 30, which says: "The question of whether these side constraints are absolute, or whether they may be violated in order to avoid catastrophic moral horror, and if the latter, what the resulting structure might look like, is one I hope largely to avoid." My model might be viewed as an attempt to stop avoiding this question.

7. This view is suggested by some language in W. D. Ross, *The Right and the Good* (Oxford: Oxford Univ. Press, 1930), chap. 2, particularly on p. 41 when he speaks of the "greater balance of prima facie rightness." Elsewhere, when he compares them to judgments of beauty (p. 31) or when he quotes with approval Aristotle's view that they are like perception (p. 42), it is clear that Ross sees judgments about which appeals take precedence as judgments not based on any weighing on a common scale. To that extent, Alan Donagan's critique of Ross, in *The Theory of Morality* (Chicago: Univ. of Chicago Press, 1977), pp. 22–24, is not entirely accurate. It would be more accurate as a criticism of Veatch *A Theory of Medical Ethics,* pp. 303–4, who does speak about balancing nonconsequentialist violations on some unspecified scales.

8. As suggested above, this is, I believe, closer to Ross's actual view. I am heavily

indebted to him on this point, although I believe that my own approach goes beyond his in one crucial respect. Ross recognized the importance of identifying all of the appeals (his "prime facie duties"), arguing for or against the alternatives open to one, and then judging which action to perform. He did not recognize the possibility that we could be aided in that process by a systematic theory of when each moral appeal has greater or lesser significance.

9. This is, no doubt, the best of Donagan's objections (see note 7 above) to Ross's view. Donagan fails to note that his own theory can equally be abused. An abuser of Donagan's theory can prohibit or permit what he or she wants by insisting on the needed specificatory premises.

10. My colleague Larry Temkin has pointed out that a compromise position is possible. Morality may at best provide only a partial ordering of actions, and the cases of epistemological ambiguity, where judgments are unsure or conflicting, may also represent cases of an objective lack of a moral ordering. This is certainly a possibility that I have not argued against. My point here is just the logical one that adopting the judgment approach to the epistemology of morality is perfectly compatible with an ontological approach that sees morality as providing a total ordering of actions.

11. Our goal, according to that way of talking, is to maximize expected utility (the utilities of the possible outcomes multiplied by the probability of their occurrence). See, for example, J. C. Harsanyi, "Morality and the Theory of Rational Behavior," in A. Sen and B. Williams, eds., *Utilitarianism and Beyond* (Cambridge: Cambridge Univ. Press, 1982), particularly section 2. That way of talking presupposes the assignment of cardinal numbers to both utilities and probabilities; my way of talking does not.

12. This suggestion is best articulated by Harsanyi, ibid.

13. Remember that it is only the final preferences before the consequences occur which count.

14. I have not found a tremendous amount of literature on these issues, and the literature I have found seems to miss the point. Allen Buchanan, in *Surrogate Decision Making for Elderly Individuals Who Are Incompetent* (prepared for the Office of Technology Assessment, November 1985), argues against the first factor as follows: "The function is, first and foremost, to sort persons into two classes: 1) those whose decisions . . . must be respected by others as binding and 2) those whose decisions will be set aside and for whom others will be designated as surrogate decision makers. . . . Persons are judged, both in the law and more informally in health care settings, to be either competent or incompetent to make a particular decision—even though the underlying capacities and skills forming the basis of that judgment are possessed in different degrees" (p. 33). While accurate about current legal—not necessarily clinical—practice, this claim seems unsupported by any good argument. The proper function of a competency analysis could be, and I believe should be, to assess the significance of a patient's refusal and of the patient's right to have that refusal respected. I suspect that the failure to see this possible function is caused by a more general failure in the literature to see that refusals of individuals can be overridden and must therefore be assessed for significance in each particular case. That more general failure is connected, I believe, with the existence of so little in the literature on the second and third factors listed here. A notable exception is B. Miller, "Autonomy and the Refusal of Life-Saving Treatment," *Hastings Center Report* 11 (August 1981).

15. This point is usually made in the course of claiming that the requirements for competency should be more stringent when the consequences of accepting the refusal of treatment are greater. It is made in this way in the President's Commission for the Study of Ethical Problems in Medicine, *Making Health Care Decisions* (Washington, D.C.: Government Printing Office, 1982), Vol. I, p. 60. Buchanan, ibid., supports that view. This point is made about standards of competency, rather than about the significance of the right to refuse, by all

those like Buchanan and the President's Commission who have not yet seen that refusals can have different significances in different cases.

16. The closest I can find to an expression of this view is the following remark by R. Faden and T. L. Beauchamp in *A History and Theory of Informed Consent* (New York: Oxford Univ. Press, 1986): "Proposals like that of the President's Commission make it clear that the model of the autonomous person is not the *only* force at work when standards of competence to give an informed consent in sense 2 are in question. The welfare of patients and subjects, broad social interests in ensuring good outcomes, and cultural views about responsibility and authority all figure as countervailing forces" (p. 293).

17. Consider some of the practical difficulties and strange consequences of provision 4C(b) of the Texas Natural Death Act, as amended in 1985, which doesn't do that:

> If the patient does not have a legal guardian, the attending physician and at least two, if available, of the following categories of persons, in the following priority, may make a treatment decision that may, based on knowledge of what the patient would desire, if known, include a decision to withhold or withdraw life-sustaining procedures:
>
> (1)  the patient's spouse
> (2)  a majority of the patient's reasonably available adult children
> (3)  the patient's parents; and
> (4)  the patient's nearest living relative

The statute gives no idea of what to do if the spouse and the majority of the children are in disagreement. Moreover, it allows the spouse and the child who has been caring for the patient to be balanced by the other children who have been uninvolved for years.

18. See ibid. It is interesting that it ranks adult children before parents.

19. However, clinicians need to be sensitive to cases in which the patient would have chosen someone else either to spare the person with the closest relationship the burden of decision making or because they assess that person as not being a good decision maker.

20. Moreover, the formally closest family member, particularly the parents, may actually have a right in that case to be a decision maker. This is part of what is involved in parental rights. On these issues, see the Rice University Ph.D. thesis of my student J. T. Thornton, entitled "Parents' Rights" (1987).

21. These issues have not been extensively discussed by common-law writers because the common law has not recognized this right to be aided. The one exception is the discussion of when a special obligation has arisen. On that issue, see W. L. Prosser, *The Law of Torts,* 4th ed. (St. Paul: West Publishing, 1971), pp. 338–50. On these issues in Jewish law, where the right to the aid and the corresponding obligation to provide it are present, see *Encyclopedia Talmudica* (Jerusalem, 1961), Vol. 10, pp. 342–51.

22. As an expression of that approach, see, for example, D. M. Feldman and F. Rosner, *Compendium on Medical Ethics,* 6th ed. (New York: Federation of Jewish Philanthropies, 1984), where the following claim is made: "A patient in deep coma, but able to breathe without mechanical assistance such as a respirator, should be afforded *all* the care and concern due to *any* ill person. The imminence of death in no way exempts the family or medical team from *fully* supporting such a patient" (pp. 101–2, italics added). The person in a deep coma is precisely the person whose care would be least mandated under a respect-for-persons approach.

23. A very different subjective notion of quality of life is based on individuals' own preferences to continue living under the circumstances in which they find themselves. That subjective notion seems more appropriate for cases in which we are evaluating their continued existence from the perspective of the appeal to consequences.

24. This bears some obvious resemblances to the right of the person to aid. But there are also differences. Because respect is not an obligation *to* the person, special relationships to that person and the fault of the person are not relevant here, even if they are relevant in determining the significance of the right to be aided.

25. One possible theory would be that the virtue of honesty is always of highest possible significance. This would be a virtue-based version of the strong view against lying held by St. Augustine and Kant, although their views seem to be based on other moral considerations. Good selections from their writings on lying are reprinted in S. Bok, *Lying* (New York: Vintage Books, 1978), pp. 265–71.

# 5

# Cases Involving Competent Adults

The goal of this book is to present and defend an appropriate model of the provider-recipient relationship and of decision making within that relationship, a model that will enable health-care providers and health-care recipients to deal with the many difficult decisions involving life and death that they now confront. Having presented this model in the previous three chapters, I will attempt to defend it in accordance with my intuitionist methodology in the cases of the remaining three chapters of this book. Each case presentation will begin with a statement of the facts of the case and of the range of questions and opinions raised by the treating team. Each will then be examined in light of the model of conflicting appeals. If the model is successful in dealing with the cases, then it will have been defended.

## 5.1   Who Is a Competent Adult?

The provider-recipient relationship and the process of decision making within it when the recipient is a competent adult are clearly different from that relationship and that process when the recipient is a noncompetent adult or a child. At the minimum, the question of who has the right to refuse treatment and what is the significance of that right is transformed by the age and competency of the patient. Therefore, the first thing we must do before we deal with specific cases is to clarify when someone is competent and when someone is an adult.

   It might be suggested that there really is only one account which needs to be presented: decision making involving children is different just because children are not competent to make medical decisions. Once they become competent, they are to be treated just like adults. According to this view, all we would need to determine is when someone is a competent decision maker. It would make no difference whether someone was incompetent because he or she was still a child or because he or she had not developed or had lost normal adult capacities. This suggestion is attractive, but I do not believe we should accept it. Some dependent adolescents or teenagers may be perfectly competent to participate in health-care decisions but still ought not to be treated as competent adults just because they are dependent children. This is for the most part the official stance of the law in most states, although that stance is now under considerable challenge.[1] It corresponds, moreover, to an intuitive feeling that the parents of dependent adolescents and/or teenagers still have some rights to make decisions for these dependent children. So we will need to look separately at the question of competency and the question of adulthood.

Two points regarding competency have been established by the standard discussions.[2] (1) Competency is related to one's abilities or capacities. Since an ability or a capacity must always be the ability or capacity to do some sort of thing, then competency must always be the competency to do that sort of thing. The competency we are concerned with here is, of course, the competency to participate meaningfully in a particular health-care decision. It is important to keep in mind that there may be people who are incompetent to manage their financial affairs but are still competent to participate in a particular health-care decision. This is often the case with geriatric patients.[3] Conversely, there may be people who are perfectly competent to handle their monetary affairs but are incompetent to participate in a particular health-care decision. This is often the case with patients who have become depressed or extremely anxious by the state of their health. We are not concerned here with global competency, only with the specific competency of a particular adult patient to participate in a particular health-care decision. (2) One thing to avoid is judging people's competency by looking at the actual decisions they make. This is, of course, what many health-care providers do. Patients who agree with their recommendations are judged competent, even if their mental status raises many questions about their competency; patients who disagree with their recommendations have their competency challenged purely on that ground. This is inappropriate. Decisional competency is the ability to participate in a certain process in an appropriate fashion. That ability may be present even if the person comes to an unusual conclusion, and it may not be present even if the person comes to the conclusion that everyone wants him or her to arrive at. Competency is a process notion, not an outcome notion. However, this point, while correct, needs to be placed in proper perspective. If a patient goes through a process of decision making and comes to an unusual conclusion about what he or she wishes done, then the patient may still be perfectly competent. This is the sound theoretical point just made. Nevertheless, health-care providers are at least entitled to use that unusual outcome as a basis for reexamining the competency of the patient in question. A patient who expresses an unusual wish may be perfectly competent, but the more unusual the wish, the more that alerts us to the possibility that, contrary to what we initially thought, we may be dealing with a patient who is not fully competent.[4]

What has not emerged from the standard accounts is a proper account of the capacities that constitute the patient's competency to participate in health care decision making.[5] They seem to be as follows. (1) *The ability to receive information from the surrounding.* There are patients who are comatose, delirious, or disoriented and who do not perceive the required information signals presented to them or do not take that received information into their information-processing centers. No one can have the capacity to participate appropriately in decision making unless they can get the required information, so such patients are clearly incompetent. (2) *The capacity to remember the information they have received.* Appropriate decision making, particularly when the decision in question is a momentous decision, is not something that can be done instantaneously. Information must be received and processed, various options considered, their advantages and disadvantages weighed, and some decision reached. Since this process requires time, patients whose short-term memory is very marginal lack the capacity to participate appropriately in decision-making processes. These first two components of competency are the two easiest to test. Being able to receive information and possessing short-term recall can be easily tested by mental-status examinations.[6] The remaining components are much more difficult to define and to assess in particular cases. (3) *The ability to make a decision and give a reason for it.* There are some patients whose incompetency consists precisely in the fact that they continue to waiver concerning what they wish. Decisions eventually have to be made, and people who are unable to come to some decision or who are continually changing their minds are incapable of participating appropriately in decision-making processes. The difficulty is, of course, distinguishing those who are simply being careful and not rushing into a decision from those who either can make no decision or continually vacillate. (4) *The ability to use the relevant information in making the decision.* Some patients can receive information relevant to their case and can remember it but do not take it into account in making their decisions. Sometimes, this is because the information, while relevant from the perspective of the health-care provider, is not relevant from the values and perspective of the health-care recipient. This poses no challenge to the competency of the patient. In other cases, however, the patient doesn't take the information into account, either because he or she doesn't understand the implications of the information or because he or she is denying the validity of that information. The greater this lack of understanding or denial, the less competent the patient is to participate in decision making. The difficulty, of course, lies in distinguishing between the patient who doesn't understand or denies the information and the patient who fully accepts the information but doesn't take it into account because, from the perspective of his or her own values, the information is irrelevant. (5) *The ability to appropriately assess the relevant information.* There are patients who are depressed because of their illness. They place excessive emphasis on bad outcomes (thinking that they will surely occur and/or that they will be terrible) and underestimate the significance of possible favorable outcomes (thinking that they won't occur or that they won't be so good). Other patients deal with their anxiety by becoming excessively hopeful about the possibilities and merits of a successful outcome. These reactive depressions and anxieties weaken a patient's competency because they lead to a misjudging of the situation. The difficulty here is in distinguishing the patient who competently comes to a decision that the health-care provider disagrees with, because the patient is more or less optimistic than the provider and/or has different values, from the patient whose decision is arrived at incompetently because he or she cannot appropriately estimate probabilities and/or assess outcomes in light of his or her own values.

All of these capacities are ones that people can have to a greater or lesser degree, and all of the impairments can be present to varying degrees. Someone's short-term memory, for example, can range from mildly impaired to totally destroyed. Depressed patients can range from pessimistic to devastated. Every judgment about competency is a judgment about the degree of competency rather than an all-or-nothing judgment.

We now need to examine who is an adult. The hard cases will be those involving adolescents (ages 11 to 14) and those involving teenagers (15 to 17).[7] These individuals are old enough to have wishes and/or values that might be taken into account, particularly (but not only) when dealing with the question of the right to refuse treatment. The question of who is an adult becomes (at least in part) the question of whether one or one's parents has the right to make decisions.

Consider the radical claim that all children ought to make decisions about their health care in consultation with their health-care providers and without parental involvement (unless they want to involve their parents).[8] Why would most people reject that claim? Why do they think that parents must play a more central role, leaving the role of even adolescents and teenagers unclear? Two answers come immediately to mind.

The first answer emphasizes the relative incompetency of children. Children often lack the background information required to understand their condition and the options open to them. Children often lack the reasoning ability to calculate which of the options would maximize the expected outcome. Children often are excessively prone to depression or optimism, and this often leads them to weigh inappropriately the benefits and losses which follow from the options open to them. Someone who adopts this first answer should be interested in the results of psychological studies which test the abilities and competencies of adolescents and teenagers in these areas.[9] The results of these tests should be used as the basis for determining the age at which people generally acquire these abilities and competencies and at which they should be decision makers. Secondly, someone who adopts this first answer needs to remember that abilities and competencies are not all-or-nothing matters. People, including adolescents and teenagers, have them to a greater or lesser degree. So, looking at the results of these studies, an adherent of this first answer would either choose a point of minimum competency from which time on adolescents and teenagers should be recognized as having the right to be a decision maker or (more plausibly)[10] introduce a theory of an increasing role for adolescents and teenagers in decision making correlated with their increasing competency. There are certain legal doctrines, particularly the mature-minor rule,[11] that have emerged in recent years and reflect this way of thinking about adolescents and teenagers. The general legal rule is that physicians can provide health care to minors (those under the age of 18) only with the consent of their parents. There are a number of exceptions to that rule, one of which is the mature-minor rule. This rule allows physicians to provide care with the consent of a minor patient if the minor has demonstrated sufficient maturity of understanding and intelligence. This rule is usually applied to teenagers aged 15 to 17, although it has occasionally been applied to younger adolescents.

The second answer to why parents normally play the central role in decision making emphasizes parental responsibility. It reminds us that parents have a responsibility to care for their children, including dealing with the consequences of decisions made about their children. Because they bear these responsibilities, it might be argued, they are entitled to make the decisions that lead to these consequences. Whatever the decisional abilities of their children, those who must accept the consequences of the decisions should be allowed to make them. Someone who adopts this second answer should be sympathetic to a different legal doctrine. It is also an exception to the standard rule that physicians must obtain parental consent before they can treat minors. This is the emancipated-minor rule. It allows physicians to proceed with the consent of a minor patient if the parents are no longer responsible for the minor. If the minor has truly accepted responsibility for himself or herself, it is the minor who should function as decision maker.

What does all of this mean for the question of who is an adult? (1) Parents together with health-care providers clearly should make health-care decisions for a minor when the minor has not yet demonstrated a reasonable amount of the abilities required to be a competent decision maker and when the minor is totally dependent on the parents. (2) An adolescent or teenager together with health-care providers clearly should make health-care decisions when the adolescent or the teenager has clearly shown the maturity required to be a reasonably competent decision maker and when he or she is totally responsible for his or her own affairs. (3) The hard cases will be those involving (a) adolescents or teenagers who have shown that maturity but are dependent on their parents, and (b) adolescents and teenagers who have not shown that maturity but who are independent of their parents.

Another crucial issue is that all of the discussion until now has presupposed that there is parental agreement about some health-care decision. Suppose there is a case in which the parents have decisional authority but the parents disagree. Whose wishes should prevail? When, if ever, should the wishes of the minor help determine which parental wish should prevail? Furthermore, we have said nothing about the extent to which parents, even if they have sole decisional authority, should consider the wishes of their children in making decisions. A particularly difficult question is the question of the extent to which parents should be guided by the wishes of their adolescent and teenage children in making hard decisions for these children. Finally, there is also the question of whether there are some forms of health care which are special (e.g., abortion, contraception, treatment for substance abuse) and should always be left in the hands of adolescents and/or teenagers.[12]

It is clear that the discussion in this section has not created a complete and unambiguous theory of competent adulthood. It is hoped, however, that it has provided a framework for dealing with the specific cases that follow.

## 5.2  Competent Adult Patients Who Wish Not to Be Treated

*CASE NO 1.  "I'm old and tired, so let me alone":*
*The significance of a wish to be allowed to die*

FACTS    Mrs. A is an 84-year-old woman who was widowed in her early thirties. She was left with three small children whom she raised on her own. Raising these children was very difficult because of her lack of education and vocational experience, but she did it, never asking for any help, either from family and friends or from social agencies. In general, Mrs. A was a very independent lady who always did things on her own. Her health had always been good. She had no significant history of illness and had not been hospitalized previously. She was admitted to the hospital after sustaining a compound fracture of the tibia in an automobile accident, because people weren't quite sure that a woman of her age in a cast could handle her daily needs. Since entering the hospital, she has clearly been depressed. She doesn't like the nurses caring for her because she resents the dependent role in which she is placed, and she has become progressively withdrawn. Her family reports that she is listless and nonresponsive and spends most of her time lying in bed and staring out the window. From the beginning she ate very little and has therefore become progressively weaker. Recently she stopped eating. While she speaks very rarely, Mrs. A has said on more than one occasion something like the following: "I am old and tired. I am ready to die. If you will just let me alone, I will stop eating and die. I am ready to go to God." Psychiatry was called for a consultation concerning her mental status. They report that she is clearly oriented, has good short-term recall, understands what she is doing, and has made a decision to die. They therefore evaluate her as competent, although they recognize that she is also showing significant symptoms of a reactive depression, presumably caused by her hospitalization and dependency. The medical and nursing staff like this woman, although she is making life hard for them, and they are very ambiguous in their feelings about whether they should respect her wish and let her die or whether they should restrain her and force-feed her. Her three daughters have equally ambiguous feelings. It is clear that they love and respect their mother and are reluctant to go against her wishes. At the same time, they don't want her to die, and they think that if she eats and gets stronger, she will be able to go home to live on her own.

QUESTIONS   A great many questions are raised by this case. The major reason for not force-feeding this lady must be her own expressed wish that she be allowed to die. She is suffering from no significant illness and is not experiencing a great deal of pain. So she is not like those patients who are allowed to die because their death is imminent anyway and we want to avoid prolonging their painful suffering. If she eats and gets stronger, she can go home and live as she did before her hospitalization. The quality of her life before her hospitalization was certainly quite satisfactory both to her and to outside observers. So she is not like those patients who are allowed to die because they can only continue to live with a very low quality of life. In her case, it is a matter of her having decided that she is tired and ready to die. It therefore becomes crucial for us to ascertain whether she is competent to make such a decision. Her history and the psychiatric evaluation indicate both the basis for a reactive depression and symptomatology of such a depression. But is that enough to say that she is incompetent? This is not the only question. Suppose that she is competent. Suppose, therefore, that her wishes to be left alone and allowed to starve herself to death are the wishes of a competent adult. Does that mean that they should be respected? Isn't this a case of someone passively committing suicide? The cause of her death, after all, would not be any underlying illness but simply her decision to die at this time. Are we prepared to acquiesce in that decision and allow her to commit suicide? We have laws against aiding and abetting a suicide. Doesn't this express a social decision that suicide ought to be prevented? Still further questions are raised. What is the role of the family in this case? Can they play any role at all if we assume that the patient is competent? And if we assume that the patient is not competent, ought the decision to be theirs? In any case, what can their role be in light of their own ambiguities and vacillations? Finally, the following compromise strategy has been suggested by several members of the team: Why don't we ensure that she eats, either by force-feeding her or by talking her into eating, and see that she goes home? If she still wants to die, she can always stop eating and die at home. Might this not be the best way to reconcile respecting her wishes with protecting her life?

THEORETICAL ANALYSIS    In the case of Mrs. A, it is clear that there are several moral appeals that support getting her to eat so that she can recover her strength and go home. Moreover, it is clear that they have considerable significance in this case. The two most prominent of these appeals are as follows. (1) *Respect for persons.* Mrs. A is currently engaged in few of those activities we value so much. She is just lying in bed and staring at the window, nonresponsive to her family and health-care providers. Nevertheless, there is every reason to believe that if she can be persuaded to eat, restoring her strength, she can go home and resume her prehospitalization life, which included many of those activities. From the perspective of the appeal to respect for persons, we have substantial reasons for wanting to save Mrs. A's life by ensuring that she eats. (2) *Consequences of our action.* Let us begin by examining the consequences for her family members. We know that they want her to be able to resume her previous life. Getting her to eat therefore has consequences that they value greatly. This is also true to some degree of the consequences for Mrs. A. She does have a strong preference at this point to be left alone and allowed to die. Any action that does not lead to the satisfaction of that preference would therefore result in negative consequences from her perspective. Still, there is every reason to believe that there are many preferences that she will be able to satisfy if she returns home and resumes her normal life. The fact that feeding her will result in her being able to satisfy the preferences that she will then have then provides an additional reason for feeding her. Therefore, there are major aspects of the appeal to consequences which offer reasons of considerable significance for feeding her. Note, by the way, that the appeal to consequences, even when the consequences are evaluated in terms of the preferences of the person involved, does not necessarily lead in this case to doing what the person wants. (The existence of this possibility was noted in section 4.1.)

There is one important presupposition of these two arguments. If Mrs. A is fed, she will recover her strength, return to her home, and resume the quality of life which she had before she was hospitalized. One can certainly imagine her remaining depressed instead and not resuming that life. If that were the case, neither the appeal to respect for persons nor the appeal to consequences would justify force-feeding her. But there is nothing in her history to indicate that this would be the likely outcome. All the information we have points to her problems as being reversible if only she can recover enough strength to go home.

It might be suggested that there are additional arguments for feeding Mrs. A. What about her right to be aided in life- or health-threatening situations? Mrs. A's refusal to eat is certainly threatening to her life and health. Doesn't she have a right to be aided against that threat? This suggestion, while initially very promising, faces a crucial difficulty. Mrs. A, in the very act of saying that she wishes to be left alone, is waiving that right to be aided. To be sure, because Mrs. A is less than fully competent, her waiver of that right is less than completely efficacious, so that right and our corresponding obligation to help her through this crisis continues to have some significance. But we cannot give that right substantial significance without misestimating the degree of her incompetency. Parenthetically, the fact that her competency, while incomplete, is present to a considerable degree means that her family would have at most a modest right to participate in any decision making.

What about the other substantive rights of Mrs. A, such as her right not to be killed and our corresponding obligation to avoid killing her? Isn't it relevant here? I think not. If we provide food to Mrs. A and she refuses to eat it, we can legitimately say that it is she who starved herself to death, thereby committing suicide, and that we have in no way caused her death. This is not like the case of withholding food from somebody who cannot feed himself or herself, where it can be said that we have starved the person, thereby violating his or her right not to be killed.

There are, of course, value considerations that support letting her die. The most important of these appeals to her right to refuse the care that she doesn't wish to receive. There are several reasons for thinking that this right lacks its usual significance in this case: (1) *Her impaired competency.* The staff, in discussing the case of Mrs. A, supposed either that she was fully competent or that she was totally incompetent. We have learned that this supposition is a mistake. There are aspects of competency (orientation, unimpaired short-term memory, the ability to understand facts and come to decisions) which Mrs. A fully displays. Her depression casts considerable doubt, however, on another aspect of competency: her ability to properly assess the relevance of various facts. So Mrs. A is less than fully competent, even though she is hardly totally incompetent. (2) *The duration of this decision.* Mrs. A's refusal of treatment is not a long-standing refusal of a certain form of care. It has arisen just now in response to the sad circumstances in which she finds herself. This does not mean that her right to refuse treatment has no significance, but it certainly means that it has less significance than it would have if it involved a more long-standing refusal. (3) *The source of her refusal.* Although Mrs. A speaks of being old and tired and ready to die, she didn't say anything like that until she was hospitalized and became dependent. It seems reasonable to suppose that the real source of her refusal to eat is her strong personal value of independence combined with her belief that she is never going to be able to escape her dependency. This belief and this value lead her to the conclusion that she would prefer to be dead. The value in question is very central to Mrs. A's existence, but the belief in question (besides being improbable) is peripheral. Mrs. A's refusal to be treated is at least partially rooted in peripheral beliefs and has therefore less moral significance than other refusals of treatment.

In summary, then, the appeal to respect for persons and the appeal to consequences provide significant reasons for seeing that Mrs. A eats so that she can recover her strength, be discharged from the hospital, and return to her previous life at home. A major consideration raised on behalf of respecting her wish not to be fed—the claim that she has a right to refuse treatment—lacks the significance it has in other cases for a variety of reasons. It seems reasonable, therefore, to judge that we ought to go ahead and feed Mrs. A.

There is, however, one further issue that needs to be looked at. There are two ways we can feed Mrs. A. The first is to force-feed her. The second is to persuade her to eat on her own. Those members of the team who offered the compromise strategy have offered a strategy for getting her to agree to eat: convince her that she can resume control of her own life by eating until she is strong enough to go home and by then deciding when she returns home whether she wants to die or to live. Powerful considerations of compassion argue for attempting that second strategy before force-feeding Mrs. A. Moreover, if successful, it will eliminate the unfavorable consequences of force-feeding her. If the strategy is successful, we will have found a compassionate and benevolent way of producing the desired consequences and respecting her personhood. If it is not successful, we will have to rely on force-feeding her.

*CASE NO 2. "I've been in the hospital too many times":*
*The significance of pathetic wishes of tragic patients*

FACTS    Mr. B was born 32 years ago with spina bifida. It was a little too early for the more effective procedures for treating such patients that have developed in recent years. He suffered all the traditional problems of the midlevel spina bifida patient, including paraplegia and loss of bowel and bladder control. As a result, he has been hospitalized many times for surgical and medical treatments, and his life has been limited in many ways. One of his major problems has been recurrent pyelonephritis and renal insufficiency. Six years ago, his left kidney was removed. Renal function continued to decline, and this led to his current hospitalization. It is now clear that he can continue to live only if he is regularly dialyzed. When that was explained to him and his family, his initial reaction was extremely negative. He said that he was tired of being in the hospital all the time, that his life was no joy even before the current crisis, and that he wanted to go home to die rather than spend even more time receiving health care. His family is strongly supportive of his wishes, claiming that he has been unhappy for so long because of his unending set of medical problems. Their support may, however, be partly a result of the fact that they too are tired of the many burdens resulting from caring for him. Several people have suggested that Mr. B try dialysis for a period of time. They point out that he would have the option of not showing up for treatment later on. He has refused. He wouldn't even go up to the dialysis unit to see what's involved and to talk to other patients. Psychiatric evaluation of this patient has revealed that he is oriented and that there is no problem with his short-term memory. He is clearly very anxious about having to come to the hospital regularly for dialysis. There is also the suggestion of some denial of the prognosis that he will die shortly without dialysis, since he regularly talks about his faith in God and his belief that God will save him. Unfortunately, it is hard to find out whether this means that he believes that God will miraculously intervene and keep him alive without the dialysis or simply that he has faith in God's eternal salvation.

QUESTIONS This case, like case 1, presents a question of competency. There is evidence of anxiety and perhaps of denial, although there are none of the clinical signs of depression which were present in case 1. Furthermore, the family is strongly supportive of the patient's wishes. In case 1, we might be persuaded to keep the patient alive in light of the family's vacillation about respecting the patient's wishes. In this case, however, the family is very supportive of the patient's desires. However, to complicate matters, there is some question about the motives of the family. Are they really thinking of the best interest of the patient, or are they more concerned with their own exhaustion from dealing with his many medical problems? There is a further complication. In case 1, the patient was already very old, and accepting the patient's wishes might not have that much of an impact on how long she lived. In any case, the patient had already had a long and good life. In this case, however, the patient is much younger. He could live for many years on renal dialysis, and he has not lived a long life. Many members of the health-care team are swayed by that factor and therefore believe in dialyzing him. Still more complications abound. Mr. B's quality of life has always been considerably lower than the norm because of his recurrent medical problems dating back to his initial spina bifida. Those who argue for respecting the patient's wishes make this point and urge that we respect the patient's wishes in light of the poor quality of his life. Other arguments are appealed to by those who would respect the patient's wishes. Even if we forcibly dialyzed the patient now, we couldn't keep him in the hospital permanently. The patient will go home and may not show up for the next appointment. This is different from the case of Mrs. A, whom we can force feed for a time, help to regain her strength, and send home without her current medical problems. Mr. B's medical problems would be recurrent, and the patient can't be kept in the hospital forever. What's the point of forcibly dialyzing the patient? Not everyone is swayed by this argument. Some respond by saying that if we can just get the patient over the current crisis and get him used to being on dialysis, he may see that it isn't too bad and may continue on treatment for an indefinite time.

THEORETICAL ANALYSIS The case of Mr. B represents an interesting contrast to that of Mrs. A. The resemblances between the two cases are pretty straightforward. In both cases, the major reason not to provide care is that the patients don't want the care. Moreover, in neither case is the patient terminally ill, and it is medically possible to enable both to continue to function in a manner roughly analogous to their capacity to function before the current crisis. Finally, there is some reason to suspect that each of these patients is less than fully competent. Nevertheless, a more careful analysis reveals that Mr. B's wishes should be respected, despite the fact that Mrs. A ought to be treated against her wishes.

In order to justify this claim, let us begin with Mr. B's strongly expressed wishes to be left alone and not dialyzed. One of the important moral appeals that certainly needs to be considered is the right of the patient to refuse treatment. That right had less significance in the case of Mrs. A because of her somewhat impaired competency, the recent development of her decision, and the less central source of her refusal. These factors, which diminished the significance of her right to refuse treatment, are not present to an equal extent in the case of Mr. B. We have no actual evidence of any impaired competency in the case of Mr. B. In the case of Mrs. A, there was strong clinical evidence of a reactive depression. This evidence, combined with our knowledge of the impaired competency of patients undergoing a reactive depression, supported the claim of an impaired competency. The only evidence we have here is Mr. B's anxiety about having to be dialyzed regularly and his claim that God will come to his aid. The former may represent nothing more than Mr. B's anxiety about having to undergo something that he very much wants not to undergo and cannot, by itself, be taken as evidence of impaired competency. We are not even sure what the latter means, and, in any case, it would be inappropriate to take the patient's talk about God as evidence of impaired competency. The most we can say, therefore, is that there is evidence that this patient is very anxious about his prospects and hopeful of God's grace, but those responses seem perfectly appropriate in light of his circumstances and can hardly count as serious evidence of impaired competency.

Another factor present in the case of Mrs. A that is not present for Mr. B is that Mrs. A's refusal to be treated was based, at least in part, on a rather noncentral belief of hers. Mr. B's desire not to be dialyzed seems to reflect a very central and long-standing feeling on his part (attested to by his family) that his life has come to be a burden to him in light of his many medical problems.

The only reason why Mr. B's refusal should have a lesser significance is that, like Mrs. A's refusal, it is a recently decided upon refusal of a treatment invoked by a crisis. Mr. B's refusal would have even greater significance if he continued to hold it after some period of time in which he was dialyzed regularly. Nevertheless, when all is said and done, Mr. B's refusal has to have a very substantial significance in light of the fact that it grows out of his long-standing views about his life and the fact that there is no real evidence of impaired competency. It's a sad refusal, brought about by a tragic set of problems, but that doesn't count against its significance.

Two considerations spoke strongly in favor of treating Mrs. A: a respect for persons and an appeal to consequences. The former continues to be present in Mr. B's case and with an equal degree of significance. Like Mrs. A, Mr. B is perfectly capable of engaging in a wide variety of those activities whose performance we treasure so much. Mr. B's life, however sad it may be on other grounds, continues to have a certain valuable quality. Therefore, a consideration for respect for persons argues for continuing to treat Mr. B. An appeal to consequences, however, offers less support for treating Mr. B than it offered for treating Mrs. A. The first reason for this is the crucial point, already noted by members of the team, that forcing Mr. B to be dialyzed at this time will not necessarily lead to the desired consequences. He can, after all, accept dialysis at this point and still refuse to be dialyzed at a later time, when we are not able to force him to return to the hospital to continue his treatment. While it is difficult to judge these probabilities,[13] it is clear that the likelihood of the forced treatment in the case of Mr. B having the consequences of saving his life is far less than the likelihood that force-feeding Mrs. A will save her life. If we get her over the immediate crisis, she should be able to resume her regular life without further treatment. Secondly, we have reasons to think that Mr. B's continued existence, even if he continues to be dialyzed, is going to be much less of a benefit to him than Mrs. A's continued existence would be to her. The life she led before she was ill, and which she will be able to return to if we save her now, was one that she judged to be reasonably satisfactory. From her perspective, the consequence of force-feeding her—her being able to live that life—is desirable, even if she doesn't want us to force-feed her. From the perspective of Mr. B, being able to continue living may not be a desirable outcome. There is both his statement and the evidence of his family that he finds his life an increasing burden. Even if we were to conclude that his continued living would be beneficial to him, it is likely to be far less beneficial to him than continued life would be to Mrs. A.

Another point must be taken into account. Mr. B's family accepts the idea that he would be better off dead. There is a suggestion (merely a suggestion) that they may be saying this while actually thinking that *they* would be better off if he were dead. Whether or not that is true, Mr. B's continued existence is an undesirable consequence from the perspective of others affected by his existence, either because they suffer watching him suffer or because they suffer the great burden of having to help him face his many crises.

In short, a careful examination reveals crucial differences between the cases of Mr. B and Mrs. A. A leading reason for respecting Mr. B's wishes—his right to refuse treatment—is of greater significance because his refusal grows out of his long-standing fundamental unimpaired judgment about the misery of his existence. Moreover, the arguments for continuing to treat him are much weaker than those for Mrs. A. In particular, while the appeal to consequences strongly supported treating Mrs. A, it may actually support not treating Mr. B or, at best, provide minimal support for treating him. It is not surprising, then, that these differences are sufficient to lead to the judgment that Mr. B's wishes ought to be respected.

Several members of the team have suggested bargaining with Mr. B to get him to accept dialysis for a limited period of time before he makes his final decision. I have argued that Mr. B is entitled to have his refusal of treatment respected at this point, but there is much to be said on behalf of this suggestion. To begin with, if Mr. B continues to hold his wish not to be dialyzed after a period of time, it will strengthen the significance of his right to refuse treatment; the refusal would then be a long-standing one. Secondly, his decision after such a waiting period would increase the likelihood that continued treatment would be of little benefit and of considerable harm to him. We would be more certain about our conclusion to respect his wishes if those wishes continued after a trial of dialysis. In addition, such a trial would minimize the possibility of an unfortunate set of consequences that might occur after Mr. B's death if he is not dialyzed. At some later point, when the family has recovered from the initial shock and the tremendous burden under which they have operated, they may begin to feel doubts, hesitations, and guilt about not having pushed him to be treated further. They may wonder what their motives really were, and they may wonder whether or not Mr. B really knew what he was doing. The proposed trial does not guarantee that this will not occur at a later stage, but it does minimize its probability. That is why the bargaining proposal is meritorious, even if we agree that Mr. B should not be dialyzed at all if he refuses to go along with that proposal.

*CASE NO 3. "It's so hard to breathe":*
*What to do when we don't really know what the patient wants*

FACTS    Mr. C is a 64-year-old patient with a long history of smoking two packs of cigarrettes a day. For the last ten years, he has suffered from emphysema. He had to stop working about four years ago because of shortness of breath. In the last six months, it became increasingly difficult for him even to walk across a room. Two nights ago, because of extreme shortness of breath, he was brought to the emergency room, where he underwent emergency intubation, and was admitted to the ICU. It is clear that he can be gotten through this current crisis, but his physicians estimate that he has at best six months to a year to live. His wife wants him to be treated. She is a very dependent person who will have great difficulty in handling his death. She recognizes that he doesn't have long to live, but she is trying to put off the inevitable. She is supported in her wishes by all of his children. So everyone is perfectly ready for Mr. C to be treated aggressively except Mr. C. He has pulled out his endotracheal tube twice, the second time even after he was restrained. His physicians have explained to him that it's too soon for extubation and that he will almost certainly die without respirator support. They have explained, moreover, that his family wishes him to be treated. It's very hard to assess the roots of Mr. C's actions, because he has to write his responses to questions and is reluctant to do that. The health-care team is not sure whether he wants to be extubated now simply because he hates being intubated or because he feels that breathing is so much trouble that he would prefer to be dead. Psychiatry is reluctant to do a serious assessment of his competency because of the difficulties of communicating with him. But even his family admits that he was reasonably competent before admission, and it's hard to see why he should now be judged to be incompetent.

QUESTIONS    There are new complications introduced by this case. Here, as in the last two cases, is a patient who wishes not to be treated even though he probably understands that this means he will die. Of all three patients, however, this is the first who is suffering from a terminal illness that will result in his death no matter what we do. But he will not die in the very near future. He can be pulled through the current crisis, and the best estimate is that he can go on to live for six months to a year. There is no doubt, however, that the quality of that life will be lessened by the severe restrictions on his physical activities. Still, without a clear expression of his wishes to be extubated, everyone would have treated him. This is not a case in which people would have stopped treating the patient because his death is immediately inevitable or because of a miserable quality of life. Are Mr. C's actions really an expression of a wish to die, or is he simply expressing the fact that he finds being intubated extremely painful? Can we respect his wishes to die, if that is what he wishes, in light of the fact that we can't do a full-scale evaluation of his competency? What strength should be given to the family's strongly expressed desire that he not be extubated, that he be treated as fully as possible, and that he be pulled through this crisis? Shall we accept the argument of some of those involved that it would be inappropriate to continue to treat him against his wishes whatever their roots, in light of his short life expectancy and the poor quality of his life? Another theme has emerged in the thinking of some members of the health-care team. This is a man whose illness is self-induced. Against all sound medical advice, he has smoked for many years. Why, they argue, should we invest so much energy and resources, against the wishes of the patient, to pull him through an acute crisis induced by a self inflicted illness? As one team member put it, "He assumed responsibility for his smoking. Now let him assume responsibility for his dying." Is that a legitimate expression, or does it represent an inappropriate judgment? Finally, at least some members of the team would have had no trouble with the idea of not intubating Mr. C when he arrived in the emergency room if they had known then about his wishes. However, they cannot accept the idea of extubating him at this point. They feel that would be killing him, not just allowing him to die, and they are not prepared to do that. Other members of the team don't see any difference between not intubating him before and extubating him now.

THEORETICAL ANALYSIS    The case of Mr. C is different from the cases of Mrs. A and Mr. B primarily because we really don't know what Mr. C wants done for him. With Mrs. A and Mr. B, there was no question about what they were requesting, even if there were doubts about following their requests. Mr. C has made no request at all, only some actions on his part which need interpretation. This case therefore needs an entirely different analysis.

Let us first examine the claim made by some members of the team that extubating Mr. C is not a licit option because it would be killing him rather than just letting him die. This argument clearly appeals to the right of the patient not to be killed. This is a very strong right, possessed by all living members of our species. One possible response, compatible with the theory of rights presented earlier but not compatible with the current state of Anglo-American law,[14] is that this right not to be killed can be waived by the patient. When a competent adult patient has waived that right, then it is permissible to take those actions that result in his or her death without violating his or her right not to be killed. This point, while theoretically sound, cannot be applied in our case. Given the difficulty in interpreting Mr. C's action, given that we really don't know what he wants or what he is trying to say to us, we can hardly assume that he is waiving his right not to be killed. So if extubating Mr. C is killing him, there would be a very powerful moral argument against it.

I would like to challenge the assumption that extubating Mr. C is killing him, whereas failing to intubate him would just be letting him die. The crucial distinction between the two, as we saw in chapter 2, is about the causal chain in a given case. You kill someone when your action or inaction is the cause of his or her death, whereas you merely let the person die when his or her disease process is the cause of the death and you are just allowing that process to produce the result in question. If Mr. C, when extubated, has trouble breathing on his own and dies from respiratory failure, then the cause of his death will be his long-standing emphysema. To be sure, by extubating him one has acted so as to take away something that interferes with the effects of the disease process, thereby allowing it to cause his death, but this is not equivalent to being the cause of his death. It would certainly be easier to make this claim if we had a satisfactory full-fledged theory of causality, something which is greatly needed for the development of moral theory. Lacking such a theory, we can only rely on our intuitions about causality, which tell us that it will be Mr. C's emphysema that will cause his death.[15] So there are reasons, even without invoking Mr. C's waiving his right not to be killed, for dismissing the claim that extubating Mr. C would be wrong because it would be causing his death.

The other arguments in favor of continuing treatment for Mr. C include the following. (1) *The appeal to the right of the family to be decision makers.* The family wishes that Mr. C be supported through the current crisis if at all possible. They have made that absolutely clear. Doesn't the appeal to the right of the family to be a decision maker for the patient have some significance here? Perhaps, but it must be remembered that the family is not testifying to what they believe Mr. C would have wished, providing evidence of Mr. C's wishes when we are incapable of getting the information from him. They are attempting to assert their right to be decision makers. But we have no reason to believe that they have this right because we have no reason to believe that he is incompetent to make a decision. (2) *Respect for persons.* It is true that Mr. C has had a poor quality of life for some time now and has a dim long-term prognosis. Still, if he is pulled through the current crisis, he can return to his prehospitalization condition, which, however limited, still involved his being able to perform a wide variety of those actions we greatly value. To be sure, that capacity will not exist for as long as it would in the case of Mrs. A or Mr. B, but it will exist for some period of time. (3) *The right to be aided.* Mr. C is certainly facing a life-threatening situation. People have a right to be aided in such situations. To be sure, this right can been waived, but it continues to exist as long as it has not been waived. Mr. C's equivocal actions cannot constitute a waiver of any right. The significance of that right will not be very great, however, in light of the fact that the aid would provide only a modest benefit to Mr. C, at most keeping him going for a few months at a low level of functioning. Still, unless we are prepared to say that he is better off dead than alive, we must conclude that it would be aiding him to provide that care and that he has a right to that aid because he has not waived it. (4) *An appeal to consequences.* The very same point just made provides some reason for thinking that pulling Mr. C through this acute crisis would produce consequences that are desirable from his point of view. This may be true even if Mr. C does not wish to be intubated. Remember that doing what will lead to what is best for patients (even in light of their preferences) is not the same thing as doing what they want at the given moment to have done to them. Moreover, there is no doubt that pulling Mr. C through this current crisis will have desirable consequences for the family; it will produce those results they clearly want.

In short, some appeals certainly speak on behalf of continued treatment for Mr. C. However, none of these appeals has the force it would have if Mr. C did not have a terminal illness from which he will die in the not too distant future and which will greatly limit his life prospects until then. That fact weakens the significance of all of the reasons on behalf of his continuing to be treated. The whole situation would look very different if we had an unequivocal statement from this clearly competent patient saying that he finds life unbearable and prefers to be extubated so that he can die. But we don't have such a statement, and that must lead us to continue treatment.

Finally, Mr. C's physicians need to make clear to him that, despite the fact that he has twice extubated himself, they will continue to treat him by keeping him intubated and by restraining him. They need to explain that they are doing this because they are not sure whether his attempt to extubate himself represents a reflective decision that he prefers to die or is simply an expression of his discomfort with the intubation. They need to stress that he can help them come to a different decision, if that is what he wants, by clearly indicating what he wants. They need to press upon Mr. C the importance of his clarifying his desires. References to the virtue of courage are appropriate here. Part of the frustration of this case is that Mr. C may have made a decision that he wants no further treatment but lacks the courage to communicate it to us. It must be explained to him that if this is what is going on, he needs to find the courage to convey his wishes so they can be acted upon. Naturally, when dealing with a terminally ill patient, one does not want to preach sermons about courage. None of this prevents, however, telling the patient that if he or she does have some strong and settled feelings against further treatment, he or she needs to find the courage to convey them.

These first three cases are different, but they all represent cases in which adult patients who are arguably competent are requesting that they not be treated any further, with the result that they will die, and in which the major argument for discontinuing treatment is precisely that it would be following the wishes of the patient. These cases are further complicated by factors which argue for or against respecting these wishes. These include the patients' underlying medical conditions, the roots of their wishes, and the concurring or dissenting wishes of their families. The next set of cases will also concern patients who no longer wish to be treated, but in these cases there are other major arguments against treatment having to do with the futility of further treatment and/or with the suffering that further treatment will impose.

*CASE NO 4. "I don't want to be treated, but I'm not ready to die":*
*The danger of speculating beyond what the patient says*

FACTS   Mr. D presented nearly five years ago with testicular cancer. At that time he was 31 years old. His right testicle was removed surgically. Since local lymph nodes showed no evidence of disease, there was considerable optimism about his prognosis. Unfortunately, about two and a half years later, he presented with metastatic disease. This was treated very aggressively with both radiation and chemotherapy. Following this, the patient went into remission for more than two years, and there was modest optimism about his prognosis. This optimism was dashed again when further metastatic disease to the lung was discovered. He was then enrolled in multiple courses of chemotherapy and suffered from nausea, vomiting, and high fevers. For the first time, he was unable to work, and this depressed him considerably. He stayed at home; since he has no close family, he spent many hours alone. Though he did show some response to his treatment, his symptoms were so frightening that he increasingly began to fear the treatment and to desire not to be treated. Now all that is available to treat his tumor are last-hope experimental protocols. Nobody is very optimistic about what can be done for this patient, although these protocols probably will prolong his life for a short period (weeks, maybe a few months). Mr. D says that he doesn't want to be enrolled in these protocols, primarily because he fears the side effects of the treatment. At the same time, he says that he is not ready to die and that he would take any treatment that offered him any hope for prolonging his life even for a short time. There has been no formal psychiatric consultation, but there is little reason to doubt the patient's competency. Mr. D is anxious about the proposed treatment and depressed about the prospects both of being treated and of dying, but these anxieties and depressions are not out of the normal range. Those treating him have had several very thoughtful conversations with him about whether he should allow himself to be enrolled in the new experimental protocols. They find him unwilling but scared about not being treated. He has no close relatives, so there is no one else the health-care team can turn to for help in resolving this patient's ambivalences.

QUESTIONS    What does it mean to respect the wishes of this patient? At one level, we have a patient who is refusing therapy. Respecting his wishes might mean respecting his desire not to receive further chemotherapy and simply providing symptomatic relief to keep him comfortable (palliative care) until he dies. However, this patient also says that he is not yet ready to die and that he wants any treatment that holds out some prospect of prolonging his life. The proposed chemotherapy holds out the only prospect of a modest prolongation of life. Isn't there an argument for pressing this patient to accept chemotherapy at this point? That is the view of some members of the team. Others think that this patient's wishes are not the major factor to take into account. They call attention to the fact that, even with the proposed chemotherapy, this patient is going to die shortly. Further treatment, they argue, would be a futile attempt to prolong life in a patient who has already demonstrated very bad reactions to a wide variety of chemotherapy regimens. They argue that the costs to this patient of being enrolled in this further chemotherapy trial are very high and the gains very few. They challenge the legitimacy of enrolling this patient in the experimental course of chemotherapy. Some go so far as to say that they would not want to enroll such a patient even if he were eager to volunteer, either because of his desire for any possible chance for prolongation of life or because of a willingness on his part to help advance scientific knowledge in this area.[16] Not all would go that far, but this whole group feels that there can be no justification for further attempts to encourage the patient to undergo more chemo-therapy.

THEORETICAL ANALYSIS    Mr. D represents an interesting contrast to Mr. C. We have no clear-cut statement of what Mr. C wants. He has pulled out his endotracheal tube twice, but he has failed to explain his behavior, and we don't know whether it merely represents discomfort from being intubated or a decision on his part that he prefers to be dead. Mr. D has explicitly refused further chemotherapy. To be sure, he has also said that he is not ready to die and that he would take any treatment which offered him any hope for prolonging his life even for a short time. But that can be interpreted in many ways. Perhaps all he is really saying is that he would accept a treatment that would give him a chance at some prolongation of life as long as the treatment didn't produce the terrible symptoms he suffered after his earlier courses of chemotherapy. We cannot therefore justify the claim that he is retracting his refusal of treatment. Mr. D is a patient who has refused care.

What are the arguments for accepting that refusal? One is, of course, the right of the patient to refuse treatment. That right has a reasonably great significance in a case like this, but not as great as it might have in other cases. One reason for this is the force of the refusal. It is true that the patient refused the care after several discussions, but his other claims and his anxiety about the decision suggest that it isn't quite the firm refusal of care that other cases might present. He hasn't retracted his refusal; he has weakened its significance. Still, it is the refusal over time of a patient whose competency we have no reason to suspect. The source of the patient's refusal of care does not strengthen or weaken the appeal in this case. On the one hand, it isn't rooted in a special fundamental belief or value of the patient; on the other hand, it is rooted in the patient's no doubt reasonably central desire to avoid terrible discomfort.

There may be cases in which a patient refuses care and in which his right to do so has a reasonable significance but is overridden by other moral factors. Some of those other moral factors played a major role in the decision to continue treating Mr. C. But many of them are not present here. Consider, for example, the appeal to consequences. In light of the likely horrendous side effects of the chemotherapy and in light of Mr. D's clear feeling that these side effects are unacceptable to him as a way of obtaining a minimal extension of life, it seems that the appeal to consequences reinforces the decision not to treat Mr. D rather than challenging his right to refuse treatment. In Mr. C's case, where we had no decision from him, we might (although, I have argued, we should not) be tempted to appeal to his family and their wishes, and this might provide a reason for treating Mr. C. There is no family present in the case of Mr. D, and even if they were present, their wishes could not provide reasons for overriding his in light of his competent decision against care. Families have at least some right to be decision makers only when patients are at least somewhat incompetent to make decisions. No appeal to the right to be aided could argue in this case for continued treatment for Mr. D. To begin with, it is very unclear that providing further treatment is aiding him, even if it does extend his life for some period of time. Moreover, in light of his competent refusal of treatment, he has clearly waived that right to be aided. At best, we have respect for persons as an argument for continuing to treat him. After all, if we can prolong his life for some short period of time, and if he can continue to engage in those actions which we greatly value for that period of time, the appeal to the respect for persons would certainly argue for continued treatment. But that appeal is much weaker here, in part because he will have that capacity only for a short period of time and in part because, given the horrendous side effects, he will be able to engage in far fewer of those valuable activities.

In short, the right to refuse treatment and the appeal to consequences jointly provide powerful arguments for not treating Mr. D. The only serious argument for treating him is an appeal to respect for persons. If that were an appeal to the sanctity of life, then it might justify treating Mr. D. Given that it is not, given that it is an appeal that has various degrees of significance, and given that this is one of the cases in which it has a lesser significance, it cannot take precedence over the powerful reasons for not treating Mr. D.

One question remains to be considered. Should the team push Mr. D about the meaning of the apparent contradiction between his decision not to be treated and his claim that he would do anything to prolong his life even for a short period of time? We have two reasons for not treating him. One is his expressed wish that he not be treated. The other is the appeal to consequences that suggests that he would be better off, in light of his own judgment about the horrendous nature of the side effects, if he were not treated. If he were to retract his decision when it is pointed out to him that it contradicts his expressed statement that he wants to be treated so that his life can be prolonged, we would have strong reasons for treating him. Respect for persons would still argue for treating him. Moreover, in changing his mind, he would be telling us that the side effects are less horrendous than dying prematurely. Given the principle of consumer sovereignty, we would have to assess the consequences of treating him as favorable. Finally, there would be no argument against treatment from his right to refuse treatment. I am inclined to conclude therefore that he ought to be approached one more time and have the apparent contradiction pointed out to him. He should be asked very specifically whether his statement that he would do anything to continue living really means that he would accept the chemotherapy despite his expressed wishes otherwise, or whether it only means that he would accept some treatment that didn't have horrendous side effects. It must be pointed out to him that his answer to this question is very crucial in the minds of those treating him. If he responds by reiterating his wishes not to receive chemotherapy, then he should certainly not receive it. If he responds by changing his decision, then, after allowing him a little time for suitable reflection about whether that's what he really means, his new wishes should be followed, and he should be treated. In the absence of any such discussion with him or if it becomes impossible to have that discussion because his condition deteriorates, the arguments favor not treating Mr. D, primarily because we are not justified in reading into his ambiguous remarks a retraction of his unambiguous refusal of treatment.

## CASES NO 5, 6. Different ways of pulling the plug: The ethics of keeping a dying patient comfortable

FACTS    Mr. E is a 62-year-old man who presented a few weeks ago in a confused state, with difficulty walking. He was found to have oat-cell carcinoma of the lung with brain metastases. He received X-ray therapy for the metastatic disease in his brain to help relieve some of the symptoms (a palliative measure). However, since the chance of obtaining a remission was judged to be slight, the patient was not given any therapy for his lung disease. This decision to treat only his symptomatic disease was made with his concurrence, but, because of his confused state, it was made primarily by his family, which consists of a wife and three grown children. The X-ray therapy provided significant improvement in Mr. E's mental status, and he retroactively concurred with the decision. He then became increasingly short of breath, so he was intubated. The hope was that intubating him would get him over this acute episode of difficult breathing, thereby avoiding an agonizing death. Again, all of this was done with the concurrence of Mr. E and his family. However, things have not worked out as well as anticipated. Mr. E's respiratory status has progressively worsened, he has developed a pneumonia, and he requires higher and higher oxygen settings for his ventilator. He has also developed gastrointestinal bleeding. He is still alert and oriented and able to follow the discussion about his treatment, and he feels that everything should be stopped and that he should be allowed to die. What he wanted when he was intubated was relief from his symptoms and a few good months of life. He now knows that he won't get that, so he wants it all over with. His wife and at least one of his children seem willing to go along with not treating his pneumonia and his GI bleed, but they have difficulty with the idea of withdrawing his respirator. They view it as actively killing him. The other children see it differently. They find it hard to accept that he won't get normal medical treatment for his pneumonia and his GI bleed, but they are perfectly willing to accept the idea that he be disconnected from his respirator, which they view as "unnecessary heroics." His views have become increasingly unclear. The team caring for him is about as divided as the family and Mr. E.

QUESTIONS   From the beginning, the team was guided by the decision that in light of the slim chance of reversing Mr. E's underlying disease, no attempt should be made to do so, and he should simply be kept as comfortable as possible. Many of them now wonder whether they shouldn't have attempted to treat the primary oat-cell carcinoma. If they had done so, they feel, there is a good chance that Mr. E could have been spared this very difficult process of dying. Others, however, feel that a roughly similar process of dying was inevitable for Mr. E at some point or other and that the decision to avoid chemotherapy for the primary disease in his lung was appropriate in light of his wishes. One might look at this debate as an irrelevant ex post facto discussion, but it seems to be strongly influencing people's current feelings, so it needs to be kept in mind. Turning to the current debate, the case raises still another question. When a decision is made to let him die, in light of the patient's wishes and in light of the inevitability of his death in the relatively near future, what are the limits of that decision? Is it, as some members of the family feel, only a decision to forgo heroic, extraordinary, high-technology medicine? Or can it also be a decision to forgo ordinary medical care for his pneumonia and his GI bleed? And how, if at all, can any of these withholdings and/or withdrawings of care be distinguished from active euthanasia? Procedural questions have also arisen. A growing number of providers, frustrated by the difficulties of the case, think that the whole decision should be thrown into the lap of Mr. E and his family. Their wishes have guided the health-care decisions from the beginning, so they must now decide which, if any, medical care he should continue to receive. Others resist this suggestion, saying that it is too much of a burden to throw on the patient and his family. Can they really understand all of the technical issues and make concrete decisions in a thoughtful fashion? Should they be burdened with that responsibility? These providers feel that while the staff should be guided by Mr. E's goals, they must make the technical decisions.

FACTS   Mr. F is a 79-year-old man with severe congestive heart failure. His prospect of recovery and leaving the hospital is null, although at the moment he has no problems with either infection or arrhythmias. Acceptable cardiac output for this patient can be maintained by using intravenous dopamine, a drug which improves the strength of ventricular contraction. Adequate breathing is maintained only because the patient is intubated. The patient, who is oriented and responsive but on whom no formal psychological evaluation has been performed, is in a fair amount of pain and discomfort but is being treated for that. Before he was intubated, the patient was not very responsive to questions about level of treatment, but he did say that he simply wanted to be kept comfortable. The family also knows that the patient is going to die, and they agree with the patient's wish that he just be kept comfortable. They are not very responsive to further questions. The team is unclear about what an instruction to merely keep the patient comfortable means in a case like this.

QUESTIONS    This case, perhaps even more strikingly than the previous case, raises the question of what it means to accept the judgment that further treatment is futile and that the patient should just be kept comfortable until he or she dies. The team wants to know whether that means that dopamine should be discontinued. Isn't the continued use of dopamine equivalent to prolonging the life of the patient, and hasn't it been agreed that the only goal is to keep the patient comfortable? Others don't see it this way. Withdrawing the patient's dopamine, they say, would just be killing the patient. Another question that the team strongly disagrees about is what to do if the patient develops an infection. Some believe that the merciful thing to do would be to keep the patient comfortable by treating the symptoms but not the underlying infection. This means no antibiotics. Others view infections as requiring treatment and cannot accept the idea of letting the patient die from an infection that is easily treatable.

THEORETICAL ANALYSIS    These cases lead to a new set of issues which we have not yet explored extensively. The cases of Mr. E and Mr. F differ from the preceding ones in that everybody is in agreement that the patients should simply be kept comfortable and allowed to die. The patients think so, their families think so, and the teams treating them concur. There are, moreover, no significant appeals that argue for trying to keep them alive. What are the implications of the decision for continued treatment? Does that decision mean that one should consider active euthanasia? Does it mean that everything can be withdrawn and that only active euthanasia would be wrong? Does it mean that only extraordinary, high-technology care such as respirators can be withdrawn? Can we only withdraw all those treatments whose withdrawal will not produce a quick death? Can we only withhold new care but not withdraw any care already started? And who should decide this?

Active euthanasia is causing the death of the patient. Passive euthanasia is allowing the patient's disease processes to kill the patient without intervening to prevent that from happening. This distinction, while clear conceptually, is not always clear in practice. The root of that unclarity is the lack of an adequate theory of causality. Still, we need to use these distinctions to the best of our ability in each case.

What is wrong with active euthanasia? The primary answer is that it violates the patient's right not to be killed. This right is possessed by all living members of our species and is possessed by them in each case with a high degree of significance.

Contrary to what Anglo-American law currently says, however, it can be waived. If Mr. E really meant that all that he wants now is to be done with it, then from the moral point of view (leaving aside the question of the morality of disobeying the law) there would be nothing wrong with active euthanasia. But that is reading too much into Mr. E's claims. He has not clearly waived that right. Mr. F certainly has not. There are, therefore, strong arguments in both cases against active euthanasia. Moreover, keeping in mind independent moral considerations having to do with respect for the law, there are strong reasons for not even raising the question of active euthanasia with either patient.[17]

What about the various issues concerning withdrawing care? Would withdrawing the dopamine from Mr. F be active euthanasia? Would withdrawing the respirator from Mr. E be active euthanasia? No, because neither of these would be causing the death of the patient. Both involve withdrawing forms of care that are preventing the disease process from killing the patient. That some forms of care (dopamine) are more ordinary than others (respirators), whatever exactly that means, seems irrelevant to the question. This is equally true of withholding antibiotics from both. Since withdrawing or withholding these forms of care would not be killing these patients, the only substantive right that might be violated is the right to be aided. But these patients have certainly waived that right. So there seems to be no violation of anyone's rights in withdrawing and/or withholding any of these forms of care, and there are powerful moral arguments (including compassion, respecting the patient's right to refuse care, and the appeal to consequences) for doing so. To be sure, respect for persons argues for continuing to keep these patients alive, but that argument cannot be very significant in light of their minimal capacities for action in the time that remains for them, no matter what we do.

We have a variety of options for withholding and/or withdrawing care, each of which is morally licit since they are supported by a number of moral appeals and opposed by no significant moral appeal. Which of these options should we adopt? And who should decide? Perhaps the best way to deal with these questions would be to invoke the appeal to consequences. It is crucial to secure for the patient, within the moral constraint of not killing him, the least painful and most dignified death. Another, and hopefully compatible, goal is ensuring that the patient's death does not occur in a way that causes needless suffering for the family and for the providers. From this point of view, the case of Mr. F is easier than the case of Mr. E. Withdrawing dopamine from Mr. F is likely to result in a relatively quick and painless death as cardiac function ceases. In the case of Mr. E, we face a harder choice. We can withhold antibiotics, which will produce a somewhat prolonged death for the patient (infections often don't kill that quickly) but one which can be kept relatively painless and dignified. Or we can withdraw the respirator, which would produce a relatively quick death for this patient but one which might involve some problems of discomfort both for the patient and for the family as the patient gasps for breath. These problems could be alleviated by giving the patient morphine to dull the gasping reflex, but there is the possibility of actually killing the patient if too much morphine is provided.[18]

There is, however, a procedural issue to be raised here, even if we are thinking in terms of the appeal to consequences. Should the team evaluate these consequences and make the choice, or should they put the choice to the family and/or the patient and ask them to make this decision in light of their values? After all, consequences must be evaluated in light of the values of those who are affected. And in any case, given that another argument for not treating is based on the patient's and/or the family's right to refuse treatment, don't they have to decide which treatment they are refusing? Some might claim that this is a decision that the patient and/or the family cannot make, because they lack the information required. I think this argument is incorrect. We can always put the outline of the issue to them (in Mr. E's case, for example, quicker but perhaps painful versus slower but less painful death) and see how they feel. A better argument is the claim that putting such choices in the hands of the patient and/or the family is cruel and, in the case of the family, produces the possible consequence of tormenting guilt afterward. Is this consideration sufficient to justify the team's making the decision in light of their guess about what such a patient would want?

There is a way to avoid these difficult procedural questions. We could put the following issue to the patient and/or the family (whom it is put to depends, of course, on the continued competency of the patient): "Your wishes that the patient be allowed to die are going to be respected. There are a number of ways of doing this, and they have differing implications for how long the patient will survive and for what suffering the patient may undergo. Do you wish to be provided with the full details of all of the options so that you can make the choice? Do you wish simply to tell us how you weigh avoiding suffering and prolonging life and let us choose the technically best way to meet your goals? Or do you prefer to leave this whole matter in the hands of the staff to make in accordance with their best judgment about what will lead to the outcomes you would most prefer?" If, as in the case of Mr. F and his family, the patient and the family are inclined to leave these decisions in the hands of the treatment team, that seems fine. None of their relevant procedural rights can be violated since they will be authorizing the staff to make the decisions, and the choices can be made by the staff in terms of an appeal to consequences. If, as in the case of Mr. E and his family, they wish otherwise, the appropriate issue can be put to them to decide, although, in light of their disagreement, they may in the end ask the physicians to decide.[19] There are some downside risks of guilt afterward, but there is the possible gain of their feeling a sense of control rather than helplessness. Which consequence is more likely to occur is pure speculation, and an uncertain appeal to consequences cannot take precedence over their procedural right to decide which care they wish to refuse.

CASE NO 7. *"I'm suffering from so many things":*
*When so much can be too much*

FACTS  Mrs. G is an 83-year-old woman who has suffered from circulation problems in her lower extremities for the past twenty years and who became bedridden and institutionalized in a nursing home seven years ago. Two years ago, she became incontinent; she also began to report that she suffers from constant body pain, the etiology of which is unclear. Recently, she was found in her room in the nursing home having difficulties breathing and was brought to the emergency room. There, her $PaCO_2$ was 70, so she underwent emergency intubation and was admitted to the ICU. It is difficult to communicate with her, and Psychiatry is not prepared to make a formal assessment of her competency, but she is alert and oriented and writes in response to questions that she is suffering from so many diseases that she just wants to be allowed to die. The trouble is that the etiology of her current problems is unclear. Is her retention of $CO_2$ caused by drugs? Does it indicate significant obstructive pulmonary disease? No clear answer has emerged, the team is not at all convinced that she is suffering from a terminal illness, and she has no family to consult.

QUESTIONS    This case, like several earlier cases of intubated patients, raises a special problem in getting a confident assessment of competency given the difficulties of communicating with the patient. Nevertheless, some members of the team feel that the patient's wishes should be respected, because they are her wishes and/or because of the low quality of her life in recent years and/or because she is going to die in the relatively near future no matter what is done. Other team members disagree. They find the patient's wishes to be an inadequate reason for stopping the treatment because of the difficulty of assessing her competency, partly because she is intubated and partly because she is heavily medicated in response to her chronic pain problems. Moreover, they claim, we cannot treat her as a terminally ill patient, because the etiology of her acute problem is unknown. Finally, they suggest, we have no way of assessing the quality-of-life factors influencing some members of the team—the patient is in chronic pain, is bedridden, and is incontinent. A different question has also attracted considerable attention. Should we take as another reason for not treating the patient the fact that she is alone, institutionalized, and a burden? Or, as one member of the team strongly argues in response, should we treat this patient precisely because we want to avoid prejudices against the elderly institutionalized patient?

THEORETICAL ANALYSIS    The case of Mrs. G brings together in a very useful fashion many of the themes we have been discussing. It forces us to confront once more the meaning of competency, the significance of the right of patients to refuse care, the problems with evaluating consequences not merely to the patient but to others, the upper limits on what respect for persons can demand from us, and the meaning of compassion for suffering patients.

Mrs. G is not like Mr. C and Mr. D in that there is no question about what she wants. She wants care to be stopped so that she can die. This gives rise, of course, to the first argument for not treating Mrs. G, that she ought not to be treated because we should respect her right to refuse care. We have seen, however, that the significance of that right depends on a number of factors.

The first factor is, of course, the competency of the patient. In this respect, Mrs. G is like Mr. B and unlike Mrs. A. There is no clear-cut evidence of clinical depression present in the case of Mrs. G. Any talk of impaired competency caused by a reactive depression seems unjustified; all evidence testifies to at least a fair degree of competency. Nevertheless, other considerations lessen the significance of her right to refuse treatment in this case. To begin with, Mrs. G's refusal is a relatively recent one occasioned by the current crisis. This does not mean that it has no significance; it merely has less significance because it is not a long-standing decision to refuse care. Moreover, unlike Mr. B's refusal, Mrs. G's refusal grows out of no long-standing central belief about the negative quality of her life.

There are additional considerations on behalf of not treating Mrs. G. Suppose we consider the question of not treating her from the point of view of the consequences of the action. Treating her may well result in her staying alive, and, given her condition and her evaluation of it, we have reasons to suppose that this is an unfavorable consequence. The appeal to consequences has several forms, only one of which is the appeal to the consequences for the patient. Another is the appeal to the consequences for society. Keeping Mrs. G alive against her wishes is imposing costs on society—the costs of caring for her in the hospital and in her institution afterwards—without any clear-cut offsetting benefits (since, as we have seen above, keeping her alive may be of no benefit to her). The only possible offsetting benefit is the one suggested by those who view further care as a way of resisting the prejudice against elderly institutionalized patients.[20] But this point cuts both ways. One prejudice against elderly institutionalized patients is the view that they are of no worth and that we should just let them die. Actions such as keeping Mrs. G alive certainly oppose that prejudice. Another prejudice against elderly institutionalized patients is that they are incapable of making decisions for themselves and that we must impose our judgments upon them.[21] Keeping Mrs. G alive actually encourages such prejudices against the elderly institutionalized patient. So, from the perspective of avoiding prejudice, there probably are offsetting benefits and losses. The only appeal to consequences that seems to generate a clear-cut argument is that the costs to the patient and to society (which pays for her treatment) argue against treating her.

There is also an appeal to the virtue of compassion. This is a suffering patient who is begging to be allowed to die so that she can stop being miserable. Would it not be a compassionate act to respect her wishes?

Those who propose these arguments for letting Mrs. G die should not be moved by certain considerations offered by some members of the team and summarized above. They have pointed out that there is no justification for viewing her as a terminally ill patient. But none of the arguments for stopping treatment makes reference to the claim that she is a terminally ill patient. They justify not treating Mrs. G whether or not she is terminally ill. They have also pointed out that we have no way of assessing her quality of life. Even if this is true, none of the arguments for stopping treatment supposes that *we* can evaluate these quality-of-life factors. They all appeal to *her* assessment of these factors, an assessment that leads her to want not to be treated (and to demand that her right to refuse treatment be respected), that leads her to the conclusion that her continued existence is a loss rather than a gain (and to an appeal to consequences to justify not treating her), and that leads her to the conclusion that her continued existence is a form of suffering and loss (and to an appeal to compassion as a reason for not treating her). So the fact that we have no way of assessing the quality of her life is irrelevant; none of the arguments against treating her presupposes that we can.

What are the arguments for continuing to treat Mrs. G? The first is her right to be aided against life-threatening situations. But she has clearly waived that right. Moreover, even if we disregard her waiver, the appeal to that right cannot have a lot of significance in this case, because it is not clear that keeping her alive is aiding her in light of her evaluation of her condition. The only argument left for treating Mrs. G is an appeal to respect for persons. However low the quality of her life may be in terms of her being bedridden, incontinent, and in constant pain, she still does maintain the capacity to perform some of those actions whose performance we value so much. She can still engage in a variety of intellectual processes, interact with other people, form evaluations, take pleasure in various daily events, and so on. Moreover, because she is not definitely suffering from some terminal illness, we cannot say that the appeal to respect for persons is of little significance in this case in light of the fact that she will soon be dead anyway. So it stands as a significant argument for continuing to treat her. But it stands alone, against all of the other considerations, most of which have rather considerable significance in this particular case. It seems best, therefore to judge that her wish to be allowed to die should be respected.

There are many who have accepted the right of a terminally ill patient to refuse care and to be allowed to die but who are not willing to extend that right of refusal of live-saving therapy to patients who are not terminally ill.[22] Those people would reject the idea of not treating Mrs. G and allowing her to die. Their view cannot be based on a sanctity-of-life position, however, since the sanctity-of-life position claims that the value of human life is so significant that it must be kept going as long as possible, even if the patient is terminally ill and will shortly die. What, then, can be the basis of this view? One possible basis is the judgment that respect for life should take precedence over the many factors arguing for allowing a patient to die as long as the patient is not terminally ill, but it should not take precedence in the case of the terminally ill patient. I would argue instead that a case such as Mrs. G illustrates the reasons for judging that at least in some cases of nonterminally ill patients, we should respect their wishes and allow them to die even against the dictates of respect for persons. But not all cases will be similar to Mrs. G. There will be cases in which the patient's competency is less clear, and that will count against the right to refuse treatment having such great significance. There will be cases in which the patient's evaluation of the consequences of continuing to exist will not be as dismal as Mrs. G's evaluation of her circumstances, and that will give the appeal to consequences and the appeal to the virtue of compassion less significance. In those cases of nonterminally ill patients, one might agree with the judgment that they ought to be kept alive, even while maintaining that the appropriate judgment would be to allow Mrs. G to die.

None of the members of the team focused on the question of exactly what we should do in allowing Mrs. G to die; their attention was focused on the question of whether her wish to be allowed to die ought to be respected. A final point is that we need to apply to this case the very same analysis that was applied in cases 5 and 6 to help settle both the procedural and the substantive questions which arise when a decision is made about which forms of health care should be withdrawn from Mrs. G.

These last four cases have caused us to look at the meaning of futility of further treatment for the decision to just keep patients comfortable and let them die. The final two cases in this section will also involve competent adult patients who wish not to be treated. But these patients have very special reasons for wishing not to be treated, and these cases raise very different questions.

*CASE NO 8. "I just don't like doctors":*
*The need to save salvageable lives*

FACTS   Mr. H is a 73-year-old man with a long history of significant medical problems, including both chronic obstructive pulmonary disease and heart disease affecting his aortic valve. He has consistently refused surgery for the latter and treatment for the former, despite strong family requests, saying that he doesn't trust doctors and won't put himself in their hands. This has not prevented his family from bringing him to the hospital emergency room several times a year for the last few years to treat acute crises. He presented last week with a third-degree heart block. For the first time, he agreed to surgery (pacemaker placement), although it was done under family pressure, and whether he voluntarily consented is an open question. The surgery has not been performed because it is believed that his pulmonary problems, which have worsened, must be dealt with first. The physician treating him, who is doing his best despite the fact that Mr. H is a very difficult patient, had a long talk with him about intubation. Mr. H insisted that he did not wish to be intubated. At that time, the physician found him oriented, responsive to questions, but lethargic. When asked for reasons for his refusal, he repeated his familiar refrain that he just didn't trust doctors. The physician has continued to treat him with medications and pulmonary toilet, but that was not completely successful. Later that same day, Mr. H became hypoxemic (Pa $O_2$ = 30). The physician does not wish to intubate him, in light of Mr. H's instructions given just a few hours earlier and in light of the physician's judgment that Mr. H is competent. The family is furious, insisting that he be intubated if it is medically indicated. They say that Mr. H really doesn't want to die, and they certainly don't want him to die.

QUESTIONS   We have, to begin with, an extremely clear-cut case of the conflict between different ways of thinking about competency. From the point of view of orientation, short-term memory, ability to make a decision, and ability to give reasons for a decision, Mr. H is competent. But the reasons he gives for his decisions are bizzare, and there is a significant group of people, including his family, who view the patient as incompetent. Furthermore, if the patient is judged to be competent, why was he regularly admitted to the hospital against his wishes, and should his consent to surgery under heavy family pressure be taken seriously? If the patient is judged not to be competent, why has there been a deference to his wishes up until now? Still more problems abound. Should we take seriously a patient's refusal of treatment, even if the patient is competent, if the reasons are simply the repeated claim that he doesn't trust doctors? The patient is not saying that in this particular case, given his analysis of the benefits and the risks of trusting these doctors, he judges it better not to put himself in their hands. It is just a general fixation on the part of the patient. Should that basis for a refusal of treatment be respected? But if not, why not, unless it is being taken as conclusive evidence against competency?

THEORETICAL ANALYSIS   The case of Mr. H presents a very valuable comparison to the case of Mrs. G. Neither patient is terminally ill, although both are facing a life-threatening illness. Despite the important similarities, there are substantial reasons for treating Mr. H even if we do allow Mrs. G to die. These reasons will help us understand the point that emerged at the end of the discussion of Mrs. G's case, namely, that there will be cases of nonterminally ill patients who don't want to be treated but who ought to be treated anyway.

The major reasons for not treating Mrs. G were (1) an appeal to her right to refuse treatment, (2) an appeal to the detrimental consequences to her of being kept alive, and (3) an appeal to compassion. Some of these reasons are not present in the case of Mr. H; others are present only to a lesser degree of significance.

Mr. H, like Mrs G, is now refusing intubation, even though he did very recently consent to pacemaker placement. This refusal provides a reason for not treating him, namely an appeal to his right to refuse treatment. But how significant is that right in this case? Counting in favor of its having great significance is the fact that it is part of a relatively long-standing pattern of refusal and seems to grow out of a relatively central belief of this patient that physicians are not to be trusted. But that pattern had been broken by his consenting to pacemaker placement, so his refusals no longer have their full significance. Moreover, there are reasons for supposing that this patient is less than fully competent, and that gives this right less significance here than it might have in other cases. As pointed out earlier in this chapter, part of competency to make a decision is the ability to use the relevant information in making a decision. This patient seems to partially lack that capacity. We need to be very careful about this point. The reason for doubting Mr. H's competency is not that he is disagreeing with the recommendations of his physician and his family. To say that would be to turn competency into an outcome notion instead of a process notion. Rather, it is the sort of reasons he gives, reasons that indicate that he is not attending to the seriousness of his condition and/or that he is focusing on some imaginary vision of a threat that physicians pose to him. So his right to refuse treatment, while of some significance in this case, certainly is not of overwhelming significance.

What about the appeal to consequences? In the case of Mrs. G, the appeal to consequences provided additional reasons for not treating her. In this case, on the contrary, it provides reasons for treating Mr. H. To begin with, we have no reason to suppose that he wants to die, and his agreement to pacemaker surgery (to the extent to which he did agree) and the testimony of his family are evidence that he does want to live. So intubating him so that he can be pulled through this crisis, implanting the pacemaker, and sending him home gives him the best chance of obtaining the consequences he wishes, even if these steps do not produce them in the way he wants. Moreover, the treatment will certainly produce consequences that are desirable from the family's point of view, and they are also an affected group. All of this contrasts sharply with the case of Mrs. G, where the consequences for her and her family of her continued living were very bad.

A very similar point needs to be made about the appeal to the virtue of compassion. To the extent that the consequences of pulling Mr. H through are beneficial to him, in that they prevent the loss of his life (which would be a loss in his own estimation), an appeal to the virtue of compassion calls on us to intubate him and to attempt to resolve his current crisis so that he can go to surgery.

What has emerged so far is that many of the factors that argued for not treating Mrs. G argue for treating Mr. H. All that can be said on behalf of not intubating Mr. H is that it would be respecting his wishes, but that appeal cannot have the significance it might have in other cases given the facts about the pattern of his choices and the extent of his competency. So there seem to be better reasons for intubating Mr. H than for letting him die.

All of these reasons are fortified by an appeal to respect for persons. Mr. H, in his baseline situation, was certainly capable of engaging in the wide variety of activities whose performance we value. Given that his condition may be reversible so that he can return to that baseline condition, there is a significant appeal to respect for persons for doing so. This appeal adds to the many other reasons for treating Mr. H.

All of the arguments for treating Mr. H presuppose that there is a reasonably good chance that he will be pulled through, have his surgery, and go home in better shape. If his condition deteriorates so that this no longer seems so likely, then things will be very different. The argument for intubating him from the appeals to consequences, compassion, and respect for persons will become far less significant, and his right to have his wishes respected may come to take precedence.

Mrs. G was a good example of a patient who is not terminally ill, who wishes not to be treated, and for whom it is morally appropriate not to give treatment. This is a criticism of those legal systems which have extended the right to refuse life-saving therapy only to the terminally ill. We have also seen that there are cases in which one should not respect that right, cases in which life-saving therapy ought to be provided to nonterminally ill patients who don't want to be treated even if they are at least somewhat competent. This would be in accord with the view embodied in the laws of those legal systems. Mr. H is a good example of such a patient. When there are many moral appeals that need to be considered in resolving cases, a simplistic rule that either extends the right to refuse life-saving therapy to the nonterminally ill or denies it to them is going to be inadequate. A more adequate rule will have to respect that right in some cases and reject it in others.

*CASE NO 9. "I'd rather live with God than live in sin":*
*When a hard case is really hard*

FACTS    Mrs. I is a 53-year-old woman who presented to the hospital with a long history of problems related to a mitral stenosis. She had developed problems with blood backing into her lungs and resulting pulmonary congestion. She received a mitral valve replacement. This surgery seemed successful, and she was allowed to go home. Several days later, she began having difficulty breathing, and by the time she arrived at the hospital, she required emergency intubation and was placed in the ICU. By day three, she was making some progress, although it was clear that her left ventricular functioning was still impaired. On day four, she spiked a fever, became agitated, and was difficult to understand. Sepsis was suspected, and a sepsis workup was ordered. In addition, significant GI bleeding was noted. Blood transfusions would be part of the normal regimen for managing such a patient and are viewed by the staff as essential in this case. They note, however, that when she was admitted for her original surgery, she indicated that she was a Jehovah's Witness who did not want any medical care that involved blood products. She said that her relationship with God was more important than her earthly existence. Her initial surgery was performed in accordance with her wishes, and she received only some autotransfusions. The physicians have consulted her family members. Her husband has said that she was a recent convert, who joined the Jehovah's Witnesses less than a year ago, but that she is a very strong believer in the teachings of the church. He is sure that even in the current life-threatening situation, she would not wish blood transfusions. Her children disagree. They question the depth of her commitment to these beliefs, pointing out that she is a recent convert, with the enthusiasm but lack of depth of commitment often found in such converts.

QUESTIONS    Should we respect the wishes of competent adult patients who refuse certain forms of medical treatment for curable problems on the grounds that these forms of medical treatment go against their religious beliefs, even if respecting their wishes means letting them die? Some members of the team feel that we are required to respect the wishes of such a patient, even if they are based on unusual religious beliefs (e.g., that one sins against God by accepting blood transfusions), since people have a right to follow their religious beliefs even at the cost of their lives. Other members of the team view this claim with great suspicion. They argue that people have no right to commit suicide even if it's based on their religious beliefs and that health-care providers are obliged to prevent them from doing so. There are additional questions raised by the special facts of this case. How seriously should we take Mrs. I's wishes not to receive blood products in light of the family's conflict about the seriousness of her commitment and her beliefs? Does it make a difference that she is only a recent convert to that particular religious faith and that her wishes may express only a passing commitment rather than a long-standing one? Would we feel differently if she had been a Jehovah's Witness for the last twenty years? Does it make a difference that her wishes were expressed when she was not facing a crisis and that we do not have an expression of her wishes when the crisis is real? Finally, to what extent are providers of care bound by commitments made not to use blood products? After all, when Mrs. I was admitted to the hospital for her surgery, a promise was made that she would receive no blood transfusions. It seems likely that she understood that promise to include her postoperative care and that the promise was made with that understanding. Should such a promise ever have been made? More crucially, given that it was made, are the current health-care providers, who are not the surgeons who made that promise, bound by that promise?

THEORETICAL ANALYSIS    Patients such as Mrs. I have posed tremendous difficulties for clinicians and writers in this field.[23] The arguments on both sides of this case are very powerful, and our model helps to explain why. A very careful analysis must be done before one can begin to make a judgment about this case.

The most crucial argument for not providing blood to Mrs. I, even if this means that she will probably die from the loss of blood, has to be that not treating her will be respecting her right to refuse the health care that she does not want. Many factors need to be examined when we assess the significance of that right in a particular case. To begin with, Mrs. I's refusal of blood products is based on a very central belief of hers, her belief in the religious teachings of her church. To be sure, as some members of the family have pointed out, she is a recent convert to those religious beliefs. Be that as it may, in her current belief system, these are central beliefs, and refusals based on them have great significance. Secondly, Mrs. I's refusal is not a sudden or hesitant refusal. She made it clear when she entered the hospital originally for surgery that she wanted no blood products, and that refusal was a firm refusal. This refusal has additional significance because it is both long-standing and firmly held. The third factor we need to consider is her competency. This is a more complicated matter. At the current moment, when the issue of her getting blood has become so central, she is no longer competent because of her agitation and other disturbances caused presumably by infection and fever. But when she initially made it clear that she didn't want blood products, she was completely competent. So her refusal represents the latest information we have about the competent wishes of the patient. In short, with the exception of the fact that Mrs. I's competent refusal is not contemporaneous with the acute crisis, it has all of those features which give respect for her right to refuse treatment the greatest possible significance. There is therefore a powerful argument for respecting her wishes and not transfusing her. Cases of Jehovah's Witnesses who are still competent at the time of refusal are the only ones where that right rises to a higher significance.

Additional arguments might be given for respecting her wish not to be transfused. One appeals to supposed unfortunate consequences of forcibly transfusing her. Even if she does survive, won't she survive with a great sense of sin? She will feel that she is alive only because she has violated God's will, and that will cause immense suffering to her, based both on a sense of sin and on anxiety about her ultimate salvation. This appeal to consequences is often reinforced by the claim that it would be compassionate to respect these factors and not impose this suffering on her. I have my doubts about these arguments. The crucial point is that we are considering forcibly transfusing her. If she is forcibly transfused, then she will not have sinned, although she will think that others have sinned when they forcibly transfused her. That being the case, these undesirable psychological consequences might not eventuate. No real study has even been done on this topic, but court cases and physician anecdotes inspire no clear confidence that these consequences will come about. And even if they do, they might well be less significant than the positive consequences of her being able to live a life which is still worth living.

Another argument is that integrity calls upon us not to transfuse her. To transfuse her would be for her to act in violation of her own convictions. That is a moral failing, the failing of not exemplifying the virtue of integrity. This argument is, I believe, just a non sequitur. If she were forcibly transfused, she would not be acting against her convictions, so there would be no failing on her part to exemplify the virtue of integrity. An appeal to integrity provides no reason for not forcibly transfusing her.

What about the promise made to her? Leaving aside the question of whether the promise should have been made, a question that is closely connected to but not identical with the question of whether she should now be transfused, the question I'm concerned with here is whether we are under an obligation not to transfuse her now because of the promises made by others earlier on. It is hard to see what the basis of that obligation can be. How can promises made by one person bind the actions of others? There is, however, an argument for respecting that promise, which appeals to consequences. Mrs. I entered the hospital to have the needed surgery only because this promise was made to her. Suppose that the physicians who are currently treating her violate that promise, arguing among other things that they didn't make it. What are the implications of this for the willingness of Jehovah's Witnesses in the future to enter the hospital for needed surgery? Will they trust the promises made to them? And if not, isn't that a reason for not transfusing her? I think it is, although this is one of those appeals to consequences whose significance is very hard to assess; it is very difficult to know how probable it is that breaking the promise will have the bad consequences in question.

We have seen that there is one major argument for respecting her wishes and not transfusing her. This is the appeal to her right to refuse treatment, an appeal that has a great deal of significance in this case. There is also a somewhat speculative but real argument that appeals to the detrimental consequences of breaking the promise to her for the health of other Jehovah's Witnesses who require surgery but may not enter the hospital when they recognize that doctors may forcibly transfuse them even if they receive a promise that they will not be transfused.

There are, on the other hand, important arguments on behalf of transfusing Mrs. I and saving her life. Some of them rest on two important facts about this case: that this is a woman who has every likelihood of living a long and meaningful life if she can get over her current crisis, and that she is a woman who would like that to happen if only it can be done without violating her religious conscience. These two considerations give rise to the following arguments. (1) *An appeal to consequences.* If we do transfuse her and pull her through the current crisis, she can go on and lead a normal life. It may be somewhat troubled by her feelings about this incident, although there are reasons that we have given above for not being overly moved by this consideration. On the whole, then, we have reason to believe that her life will be (in her estimate) a life worth living; we have reason to believe that the consequences of saving her life will be something that is good from her perspective. Moreover, even from her perspective, the price of her life being saved will not be her eternal damnation because she will not have sinned if we forcibly transfuse her. So the appeal to consequences speaks on behalf of saving her life, since the consequences of doing so are, from her perspective, very good. (2) *An appeal to respect for persons.* There is absolutely every reason to believe that if Mrs. I can be pulled through the current crisis, she can go on to lead a normal life in which she is perfectly capable of engaging in the wide variety of activities whose performance we value so greatly. So an appeal to respect for persons argues for saving her life. This appeal is particularly strong in a case like this, as compared to some of the cases examined earlier, precisely because she is a person who can live a full and meaningful life for many years.

An additional argument for transfusing Mrs. I appeals to the virtue of integrity.

One of the values shared by members of the team treating Mrs. I, and by most health-care providers, is the commitment to save salvageable lives, lives which can be prolonged with a meaningful existence for a considerable number of years. From that perspective, sitting by and allowing this patient to die when her life could be saved would be violating a fundamental value, one connected to a belief in the respect for persons. There is, therefore, an appeal to integrity, an appeal that has considerable significance in this case, which calls upon the physicians to transfuse the patient and save her life.

We have here the very sort of case that we were most concerned about when we first articulated the model of conflicting appeals, a case in which a careful examination of the various moral appeals on either side leads to results that make a firm judgment very difficult to defend. There are powerful moral considerations on either side. I note, parenthetically, that some of the clinicians whose sense of values I have come to most appreciate are themselves badly split on cases like this, feeling the appeal of both approaches.

One thing seems clear. If we decide on behalf of saving Mrs. I's life (emphasizing the appeals to consequences, to the respect for persons, and to integrity), we would do best to do so by forcibly transfusing her rather than by tempting her and/or her family to consent to the transfusions. This would avoid obvious bad consequences of guilt feelings on her part and/or family feuding later on. Moreover, if we transfuse her, this would be the sort of case where an appeal to honesty would call upon us to tell the family (and the patient) what had been done, rather than attempt to hide what had been done.

My own tentative judgment in this case is that these appeals to consequences, to respect for persons, and to the integrity of the health-care providers in question should take precedence over Mrs. I's right to refuse treatment and over possible detrimental consequences and that she should be transfused. I say this, however, with no great conviction. I am continually amazed by people who find this case easy. This is the sort of moral ambiguity whose existence offers an uncomfortable but real argument for the validity of the model of conflicting appeals.

## 5.3   Competent Adult Patients Who Wish to Be Treated

*CASE NO 10. "Treat my Hodgkin's disease":*
*Above all, do no harm*

FACTS   Miss J presented several months ago with progressive neurological deficits. She had developed a variety of abnormalities in both her motor function and her vision, and her speech was slightly impaired. It was clear that she was suffering from progressive multifocal leukoencephalopathy, an inevitably fatal disease of the central nervous system. During various diagnostic studies, it also became clear that she was suffering from Hodgkin's disease. All of this was explained to the patient, who was awake and reasonably oriented and who usually displayed good short-term memory. The patient and her family are aware of the fact that there has been significant progress in the treatment of Hodgkin's disease by use of a four-drug combination chemotherapy known as MOPP. The patient and her family wish to have her Hodgkin's disease treated. The physicians are reluctant to do so, in part because the patient is probably going to die from the leukoencephalopathy before her Hodgkin's disease produces significant symptoms and in part because they believe that the chemotherapy will actually worsen the patient's immune system and cause more damage than good. This has been explained to the patient and her family, but they insist that the patient has a curable cancer and they want it treated. It's almost as though they don't hear the reasons for not treating the patient, although when you ask them to repeat why the doctors don't want to give the patient MOPP, they certainly can repeat what has been said.

QUESTIONS    The first question that this case raises is that of the patient's competency, which is challengeable in light of her leukoencephalopathy, although she doesn't do badly on the basic tests for competency. There is another reason for questioning the competency of both the patient and her family. It seems to many members of the team that the patient and her family are simply denying the existence of the more serious disease and focusing entirely on the Hodgkin's disease, probably because they know of the considerable success in treating Hodgkin's disease in recent years. Some would conclude that the patient and her family are therefore incompetent. Others don't see it that way. They see the family and the patient facing a desperate situation, requesting such treatment as is available, and hoping for the best. Is this a case of a patient, supported by her family, making a tough decision in an impossible situation, or is it a case of an incompetent request based on denial? Furthermore, many members of the team feel that, whether or not the patient and/or her family are competent, she should not receive MOPP for her Hodgkin's disease. They feel that a physician should never provide a form of treatment that is harmful to the patient, even if a competent patient requests the treatment. Others feel that it is the patient's life that is severely threatened at this point, and it should be the patient's choice, if she is competent, about whether or not she should be treated. As might be expected, a third compromise position has emerged. Some claim that in light of the patient-physician disagreement, the physicians should strongly recommend to the patient that she seek medical help from another physician who will give her what she wants. Still others argue that the physicians' real job in this case should be to continue to work with the patient and the family to understand why their choice is inappropriate rather than try to pander to their wishes by finding someone else who will go along with them.

THEORETICAL ANALYSIS    The case of Miss J is the first of our examples involving an arguably competent adult patient who wishes to receive a certain form of treatment but whose physicians do not think they should provide that treatment. This fact sharply distinguishes this case and those that follow from the earlier cases in this chapter, and it has a profound implication for the question of which moral appeals are relevant. In order to see why, we need to review an important point that emerged in the discussion of procedural rights in chapters 2 and 4. In that discussion, we began with the idea that a patient has a right to determine what should be done to his or her body. Two different forms of that right are the right to refuse various forms of treatment and the right to receive various forms of treatment. While the first right is extremely important, it is far from clear that the second right even exists. Granting such a right to patients would be imposing on health-care providers an obligation to provide forms of care that they judge to be inappropriate, thereby imposing on them a form of servitude whose moral basis is very dubious. In short, while patients have a right to refuse care, even when that care might be of great benefit to them, they do not have a right to receive inappropriate care simply because that is what they want.

Miss J is not refusing care; she is demanding care. The moral question we need to consider is whether she should receive this care. She has no right to this care just because she wants it. Consequently, this case, and the ones to follow, will not involve an extensive appeal to the patient's procedural rights.

One appeal that we certainly do need to consider is the appeal to the consequences of providing Miss J the desired course of chemotherapy. That appeal provides arguments in two conflicting directions. On the one hand, there are good reasons to believe that treating Miss J would actually worsen her condition and perhaps even hasten her death. These are the medical considerations that lead her physicians to strongly oppose giving her chemotherapy. Since we have no reason to believe that Miss J and/or her relatives wish her condition to worsen or wish her to die, the consequences of her receiving MOPP are, from their perspective, bad. This provides us with powerful moral reasons for not following their wishes. But there is a conflicting argument resting on a different appeal to consequences. Miss J and her family very much want her to receive treatment. If we fail to treat her, we will increase the anger and frustration of the patient and the family. These are highly undesirable consequences, and they provide us with a reason for following the patient's wishes. The appeal to consequences leads us, therefore, in conflicting directions. When we consider the patient's physical well-being, we are led by an appeal to consequences to adamantly refuse her the chemotherapy she desires. When we consider the suffering and anguish felt by this patient and her family, we are led by an appeal to consequences to go along with their wishes.

Not every appeal to consequences has the same significance. It depends on how bad are the consequences in question (as they are assessed by those who suffer the consequences) and how probable it is that these consequences will actually come about. Do the family and the patient view the patient's earlier demise, if that is in fact a consequence of her receiving MOPP, as a better or worse consequence than their own feelings of frustration if the patient is not treated? Also, what is the likelihood that the patient's treatment will worsen her condition and hasten her demise, and what is the likelihood that the family and the patient will refuse to accept the point that the physicians are making and will continue feeling their current anguish about their wishes being unheeded? In short, as we look at the factors that give the appeal to consequences greater or lesser significance, we find some very difficult empirical questions which must be settled before we can decide whether the consequences of treating Miss J by giving her MOPP are better or worse than the consequences of not treating her Hodgkin's disease.

The best consequences would result from getting the patient and the family to see that their request is unreasonable and that they should not feel anger and frustration at their physicians for not enrolling the patient in a course of MOPP. One hopes that it will be possible to get them to see this, but one cannot be sure that it will be possible. An appeal to consequences would lead to the following conclusion: our first goal must be to try to convince this patient and her family that their request is unreasonable and that the patient is better off not being treated for her Hodgkin's disease. If this effort fails, then we need to settle the above-mentioned empirical questions in order to decide whether and to what extent the appeal to consequences supports treating her with a course of MOPP.

We also need to examine the question of the integrity of the health-care providers. A fundamental value of most health-care providers, embodied in the codes of ethics of their professions, is that their primary obligation is to do no harm to the patient. Providing the requested form of chemotherapy would probably be harming the patient, even if there is some question about the full extent of the harm and about the likelihood of its actual occurrence. The physicians may therefore feel that their own professional integrity calls upon them to refuse to provide the care requested to the patient. To be sure, that decision would result in anger and frustration felt by the patient and her family. But that, it might be argued, represents self-harm (caused by a refusal to heed reasonable advice) rather than physician-caused harm.[24] So, it might be argued, the integrity of these physicians calls upon them to not provide this form of care. One of the factors that gives the appeal to the virtue of integrity its greatest significance in a particular case is the centrality of the belief or value to which the person wishes to show allegiance in a particular decision. The value of not harming a patient is just such a central value to many physicians and other health-care providers, and therefore the appeal to integrity is going to have considerable significance in this case.

No appeal to the right not be killed and/or the right not to be harmed can be relevant here because the patient is clearly waiving that right. Respect for persons might argue against treating Miss J, since the treatment may actually shorten her life, but that argument rests on the difficult empirical questions alluded to above. So it cannot be offered with great confidence.

Suppose we judge that the appeal to integrity tips the balance in favor of not providing chemotherapy. Does that allow the possible compromise, suggested by some members of the team, that the treating physicians offer a referral to other physicians who might be more willing to accede to the patient's request? I think the answer is yes. The personal integrity of the treating physicians calls upon them not to do anything that they judge will harm their patient. This does not allow them to enroll Miss J in a course of MOPP. However, that does not mean that they cannot refer her to other physicians who might see the situation from a different medical perspective or who might have a different sense of values that places less significance on not harming patients and more significance on respecting their wishes and serving as an instrument for the implementation of their wishes.

Some may find my conclusion, despite this final point, very troubling. They feel that the problem is with the values of the physicians who view their primary role as protecting the physical health and well-being of patients, without any concern to their psychosocial well being. Isn't this too narrow a view of the obligation of physicians to their patients? I don't see this objection as persuasive. The value

structure of these physicians is not such that they have no interest in the psychosocial well-being of the patient. Their causing psychosocial harm to their patient
would certainly be unacceptable to them. In their view, however, this is a case in
which the psychosocial harm is patient-induced, and that is the only reason why it is
less central.

CASE NO 11. *"I want to see again before I die"*:
*Accepting appropriate risks*

FACTS    Mrs. K is a 69-year-old woman diagnosed as having adenocarcinoma of the
lungs. Surgery to remove the primary tumor was ruled out because of local lymph-
node involvement. She received radiotherapy both for her lung disease and for more
recent metastases to the brain. She then became blind. probably because of optic
nerve compression as a result of her metastatic disease. Everyone is amazed that she
is still alive, but no one believes that she has much longer to live. She is very
depressed, more by the blindness than by her impending death, and she won't
attempt to learn any skills. All she keeps asking is whether or not she can be
operated on to remove the local compressing masses so that she can see again. Her
husband supports this request. A social worker has spent a fair amount of time
working with them, explaining that the surgeons don't wish to operate in light of her
very short life expectancy and the uncertainty of success of this difficult surgery and
that Mrs. K would do better to learn certain elementary skills so that she can make
the best of the time left to her. She and her husband refuse to accept this idea. She
says that she wants to see again. He says that all he cares about is that she can have
her chance to see, and he is very angry at the surgeons for refusing to operate.

QUESTIONS    This case raises some of the same issues as in the previous case, but
there are important differences. The question of competency once more arises, but
the issue here is depression and not denial. Some people see Mrs. K as being very
depressed by her blindness and impending death and insisting on surgery to correct
her sight as a way to avoid dealing with the thought of dying blind. Others argue
that there is insufficient evidence of depression to challenge the judgment of competency. They insist that those who challenge her competency are doing so simply as a
way of not agreeing to her wishes. Like the case of Miss J, this case raises a second
question. Are the surgeons obliged to follow her request providing that they assess
her as being competent? The debate about the relationship between a patient's
request for treatment and the treating physician's obligation to provide it also arises
in this case. There is only one special twist to the debate here. With Miss J, those
who wished not to provide MOPP argued that the treatment would harm the patient.
In this case, the surgeons who do not wish to operate on Mrs. K have as their
primary argument the very different one that she will be dead shortly anyway,
although they do also appeal to the risks of this tricky surgery. Still another question
has troubled many of the people involved in working with this family. Everyone has
a great deal of pity and compassion for this woman, who is dying blind, and her
loving husband, who wants at least some of her wishes to be fulfilled. What is the
compassionate thing to do for these people? The social worker who has worked

closely with them strongly feels that the compassionate thing is to try to get them to understand her condition and make the best of it. Others disagree, in part because that strategy isn't working. But what other alternatives are open? No one wants to see Mrs. K die with the anger and depression she now feels. But is that a good enough reason for performing the surgery she wishes?

THEORETICAL ANALYSIS   Both Mrs. K and Miss J are requesting a form of care which the physicians are reluctant to provide. This common feature of these two cases must not, however, lead us to miss the important differences between them, differences which support the conclusion that Mrs. K should receive the surgery she requests even though Miss J should not receive the course of chemotherapy she requests.

This case is not going to involve any appeal to the procedural right of the patient and/or her family to be decision makers because this is not a case of a patient and/or her family refusing care and invoking their right to do so. We can also put aside as less important the question of the competency of Mrs. K, which has been challenged on the grounds that she is clinically depressed. The question of competency would be very relevant in assessing the significance of any appeal to her right to refuse care. Since that is not going to be relevant in this case, we have no reason to assess its significance and therefore little reason to look at the question of her competency to be a decision maker.

One of the crucial moral appeals that we need to consider in this case, as in the case of Miss J, is the appeal to consequences. What are the consequences of her being operated on, and what are the consequences of her not being operated on? Not operating avoids, of course, the potential risks of the surgery in question. It has the same sort of beneficial consequences that not providing MOPP to Miss J has: avoiding potential harm to the patient from the therapy requested. What about the advantages of operating on Mrs. K? Obviously, as in the case of Miss J, there is the immediate beneficial consequence of avoiding her frustration and anger at the fact that her physicians will not do what she wants. But we come here to a crucial difference. In the case of Mrs. K, there are further potential beneficial consequences from operating on her. The operation may in fact resolve her blindness by relieving the optic nerve compression. It may enable her to be sighted until her death, and she and her husband have made it clear that this is a consequence they value very greatly. There is nothing analogous to this in the case of Miss J. So our assessment of the appeal to consequences may lead to very different results in the case of Mrs. K than it did in the case of Miss J.

I'm not suggesting that an appeal to consequences definitely argues on behalf of following Mrs. K's request. There are some very difficult but important factual questions that still need to be clarified, the most crucial of which are the probability of the surgery killing her and the probability of the surgery relieving the optic nerve compression. All I want to claim so far is that an examination of this case from the perspective of the appeal to consequences reveals that there may be (providing that certain empirical claims turn out to be correct) much stronger reasons for following the wishes of Mrs. K than there were for following the wishes of Miss J.

What about the appeal to the integrity of the physicians, which was so central to our analysis of the case of Miss J? Can they accede to the wishes of Mrs. K without violating their commitment to not harm their patient? I think the answer is yes. It is precisely at this point that our recognition that their commitment is compatible with a concern with the psychosocial needs of patients (such as the need to see again before they die) becomes crucial. If the commitment not to harm patients is a commitment to never do anything that poses some risk to the life of the patient, then operating on Mrs. K would certainly be a violation of that commitment. But there is no reason to have such a narrow understanding of that commitment, because it would rule out any risky procedure. The commitment must be understood as a commitment to avoid imposing unreasonable risks of harm. There is no reason not to see this case (if the empirical facts support this claim) as one in which one legitimately exposes the patient, at her request, to a risk of physical harm or even death in order to obtain a possible benefit for the patient which the patient desires greatly. The benefit of being able to see again before she dies is one that none of us would want to describe as unimportant or irrational, and it is one which (if the probabilities seem favorable) makes it quite likely that acceding to the wishes of Mrs. K would be compatible with the value commitments of most physicians, including the physicians who are caring for her, even if acceding to the wishes of Miss J would not be.[25] Some physicians may find themselves unable to accede to the wishes of Mrs. K. These are physicians whose understanding of the value of doing no harm to their patient is such that it rules out surgery in this case because of the potential risk to the life of the patient. Such physicians may well resolve their dilemma in this case by referring Mrs. K to a colleague.

In light of all these considerations, it seems to me that the following judgments are appropriate. (1) The very first thing that must be done is to assess as best as possible the actual risks of surgery and the likelihood that it will succeed in restoring sight to this patient. The fact that she is very ill and will undoubtedly die in the not too distant future may be relevant to assessing the risk to her, but it should play no independent role in the decisional process. (2) When that information is assessed, it needs to be combined with an understanding of the priorities of the patient and her husband so that one can determine whether the possible benefits, as judged by the recipients, justify the risk of the surgery. (3) If the judgment is that they do, then there seems to be a powerful argument from the appeal to consequences for following Mrs. K's wishes. (4) The physicians in question need to think carefully about their understanding of their commitment to the primacy of doing no harm to patients and whether that is compatible with participating in the surgery in this case. If, in light of their understanding of the issues raised here, they feel that it is, they should go ahead with the surgery. If it is not, then the referral of Mrs. K and her husband to another physician seems appropriate.

*CASE NO 12. "Stop that bleeding":*
*The difficulty of avoiding prejudices*

FACTS    Mr. L began drinking at an early age and has continued the pattern of heavy drinking since then. Despite this history, he has managed to live to his late forties, to get married and raise a family, and even to do rather well in running his family's catering business. He seems to have been able to carry on despite the heavy amount of alcohol he consumes; on those days when he is too drunk, his family steps in. Mr. L presented in the emergency room vomiting a considerable amount of blood. There is little doubt from his history and his current symptoms that he has alcoholic cirrhosis, portal hypertension, and bleeding esophageal varices. He has so far required twelve units of blood and continues to bleed. The possibility of his undergoing a portal systemic shunt procedure to reduce his portal hypertension and treat his varices was raised with him in the past, but he chose not to have the surgery done. He now wishes his acute crisis to be treated this way. There is considerable doubt about following his request, in part because people think that his prognosis may be quite dim at this point no matter what is done and in part because people have a very negative attitude toward this man in light of the fact that his disease is so clearly self-induced and that he refused needed surgery when it could have been done on an elective basis.

QUESTIONS   The point that most clearly distinguishes Mr. L's case from the last two cases is that Mr. L, with appropriate care, will not inevitably die in the very near future. Admittedly, his chances for long-term survival are very poor, but further medical care (including surgery) gives him a chance for some period of survival. Some people see that as settling the question. They feel that Mr. L's expressed wish to continue to be treated combined with the fact that the treatment offers him some hope of a reasonable period of survival is sufficient to justify treating him. They don't like him, but they don't want to sit in judgment on patients, and they think he should be treated. Others view the surgery as unlikely to make a significant difference. Moreover, they argue, blood products are in short supply and should not be wasted on people with a dim prognosis whose disease is self-induced. It's not a question of judging or punishing Mr. L, they claim; it's a question of carefully husbanding and appropriately using our medical resources. The combination of the dim prognosis and the self-induced nature of his illness makes Mr. L a bad candidate for the expenditure of resources. Still a third group approaches this case in a very different way. They feel that not giving him blood would be equivalent to killing him, and they cannot justify that. But they have no difficulty with not operating on the grounds that it's not killing him; it's just not wasting time on an inappropriate case.

THEORETICAL ANALYSIS   The case of Mr. L is in some ways very straightforward. Without replacing the blood that he is losing and without surgery, his chances of survival even into the very near future are very low. To be sure, even with all of that treatment, his chances of long-term survival are still very low. However, those forms of treatment certainly seem to provide him with a significantly greater chance of short-term survival, a consequence that both he and his family desire. It would seem that a straightforward appeal to consequences would justify a decision that Mr. L should be treated.

That appeal can be reinforced by a number of other appeals. One is an appeal to the right of Mr. L to be aided as he faces this life-threatening situation. In light of the gravity of his loss if he is not aided and in light of the significant probability that he can be helped by the medical treatment, it would seem that this right strongly supports his being treated. Moreover, he strenuously desires this aid, so he has certainly not waived this right. Mr. L has demonstrated his capacity to carry on a wide variety of those activities whose performance we value greatly during the years of his self-induced illness. There is good reason to hope that if the aggressive therapy he requests is successful, he will be able to continue to carry on with them for some period of time. The appeal to a respect for persons seems also to provide a moral basis for treating Mr. L. There are, moreover, at least two virtues which we might appeal to for still further justification for treating Mr. L. One is the virtue of integrity, which calls upon health-care providers to be true to their own value system. Many health-care providers have in their value system a strong commitment to not allowing patients to die when their lives can be saved, particularly when the patient in question very much wants his life to be saved. Standing by and allowing Mr. L to die would therefore be an act out of line with their value system. Consequently, an appeal to the virtue of integrity would argue for aggressively managing the care of Mr. L so as to give him the best chance for as long a life as possible. Moreover, an appeal to the virtue of compassion would seem to indicate that the request of Mr. L and his family for treatment not be denied.

This all represents a powerful case on behalf of aggressively treating Mr. L. Why is there some hesitation on the part of the health-care providers? Some of this hesitation is the result of a different assessment of the medical situation. Some feel that his failure to respond so far makes it likely that his life cannot be saved no matter how aggressive his care. This assessment challenges a presupposition of most of the arguments given above, namely the presupposition that the care in question could be efficacious for Mr. L. This is a legitimate clinical question which certainly needs to be incorporated into any final decision about this case.

However, additional questions have been raised by the staff about the legitimacy of continuing to treat Mr. L. Some of these refer to the self-induced nature of Mr. L's illness. Mr. L is suffering because he has been an alcoholic for many years, has refused to stop drinking despite all of the warnings he has received, and has refused needed surgery when it could have been done on an elective basis. Are these relevant facts? If we review the various moral appeals that justify continuing to treat Mr. L, this fact is certainly relevant to one. The appeal to the right to be aided when facing life-threatening illnesses is weakened to the extent that the threat is caused by one's own faulty behavior. This point, developed in chapter 4, certainly means that Mr. L's appeal to the right to be aided has less strength than it might have in some other cases. It would be wrong, therefore. to dismiss the self-induced nature of his illness as totally irrelevant. It would be equally wrong, however, to give it a greater significance than it deserves. At most, it weakens one of the many arguments that have been offered on behalf of treating Mr. L. The right to be aided still has some significance. When that right is combined with the many other arguments given above, the fact that his illness is self-induced does not seem to make much difference.

There remains the other point raised by some members of the health-care team, the fact that Mr. L has already used twelve units of blood and needs more and the fact that blood products are always in short supply. One thing is clear. If the shortage of blood products were so great that the continued care of Mr. L would mean that other very ill patients would not receive the blood they require, then the whole analysis of the case would need to be modified. To begin with, we would need to examine certain additional consequences of continuing to treat Mr. L, namely, the possible death of those other patients who might have a better chance to survive with the blood being used on Mr. L. An appeal to consequences in that extreme situation might argue against treating Mr. L. The existence of that extreme situation would also have a tremendous impact on what would be mandated by a respect for persons. After all, we might then show our allegiance to respect for persons by not treating Mr. L in order to save those other more salvageable lives. Similar points need to be made about some of the other moral appeals. But there is no evidence offered in this case that the blood supply is in fact that low; at most, we have the suggestion that this is just an expenditure of resources with modest justification and therefore a non-cost-effective form of health care.

This is a case in the private sector, and it was argued in chapter 2 that the appeal to cost-effectiveness has no place in the private sector when the patient is willing to pay for the care in question (even though most of it will be covered by his or her insurance). Moreover, the appeal to justice provides no basis for denying such care unless the care in question would then be withheld from someone else who is more entitled to it. In light of earlier remarks, there is no justification for withholding care from Mr. L on these grounds.

What if he were a public-sector patient? Should we not treat Mr. L's public-sector counterpart? This question cannot be answered with the theoretical resources available at this point. The reason is relatively straightforward. We have not developed in this book any theory about how we should measure the cost-effectiveness of a particular public expenditure for health care. It is not, moreover, intuitively obvious that the expenditure of resources on Mr. L is not cost-effective, since there is nothing intuitively obvious about whether this possible extra period of life is worth the resources required. So we cannot say for sure that treating Mr. L's public-sector counterpart would not be cost-effective and would therefore be unjust. Cases like this, and others to be examined in the next two chapters, show that the need to develop such a theory is very pressing.

Returning then to the case of Mr. L, we can conclude that providing that the aggressive care of Mr. L actually offers some reasonable chance for his surviving for even a modest period of time, there are overwhelming moral arguments on behalf of continuing to treat him as he requests. This means giving him more blood until the bleeding can be controlled and shunting him. In light of the fact that there is no absolute shortage of blood products, no considerations of justice and cost-effectiveness would justify his not being treated. Moreover, the self-induced nature of his disease only weakens one of the many moral appeals arguing for treating him. There are, then, overwhelming reasons for continuing to treat Mr. L until it becomes clear that the skeptics are right and that further treatment is futile. At that point, a new analysis will be required, comparing this case with other futile cases and based on the result of further discussions with the patient and/or the family about the futility of treatment.

*CASE NO 13. "Why aren't you treating my cancer?":*
*The need to stop a mistake*

FACTS    Mr. M is a 76-year-old, mentally alert, retired man who was diagnosed about four months ago with stage D carcinoma of the prostate. Because of the relatively late stage of his disease, he did not receive either surgery or radiation therapy. Instead, he was begun on a course of chemotherapy. The side effects of that treatment were very bad. Nevertheless, Mr. M still wishes further treatment. He says he wants to live to see his eldest granddaughter graduate from college, and she will do so in two and a half years. The trouble is that regardless of his therapy Mr. M will certainly not make it to that time. He hasn't been told this yet. He was originally told that he had advanced cancer of the prostate. His family insisted, however, that he couldn't handle the information about his prognosis, and the physicians who were treating him at that time agreed to the compromise of telling him his diagnosis but not the prognosis. Now Mr. M has metastatic disease in his bones, and he requires increasing doses of methadone to control the bone pain. Mr. M insists that, in addition to this palliative care, he continue to receive chemotherapy to keep him alive. Everyone remembers how hard it was on Mr. M, and the team is not particularly keen to put him through it again. Why should he suffer if his suffering won't get him to his goal?

QUESTIONS    Should Mr. M have been told the truth not merely about his diagnosis but also about his prognosis? Were the physicians who originally treated Mr. M right in respecting the family's claim that he couldn't handle it?[26] These questions are, of course, retrospective, but they have implications for the prospective questions. Some members of the team argue that the time has now come to tell Mr. M the truth. They feel that his chances of making it to his granddaughter's graduation are null, that he should not be put through further chemotherapy by way of pursuing this vain hope, and that he should be told the truth so that he will agree to stop. Others think that trying to give Mr. M the truth at this point would be very cruel and would diminish any trust he might have in his physicians and his family. They feel that we ought to continue further chemotherapy for Mr. M as part of continuing an approach in place, even if we should not have begun that approach. In any case, they argue, further chemotherapy does hold out hope of a modest further extension of his life. While it's true that Mr. M will not make it to his granddaughter's graduation, we can buy him some time, and if he continues to get proper pain control, the good time we can buy him may outweigh the bad time during the chemotherapy.

THEORETICAL ANALYSIS    This case is complicated because we need to consider several options which involve both the question of the medical care Mr. M will receive and the question of the information he will receive. The following options seem open: (1) Mr. M should continue to receive the chemotherapy he requests but not be told that he will not make it until his granddaughter's graduation; (2) Mr. M should be told the true nature of his relatively poor prognosis and should receive chemotherapy only if he continues to request it; (3) Mr. M's chemotherapy should be discontinued because of the harm it will do to him, and his proganosis should be explained to him; or (4) Mr. M's chemotherapy should be discontinued because of the harm it will do to him, but his prognosis should not be explained to him.

Option 1 involves his definitely receiving chemotherapy, and option 2 involves his possibly receiving chemotherapy. His previous chemotherapy indicates that the side effects of treatment are quite devastating, and this argues against options 1 and 2. To be sure, he is, with his current misunderstandings, willing to undergo them in order to obtain a goal of his. None of this means, however, that he does not find them unfortunate. Therefore, from the perspective of his preferences, continuing to treat him with chemotherapy has bad consequences. Moreover, since the continued provision of chemotherapy yields him little that he would judge as valuable (since he seems interested in the prolongation of his life only insofar as it gives him a chance to make it to his granddaughter's graduation), the appeal to consequences seems, at least at first glance, to argue for adopting option 3 or option 4. But there is a major difficulty with this suggestion. Previous physicians judged, with the concurrence of the family, that his knowing the truth (something involved in options 2 and 3) would have disastrous consequences for him. So that would seem to leave option 4. Option 4 comes, however, with its own very undesirable consequences. What will this man feel like when he does not receive the treatment that he wants in order to obtain his goal and does not have the truth explained to him? Will this not lead him to such a sense of frustration and mistrust that it will be worse than the side effects of the chemotherapy?

There is a bad mistake in the analysis up until now. It rests on the presupposition that this patient will not be able to handle the truth. What is the evidence for that? It is just his family's insistence that he couldn't handle the information about his prognosis.[27] It is always possible that they are right, but their mere insistence provides no strong reason for believing that that is so. The disastrous consequences of telling him the truth, consequences that were appealed to in the argument above, cannot have a great significance given that there is no particular reason, other than the family's mere insistence, to suppose that they will actually occur.

All of this seems to lead to the conclusion that the best consequences would seem to come from option 3. Following the option of providing Mr. M no chemotherapy and explaining to him that this is because the chemotherapy will not enable him to obtain his own goals enables us to avoid the bad consequences of continuing chemotherapy and the bad consequences of his not receiving chemotherapy and not understanding why. To be sure, we risk the possibility of his not being able to handle this information. That possibility cannot, however, have a very great significance in this case in light of the fact that we really have little reason to believe that it will occur. It is just a matter of the family's insistence, and that is often more a question of their thinking that they, rather than the patient, will not be able to handle the situation.

One further complication must be considered. It may well have been the case that the best policy to begin with would have been to tell the patient the truth, but that was not done. At this point, as some members of the team have pointed out, the patient may not believe the claim that nothing can be done for him to enable him to obtain his goal. Will telling the truth to the patient at this point lead him to so mistrust his family and his physicians that it is better to not tell him the truth? This is a difficult factual question, but the claim that he will be troubled by this new information is surely more plausible than the family's original claim. Consequently, from the perspective of the appeal to consequences, we are caught between the argument for discontinuing therapy and telling the patient the truth (option 3) with its benefits and its risks and the argument for not telling the patient the truth and continuing the therapy (option 1) with its benefits and its risks. These two options make the most sense as we examine the case from the perspective of the appeal to consequences, and there just isn't enough information to enable us to settle this case from the perspective of that appeal.

There are other moral appeals that need to be considered in this case. First is the appeal to the virtue of honesty, and that certainly argues against option 1 both originally and now. Secondly, there is an appeal to the right of the patient to refuse care. This might seem like a strange right for us to be appealing to, since the patient is demanding care rather than refusing care. But I think we need to look beyond that superficial fact. Mr. M is now demanding care rather than refusing care because he is operating under certain false beliefs about the likely prognosis. Suppose he were to obtain more accurate information. While we cannot be sure, we certainly have reason to suspect that his attitude might change. Mr. M might well insist that he no longer receive the treatment because the side effects have been so devastating to him. In other words, the patient's current consent to being treated is based on deception mutually agreed upon by the physicians and the family. It is not an informed consent of the type that both law and morality seem to demand. What we might appeal to then is not the patient's right to have his refusal respected, since Mr. M hasn't refused care, but rather the patient's right to refuse care once he has the appropriate information. Given the importance of the decision in question, it would seem that that would be a significant moral appeal, one arguing for telling the patient the truth and letting him choose. So these appeals to rights and virtues rule out option 1 and leave us only with option 2 and option 3.

As we put all these considerations together, we are led to the following conclusion: In as kind and compassionate a fashion as possible, this patient needs to have explained to him the information that he probably should have gotten a long time ago: that he will not live long enough to reach his goal of seeing his eldest grand-daughter graduate from college. When that information is clearly presented to the patient, he should then be told that in light of that fact and in light of the horrendous side effects of the chemotherapy, the doctors do not want to continue the chemo-therapy. But what if the patient insists anyway? Should we follow option 2 or 3? This leads back to the issue of patients desiring care which their providers do not wish to provide. A lot will depend on the basis of this insistence on care. This insistence may be based on unrealistic hopes and expectations and would have little force. The physicians should refuse to provide the chemotherapy and should at most offer to refer Mr. M to someone else. But it may also be based on the patient's clarifying in his own mind that he really wants to go on living as long as he can, even if he cannot obtain his goal of seeing his granddaughter graduate, and is willing to put up with the side effects of the chemotherapy. If that is what he says, then an appeal to consequences would in fact justify option 2's insistence on continued treatment. After all, the consequences of the continued treatment, insofar as it prolongs the patient's life, would be beneficial compared to the side effects according to the values of the patient, the very values which need to be considered. Moreover, providing him with continued care in such a case would be supported by an appeal to respect for persons, which argues (with some degree of significance) for prolonging his existence as long as he can still function in the appropriate ways.

In short, there are many fine nuances in this case which make it impossible for us to conclude at this point whether or not this patient should continue to receive chemotherapy. That decision must rest on what Mr. M has to say once the truth has been explained to him. But the crucial moral motif that emerges is the need to provide him with the honest information that will enable him to interact with the team caring for him so that he may receive the morally appropriate forms of medical care.


In this chapter, we have had nine cases of patients who wished not to be treated and whose physicians wished to treat them and only four cases of patients whose physicians wished to stop treatment while the patients requested further treatment. This might suggest that the former type of problem is much more common than the latter and that physicians generally want more aggressive care than patients and their families. I would urge readers not to draw this conclusion. A very different picture shall emerge in Chapter 6, where we consider patients about whom there is no doubt that they are incompetent. Families often want more aggressive care than physicians. That suggestion is moreover supported by clinical data.[28] So be careful about drawing any conclusions from the trend in the cases reported in this chapter.

## Notes

1. All of the changes in this area of the law are carefully documented in A. R. Holder, *Legal Issues in Pediatrics and Adolescent Medicine,* 2nd ed. (New Haven: Yale Univ. Press, 1985), and in J. M. Morrissey, A. D. Hofmann, and J. C. Thrope, *Consent and Confidentiality in the Health Care of Children and Adolescents* (New York: Free Press, 1986).

2. Among these standard discussions are the following: C. M. Culver and B. Gert, *Philosophy in Medicine* (New York: Oxford Univ. Press, 1982), pp. 52–62; L. H. Roth, A. Meisel, and C. W. Lidz, "Tests of Competency to Consent to Treatment," *American Journal of Psychiatry* 134 (1977); President's Commission for the Study of Ethical Problems in Medicine, *Making Health Care Decisions,* vol. I (Washington, D.C.: Government Printing Office, 1982), chap. 8.

3. This explains the development of limited guardianships for the elderly, in which the probate court explicitly delineates the types of decisions taken from the patient and given to the guardian. A good discussion of this trend is found in M. B. Kapp and A. Bigot, *Geriatrics and the Law* (New York: Springer, 1985), pp. 93–102.

4. Virginia Abernethy, in "Compassion, Control, and Decisions about Competency," *American Journal of Psychiatry* 141 (January 1984):53–58, has argued that these two standard points will not, as a matter of practice, be realized together and that we are best off insisting that people are competent, no matter how bizarre a particular decision and a particular process may seem, unless they have demonstrated global incompetency. She is certainly right in claiming that focusing on incompetency to make a particular decision makes

it easy to judge a patient as incompetent because of the content of a particular decision. I believe, however, that that tendency can be resisted and that Abernethy's approach would result in too many thoroughly incompetent decisions being accepted as fully competent.

5. Culver and Gert, *Philosophy in Medicine,* with their distinction between competency to give simple consent and competency to give valid consent, do the best job, but even they fail to bring out the difficult questions surrounding the competency of depressed and anxious individuals. Roth, Meisel, and Lidz, "Tests of Competency," properly emphasize the ability of the patient to understand, but they fail to distinguish the various aspects of that ability.

6. The classic test is the mini-mental-state examination. Its ten questions focus on whether the patient is oriented, registers information, understands simple statements. recalls simple information, and can do simple reasoning processes. Only the part of the test that assesses the ability to count backward in multiples of 7 (100, 93, 86, 79, etc.) goes beyond assessing ability to receive and remember information. An assessment of competency must therefore go beyond the use of the mini-mental. Only when the patient fails that test can it be used alone, and then only to find the patient incompetent. Finding a patient competent requires more than the patient's passing the mini-mental.

7. These terms are often undefined. I am defining them by stipulation for the purpose of this discussion.

8. The nature of such a radical claim and its defense is articulated in H. Cohen, *Equal Rights for Children* (Totowa, N.J.: Littlefield, Adams, 1980).

9. See, for example, S. L. Leikin, "Minors' Assent or Dissent to Medical Treatment," in President's Commission, *Making Health Care Decisions,* vol. III.

10. I say "more plausibly" in light of arguments in chapter 4 that competency should not be treated as an all-or-nothing matter.

11. This rule and the emancipated-minor rule mentioned below are discussed in Holder, *Legal Issues,* and in Morrissey, Hofmann, and Thrope, *Consent and Confidentiality.*

12. Abortion, contraception, and substance abuse have been the issues most discussed recently. I am also very interested in the question of who should make the decision to withhold further life-saving treatment. The 1985 Texas Natural Death Act, after allowing parents to execute a living will for their dying children, adds in section 4d(b): "The desire of a qualified patient who is under 15 years of age and who is competent shall at all times supersede the effect of a directive executed in accordance with this section." Is this an appropriate policy? What should be done if it is the child who wishes care to be withheld while the parents want further care? We will return to these questions in chapter 7.

13. The best data available are in S. Neu and C. M. Kjellstrand, "Stopping Long-Term Dialysis," *NEJM* 314, no. 1 (January 2, 1986):14–20. Voluntary dropouts reflecting a desire to die were particularly prevalent in the younger groups.

14. That is why judges, in the many cases involving withdrawing health care, have argued as I do below that withdrawing the care would not be killing the patient. See, for example, both the majority and dissenting opinions in *Patricia E. Brophy* v. *New England Sinai Hospital,* a decision of the Supreme Judicial Council of Massachusetts on September 11, 1986. On the more general background in the common law, see R. M. Perkins, *Criminal Law,* 2nd ed. (Mineola, N.Y.: Foundation Press, 1969). This common-law attitude applies not only to killing but also to lesser offenses such as maiming. This is illustrated by *The Case of the Lusty Rogue Wright* reported in *Coke on Littleton* 127a (1604).

15. Those who lack this intuition about causality will draw a very different conclusion about this case.

16. These are both legitimate motives for people volunteering to be subjects of a research protocol. I therefore don't understand why some clinicians won't allow patients—particularly adolescents and teenagers—to volunteer for altruistic reasons. On this question, see R.

Nitschke et al., "Therapeutic Choices Made by Patients with End-Stage Cancer," *Journal of Pediatrics* 101, no. 3 (September 1982):471–76. esp. 475.

17. A very difficult question, faced by both physicians and family members, is how to handle requests for active euthanasia, especially when the request seems reasonable, in light of this current illegality. Two moving accounts are D. Humphry, *Jean's Way* (Los Angeles: Hemlock Society, 1984), and B. Rollin, *Last Wish* (New York: Simon and Schuster, 1985). Neither author adequately deals with the issue of how much a law, even an unjust one, has a moral claim on us for obedience, a question that goes back to Plato's portrayal of Socrates' discussion of that issue in the *Crito*.

18. A brief introduction to the medical problems in a careful use of morphine is found in J. Lynn, "Supportive Care for Dying Patients: An Introduction for Health Care Professionals," printed as Appendix B to President's Commission for the Study of Ethical Problems in Medicine, *Deciding to Forego Life-Sustaining Treatment* (Washington, D.C.: Government Printing Office, 1983). The licitness of using morphine in this way is defended in "Declaration on Euthanasia," a statement of the Sacred Congregation for the Doctrine of the Faith dated May 5, 1980; and on p. 103 of D. Feldman and F. Rosner, *Compendium on Medical Ethics*, 6th ed. (New York: Federation of Jewish Philanthropies, 1984). The Catholic defense and (apparently) this Jewish defense rely on the use of the principle of double effect. For a critique of that principle, see A. Donagan, *The Theory of Morality* (Chicago: Univ. of Chicago Press, 1977), sec. 5.3. An alternative defense, resting on a risk-benefit analysis, is found in a recent ruling by R. Eliezer Waldenberg, printed in *Responsa Tzitz Eliezer*, vol. 13, no. 87.

19. A very difficult question for the physicians will be what to do if Mr. E and his family ask them to make the decision. The decision is supposed to be made in light of what leads to the best consequences for Mr. E, as he evaluates the consequences. That may be a realistic task if the physicians know him; it will be impossible if they do not.

20. Such a line of argument, used precisely for disabled institutionalized patients, is put forward in J. D. Hoyt and J. M. Davies, "A Response to the Task Force on Supportive Care" *Law, Medicine and Health Care* (June 1984):103–5. While they would seem to allow competent patients such as Mrs. G to refuse care, they provide extremely strict standards for when the patient is not terminally ill, and it is not clear whether Mrs. G could meet them, particularly their standard (g), which requires that environmental factors which might have influenced the patient have been considered and dealt with. I disagree with the stringency of their approach, but I think it is understandable as an attempt to avoid the type of prejudice we are discussing.

21. This point is a significant theme running through Kapp and Bigot, *Geriatrics and the Law*.

22. It is this line of thought which presumably explains why natural-death acts are typically confined to terminally ill patients.

23. The two classical conflicting court cases not complicated by considerations of other issues, such as the existence of dependent children, are *J.F.K. Memorial Hospital* v. *Heston* 279 A.2d 670 (1971), which authorized a transfusion, and In re *Estate of Brooks* 205 N.E. 2d 435 (1965), in which an order for a transfusion was expunged. The New Jersey court in the *Heston* case emphasized both the state's interest in life (appeal to respect for persons) and the hospital's rights to act in accordance with its values (appeal to integrity). The *Brooks* court appealed to the patient's right to refuse care. Unfortunately, neither court used the relevant appeal to consequences.

24. It is important to note how the appeal to causality plays a role here. This parallels the point quoted in note 24 of chapter 2 from Eric Mack about the role of the appeal to causality in defining violations of rights. Note also that the value of not being the cause of harm can be

central to the value of a physician, even if that physician agrees that causing harm is no different from failing to cause good from the perspective of the appeal to consequences. So nothing said here contradicts the challenge to the beneficence-nonmaleficence distinction in chapter 2, where that distinction was only being discussed in connection with the appeal to consequences.

25. This type of risk-benefit analysis is appealed to by R. Eliezer Waldenberg, *Responsa Tzitz Eliezer,* to justify providing the clinically required amount of morphine to dying patients suffering from gasping for breath even though doing so poses risks to their lives.

26. There is, in fact, another question about the original decision which needs to be raised, even though it will not be discussed here. The original discussions with the family clearly did not involve the patient, and the patient was not aware of them. So information went to the family without patient consent. Isn't that a breach of confidentiality? A. Jonsen, M. Siegler, and W. J. Winslade's *Clinical Ethics* (New York: Macmillan, 1982), sec. 4.3, is one of the few instances in the literature in which the issue of confidentiality vis-à-vis the family is raised.

27. D. Novack et al., "Changes in Physicians' Attitudes toward Telling the Cancer Patient," *JAMA* 241, no. 9 (March 2, 1979), present data that show that physicians are less worried than they were in the past about the ability of patients to handle bad information. That is compatible with families still saying that they are worried.

28. Some of those data are presented in A. L. Evans and B. A. Brody, "The Do-Not-Resuscitate Order in Teaching Hospitals," *JAMA* 253, no. 15 (April 19, 1985):2236–39. Other data supporting that conclusion are forthcoming from other studies already completed at Baylor.

# 6

## Cases Involving Incompetent Adults

This chapter presents another set of patients, like those in chapter 5, whose management raises significant ethical questions. All of these patients, however, unlike those discussed earlier, are clearly incapable of participating in any decisional processes. Consequently, any decisions to be made cannot involve them.

It seems reasonable that the patient's family should play a significant role in decisional processes in such cases. This chapter is therefore organized around the family's wishes. First, we will examine cases in which the patients have no family available to participate in decision making. Then we will examine patients who have family members available and who respond in different ways.

In many of these cases, there is either evidence about what the patient would have wanted done or evidence of attempts made by the patient at earlier times to have an input into these later decisional processes. An important question is the validity and significance of such evidence.

### 6.1  Incompetent Patients without Families

*CASE NO 14. "Where is her family?":*
*Proper procedures for sad cases*

FACTS  Mrs. N is a 76-year-old woman who was diagnosed eighteen months ago as having lung cancer. She has gone downhill since then and now has demonstrated metastatic disease in her liver and probably in her brain. Though she was initially treated with chemotherapy, this was discontinued on the grounds that it was having no significant impact on the patient's course. Over the last few days, she has become progressively weaker and now is noted to be hypotensive. Everyone suspects that the patient's death is imminent. A decision needs to be made about whether she should be resuscitated when she arrests. This cannot be discussed with her. For the most part, she sleeps through the day. When she is awake, she is only dimly aware of her surroundings, and it is nearly impossible to have any prolonged conversation with her, much less a conversation on such a serious topic. Her family consists of a brother and a sister, but the social worker ascertained last year that they had moved away years ago and that the patient has had no significant contact with them since then. The physicians managing the patient would like to enter a "do not resuscitate" order in the patient's chart, thereby allowing the patient to die when her heart stops beating; they believe it would be futile to resuscitate her in light of her terminal illness. Their regular practice is to obtain the permission of either the patient or the family (when the patient is no longer competent) for entering such an order. They are not sure what they should do in this case.

QUESTIONS    There are some who challenge both the decision to discontinue chemotherapy and the decision that it would be inappropriate to resuscitate the patient when she arrests. They base their challenge on one of two beliefs. A few believe in continuing to keep a patient alive just as long as they can, no matter how dim the prognosis. Most, while prepared to stop treatment when it seems futile, are willing to do so only when the patient and/or her immediate family concurs. Lacking any concurrence in this case, they cannot see how discontinuing treatment is appropriate. A suggestion has been made that the team either continue to search for the family to obtain their concurrence or seek the appointment of a legal guardian to protect the interests of the patient, a guardian whose concurrence would be obtained before the DNR order would be written. Many members of the team disagree. They don't see the point either of further chemotherapy or of resuscitative efforts, since the patient is clearly going to die shortly anyway. They see this as a medical judgment which requires no concurrence from either the family or a court-appointed guardian. There is still another viewpoint present. It accepts the legitimacy of consulting the family when the family is readily available and when the family has been close to the patient, but it challenges the idea of expending efforts in a case like this either to find a family who has had little to do with the patient for so many years or to appoint a guardian who does not know the patient. What, they ask, could the family or a court-appointed guardian contribute? So the case of Mrs. N raises questions about whether medical treatment can be discontinued on the basis of a simple medical judgment about the futility of further treatment, about the role of the patient's family in such decisions in general, about the role of the patient's family when they have been alienated from the patient for a long period of time, and about the role of guardians who don't know the patient.

THEORETICAL ANALYSIS    The major issue here is the question of the resuscitation of Mrs. N when her heart stops beating. One way to approach this case would be to appeal to the consequences of the options open to us. Resuscitating her would prolong her life for a modest period of time at a level of consciousness no better than her current level, where she sleeps through most of the day and is only dimly aware of her surroundings during the period in which she is awake. There is a widespread feeling that doing this would produce little benefit for this patient. But it is difficult to be sure that this is so in light of our commitment to assess benefits by appealing to the preferences of the patient. We do not know her preferences. How can we be sure whether or not she would see this slightly prolonged existence as being of no benefit? Perhaps she is one of those people who view mere existence even for a brief period of time as a major gain? In short, the appeal to consequences sheds little light on the decision to be made, because we have no way of evaluating the consequences from Mrs. N's perspective.

This is one reason why we would certainly prefer to have information from the family about how the patient would view this modest prolonged existence, modest both in quantity and quality. Unfortunately, in light of the family's social history, there is little hope (even if we could find the brother and sister) of getting that information from them.

This point will be of significance in many other cases, so I would like to rephrase it in a more abstract fashion. Some members of the treating team think that since the patient will be dead shortly no matter what we do, it is futile to attempt to resuscitate her. Their claim is exaggerated. The truth of the matter is that resuscitative efforts would make some difference to the probability of keeping the patient alive for a modest period of time in a very low state of conscious existence. Those who claim that this is futile can at most mean that this is of little value. But this would be evaluating the consequences in light of the team's values rather than the values of the patient, and that is not the principle of evaluation that we have adopted. The principle we have adopted is that the appeal to consequences must always evaluate consequences in light of the values of the person affected. Given that principle, we should always be suspicious of claims that medical futility settles a case *unless* the proponents of that claim literally mean that the proposed treatment has *no* chance of making *any* difference to even the short-term outcome for the patient.

A second approach would be an appeal to the right of family members to be decision makers. It is this right that lies behind the policy in this unit of obtaining the concurrence of the family of incompetent patients before DNR orders are written.[1] However, in this sad case, we cannot appeal to this decisional right to provide us with a basis for principled decision making, since there are no family members present to exercise that right. Moreover, there seems to be little point to seeking out such family members. After all, when we discussed the rights of family members to be decision makers for incompetent patients, we saw that there were really two roles they might play. They might merely act as witnesses to what the patient would have wished. In that role, it is really the patient's earlier wishes that are the basis of the decision, and the family's role is just to testify to them. In this case, even if we could find the brother and sister, there is little reason to hope that they could give relevant testimony, in light of their long-term alienation from this patient. We also identified a right of family members to be independent decision makers, rooted in the patient's wishes that those family members should make decisions for the patient. Again, in light of the long-term alienation between this patient and her family, there is little reason to see the family as having the delegation of authority from the patient. In approaching this case from the perspective of procedural rights, therefore, there is little place for a role for these long-alienated family members.

A third approach to this case—an appeal to respect for persons—is also unlikely to provide much guidance. Mrs. N is already incapable of performing most of those activities whose performance we value so greatly. If she is resuscitated postarrest, her condition will not be better, and she will still not be able to perform any of these activities. An appeal to respect for persons provides us, then, with little reason for resuscitating her. Still another approach is an appeal to the substantive rights of the patient not to be killed or harmed. These rights do not, however, generate any moral obligations to treat this patient. This is our familiar point that a failure to resuscitate her would simply be allowing her to die rather than killing her or in any way harming her. The right to be aided in life-threatening situations is also not going to be of great help here. It is not, of course, that the patient has waived this right. Rather, we have no idea whether resuscitating her would be, from the patient's perspective, aiding her, since we have no way of knowing whether the patient would view continued existence after resuscitation as a gain.

It is clear that our major problem is that we lack any relevant information about the patient's wishes and/or values. Therefore, most of the usual appeals are irrelevant. We may be required to decide in light of the implications of the decision for those affected other than the patient. The major group affected are the health-care providers, who would find it extremely frustrating to resuscitate and to continue extensive care for a patient whose death is in any case reasonably imminent and whose mental status until death is so minimal. In the absence of any other basis for making a decision, we should probably decide on the basis of this consideration against resuscitation, a consideration which is reinforced by an appeal to their virtue of integrity which challenges using their talents in ways they see as pointless.

There are, however, two morals to be drawn from this analysis. The first is the need for physicians and other health-care providers to talk to terminally ill patients when they are still competent in order to determine their wishes about their dying process, especially when there will be no family members around to be of help in the decision-making process. This whole analysis would have been very different if anyone had taken the trouble to speak to Mrs. N before her most recent decline. It was surely known beforehand that she was dying, and it would have helped immensely if the right questions had been asked. Secondly, if we make the decision not to resuscitate her on the basis of an appeal to the consequences to others—the decision makers—rather than an appeal to her interests and rights, there is a special need to see that some disinterested outsider is appointed as a guardian who will consider only the patient's interests during the decisional process. That person might find some reasons for changing the conclusions we have reached.[2] It is important to remember that the argument for not resuscitating her is only a modestly significant appeal to the consequences for others and to their virtue of integrity.

The case of Mrs. N illustrates the types of difficulties encountered when we fail to look ahead to the decisions we will need to make with some terminally ill patients. Given, however, that nobody did look ahead, it seems best to resolve the case by providing her with procedural safeguards to represent her interests and by attending to such information as we do have.

*CASE NO 15. "What are you saving him for, anyway?":*
*The use of friends rather than family*

FACTS   Mr. O is a 78-year-old man who has lived on his own for many years. He has always been very popular in his neighborhood, and his neighbors have always looked out for him. They say that he never talked about his family, and they don't know whether he has any family. About two weeks ago, one of the neighbors found him on the floor unconscious. He soon regained consciousness but remained lethargic, uncommunicative, and incontinent. After two days, the neighbor brought Mr. O to the hospital emergency room. A CAT scan showed a cerebral infarct. Moreover, during his admission workup, his chest X-ray showed a large, dense mass in the left upper lobe of his lung. A biopsy confirmed cancer of the lung. Now, by the beginning of the second week of his hospitalization, there is no evidence of any improvement in his mental status. Moreover, he has become febrile. The staff is wondering whether they should do a workup of his fever to properly treat it and whether they should make any effort to treat the cancer in his lungs. They know he can live for a while, but it seems clear that he will die in time from his cancer and will be living until then in a deteriorated mental state. Social services can't find any evidence of a family to consult.

QUESTIONS   This case, while obviously raising many of the very same issues raised by the previous one, is different in important ways and is therefore more complex. Extensive medical care could keep Mr. O alive for a longer period of time than Mrs. N. His current fever and the infection which is producing it could certainly be treated. He could receive therapy which would probably slow the progress of the cancer in his lungs, and there is no evidence so far of metastatic disease. He will die from his cancer eventually, but unlike the case of Mrs. N, the death of Mr. O is by no means imminent. Those who are thinking of withholding care at this point are not making a medical judgment about imminent death. They are taking into account the quality of life that Mr. O, who has suffered a serious cerebral infarct and has no family to care for him, will have in the time that he has left. Moreover, the treatment they are considering withholding—a sepsis workup and appropriate antibiotics—seems much less "heroic" than cardiopulmonary resuscitation, which is what is at stake in the case of Mrs. N. All of this leads to many questions. First of all, is it ever appropriate to withhold care on the basis of quality-of-life considerations as opposed to considerations of imminent death? Even if it is, shouldn't that require the concurrence of the patient, or at least the concurrence of the family? Can physicians ever be justified in withholding care on the basis of quality-of-life considerations without the concurrence of someone who speaks for the patient? Can an exception be made in a case like this because of the lack of family? Could any of Mr. O's neighborhood friends be used as alternative participants in the decisional process? If so, whom should be used? Then there is the question of infection and antibiotics. Should we distinguish between major medical interventions such as cardiopulmonary resuscitation or chemotherapy, which we may withhold, and more ordinary medical interventions such as sepsis workups and antibiotics, which we must always provide? Even if, on quality-of-life grounds, we are prepared in cases like this to withhold aggressive heroic care without any family or patient concurrence, can we withhold such ordinary care as the provision of antibiotics?

THEORETICAL ANALYSIS    The case of Mr. O represents an excellent contrast to the case of Mrs. N. They both involve patients with a terminal illness whose current mental status is very compromised, who have no immediate family members present to participate in decision making, and for whom significant choices must be made. These important similarities must not blind us, however, to the important differences, which will lead to some very significant modifications in our conclusions. Among the major differences are the following, (1) Mr. O has a large number of friends who live in his neighborhood and have helped care for him in recent years. He is not alone in the way Mrs. N is. (2) While it is likely that Mr. O will eventually die from lung cancer, this death is in no way as imminent as the death of Mrs. N. (3) While there is little hope for improvement in the mental functioning of Mrs. N, one cannot rule out the possibility of a real improvement in the quality of Mr. O's mental functioning, even if he never returns to his baseline abilities.

The question confronting the team treating Mr. O is whether or not they should work up and treat his current infection and then attempt to treat the cancer in his lungs. Let us look at that question from the perspective of the appeal to consequences. Items 2 and 3 above immediately suggest that any evaluation of this case from the perspective of the appeal to consequences must recognize that the proposed treatment is more likely to be of real value to him. After all, the proposed treatment for Mr. O holds out the hope of buying him some period of time involving a modest but real quality of life. Nothing like this was present as a possible consequence in the case of Mrs. N. Are these possible outcomes desirable from the point of view of Mr. O? And are they worth the possible bad consequences, particularly from the chemotherapy? We don't know, and he currently is in no position to tell us. Still, we have more reason to suspect that the consequences are worth it in this case than we did in the case of Mrs. N, where the treatment to be decided on—resuscitation—could at best buy her a short period of time with no restoration of mental functioning. Several suggestions immediately come to mind. One, which will be discussed below, is that we treat the current infection in the hope that Mr. O improves sufficiently so that he can give us some indication of whether treatment of the cancer, with its side effects, is worth it to him. To be sure, we risk finding out that he also doesn't think that the treatment of the infection was worth it, but that treatment brings with it fewer of the unfavorable side effects, so it is more likely to be acceptable to him retroactively.[3] A second suggestion, which will be explored first, is that we try to talk to some of those neighbors who are particularly close to Mr. O and see whether they are in a position to give us some indication of how he would evaluate the burdens of the antibiotic therapy and the chemotherapy against the potential benefits. If they can provide us with that information, it might serve as the basis for an appropriate evaluation of the consequences.

We turn now to the implications of the right to be a decision maker for this case, implications that also argue for consulting Mr. O's friends. At this point, given the patient's incompetency, he is in no position to exercise any such right. Can anyone else? There is no family present to exercise that right. But might not the neighbors be able to do so, particularly those who are closest to Mr. O? I think the answer is yes. To begin with, they may be able to provide evidence of what Mr. O would have wished in this case. He may have discussed this matter with some of his close neighbors in the past. That they are not family is irrelevant. As long as we assess them as reliable, their testimony about what Mr. O would have wished is as good as that of any family member. Secondly, at least some of them may be entitled to play the role of surrogate decision makers for Mr. O. If, for example, there are one or two neighbors on whom he has always relied and who have often played the role of substitute family member for him, then there is much to be said for their having the right to participate in this decisional process as a surrogate decision makers. After all, the right of family members to make decisions for no longer competent adult patients is based on our belief that allowing them to do so represents the wishes of the patient. In this case, these close friends may be equally entitled to play that role.

Mr. O is currently incapable of performing most of those activities whose performance we value so much. But there is a real chance that he will be able to resume at least some of that functioning. That provides a basis for saying, from the perspective of respect for persons, that efforts should be made to pull Mr. O through this current crisis.

Where does this leave us? An attempt should be made to find out from the neighbors visiting the hospital who is closest to Mr. O. That person should be approached to see if he or she is in a position to tell us either what Mr. O would have wished in this case or how Mr. O might have evaluated the potential outcomes of his continued treatment. (Note that these are two different bits of information, one designed to provide testimony about how Mr. O would have decided and the other designed to provide testimony about how Mr. O would evaluate the consequences.) Alternatively, if the person closest to Mr. O is not in a position to provide that information, we need to see whether or not Mr. O has called on him or her to act in a familylike role in the past, thereby justifying the claim that he or she should be empowered to make decisions on behalf of Mr. O. Should any of this succeed, we will be in a position to use the information provided by and/or the wishes expressed by this individual to help deal with the question of what to do in this case by appealing either to consequences or to procedural rights. Naturally, it would be desirable to formalize the use of such a friend by having him or her appointed as legal guardian.[4]

What if none of this works? What if the neighbors are unwilling or unable to play these roles? What if they say they have always taken care of Mr. O, but they really have no idea how he would feel about these matters and don't feel entitled to make a decision for him? There is a reasonable fallback strategy, one already alluded to above. That is to treat the current infection in the hope of pulling Mr. O through his immediate crisis and allowing his mental functioning to improve. Mr. O would then be able to provide relevant information about how he evaluates the consequences of the treatment of his cancer and whether he wishes to be treated, and that information may help us determine an appropriate decision. The argument for the fallback strategy is that it may provide information that will give us a principled basis for making later decisions in this case and is in any case a reasonable way of dealing with the current uncertainty. Moreover, it draws some modest support from an

appeal to the respect for persons that argues for efforts to improve Mr. O's condition. Note, however, that our arguments for it make no reference to the "unheroic"
nature of antibiotics, since it is very dubious that that makes any difference to any of
our moral appeals.

What happens if this strategy fails? What happens if Mr. O recovers from his
current infection but does not recover sufficient mental functioning to play any role
in further decisional processes? At that point, the case will closely resemble the case
of Mrs. N. We will have no appeal arguing for continuing treatment, and the modest
arguments about detrimental consequences for others and concerns for their integrity (made even more modest by the fact that Mr. O's death is not imminent)
arguing against further treatment of his cancer and for nonaggressive treatment of
further medical complications as they develop. But it will be a weak argument, so it
is to be hoped that we will not get to that point.

### CASE NO 16. "He made me his guardian": The proper role of a guardian's decisions

FACTS   Mr. P is a 72-year-old man with a history of chronic diabetes. Two years
ago, shortly before leaving the hospital after being treated for complications of his
diabetes, he asked an old friend to seek appointment as his legal guardian if he ever
became incompetent.[5] At the time, he told his friend that he was very concerned
about what would happen to him and his possessions if he had a lengthy illness,
since he had no family to take care of things. Three weeks ago, Mr. P presented to
the hospital with a ruptured appendix and underwent surgery. Postoperatively, there
was a deterioration in his renal function, and he began to have difficulty breathing.
The etiology of those problems was unclear. Eventually, he required both respirator
support and dialysis. As a result of all of these problems, his neurological status
deteriorated. When these postoperative problems developed, his friend applied to
the probate court and was appointed Mr. P's guardian. The physicians consulted the
guardian, and the guardian said that he wanted everything done for his friend. He
said that he hoped his friend would recover and that he did not see why anyone
should stop, especially in light of the fact that the exact cause of Mr. P's problems
was unclear. As a result, the patient remained in the ICU on dialysis and on a
respirator. In the last few days, the patient's status has deteriorated even further,
and he is now comatose with a marked deterioration in his EEG. The staff thinks the
time has come to step back, withdraw some of these intensive measures, and allow
this patient to die. The guardian is still hoping for a miracle. He also says that he
would want everything to be done until he was dead, and that's what he wants for
his friend.

QUESTIONS   Mr. P's case introduces a new element: the legal guardian. Many
members of the staff take the attitude that in light of the fact that Mr. P asked that
his close friend be appointed as his legal guardian and in light of the fact that he was
appointed, that friend speaks on behalf of Mr. P, and his wishes must be respected.
Others challenge continuing to treat Mr. P just because his guardian insists. Some
think of this guardian as appointed primarily to handle financial matters and wonder

whether Mr. P intended him to make this type of decision. Some question the relevance of the guardian's decision in light of the reasons he gives. It would be one thing, they say, if he were to claim that he knows Mr. P would want continued treatment. But the guardian says that he wants Mr. P to receive further treatment because that is what he would want for himself. They wonder whether that's an appropriate reason and whether a request based on that reasoning needs to be honored. There are still other issues lurking in the minds of many members of the staff which might make the wishes of the guardian irrelevant. In the case of Mr. P, it is being suggested that dialysis and/or respirator support be withdrawn. This would not be a decision to withhold initiating certain forms of treatment but rather a decision to withdraw certain forms of treatment that are already being provided. Some take this distinction very seriously and feel that the case should be settled simply on the basis of the fact that withdrawing what has already been provided to Mr. P would be killing him. Still another viewpoint is expressed by other members of the team who feel that further treatment is futile and argue that neither a guardian nor a family member can force health-care providers to continue to provide futile health care.

THEORETICAL ANALYSIS    Mr. P, like Mr. O and Mrs. N, is a patient currently incapable of participating in any decision making at a time when extremely important choices must be made. But this case is very different from the two previous cases, in part because there is a court-appointed guardian, chosen in advance by the patient, who very much wants to be involved in decision making, and in part because it is difficult to firmly describe this patient as terminally ill, because the exact etiology of his problems is unclear.

This is the only one of the three cases which involves a proposal to withdraw care already being provided to the patient. Some members of the team find this distinction crucial. Their argument is that the withdrawal of care constitutes killing the patient, killing the patient is always wrong, and therefore the patient must continue to be supported in all the ways in which he is already being supported. However, this view is in error. We need to go back again to the distinction between killing a patient and simply allowing a patient to die, a distinction which certainly has great moral significance. This, as we have already pointed out many times, has to do with the cause of the patient's death. To kill a patient is to cause the patient's death; to allow the patient to die is to not prevent the underlying disease process from causing the death of the patient. In this case, withdrawing support would result in the patient's dying from his underlying disease process. In this respect, the case of Mr. P is like the cases of Mr. E and Mr. F, where care was also withdrawn. So it cannot be settled merely by recognizing that what is at stake is the withdrawal of care already being provided.

One seemingly powerful argument for continuing to treat this patient is an appeal to the right of the guardian to participate in decision making. The guardian is firmly insisting on further care and has done so ever since the patient took a turn for the worse. Moreover, this insistence seems to represent some fundamental value of the guardian. All of these constitute reasons for giving that right considerable significance in this case. To be sure, it is not a family member who is insisting but a friend who has been appointed by the court as a guardian. But that makes no difference. As we saw in chapter 2, the basis of the right of family members to participate in decision making for no longer competent adult patients is the presupposition that they are the ones the patients would want to make decisions for them. In this case, the guardian stands in the same position. This man is Mr. P's guardian because the patient specifically said that he wanted him to be his guardian and make decisions for him. If anything, his right to participate in decision making is even stronger than the right of family members when we are just presuming that patients would want them to participate in decision making.

There is, however, a major reason for hesitating about this argument from the guardian's right to participate in decision making. This is a case of a guardian insisting on care rather than refusing care. As we pointed out in chapter 2 and also in the discussions in section 5.3, the right to have a refusal of care respected is a real right in a way in which the right to have a demand for care respected is not. Physicians are not obliged to provide care just because a guardian (or even a patient) is demanding it. That point is certainly legitimate, but its significance should not be overestimated. To begin with, this is not a case of someone demanding care which is harmful to the patient, such as case 10, where the physicians might well insist as an act of integrity that they would refuse to provide that form of care. At most, this is a case of providing probably futile care, and physicians providing that care would probably not be violating their sense of integrity by acceding to the wishes of the guardian. So there is no integrity argument against providing the care, even if there is no rights-based argument for providing the care. Moreover, the guardian would retain the right to transfer care to another physician who would be willing to continue to treat the patient aggressively.

Are there any other moral appeals that would lead us to decide for or against the wishes of the guardian? One obvious consideration is the claim by many members of the team that further aggressive care for this patient is futile. Perhaps we can best understand that argument as being an appeal to the consequences of the continued care for the patient. The claim of futility is the claim that this continued care would provide no benefit for the patient. But is that an accurate assessment of the consequences? Without this continued care, the patient will almost certainly die. With the care, the patient has at least some chance of reversal of this multisystem failure from which he is suffering. It is important to remember that we don't really know the etiology of the patient's problem; that makes it very difficult to firmly insist that the patient has no chance of recovering (even though we can agree that the steady downward course certainly is very worrisome). So perhaps an appeal to conseqqences justifies the continued treatment of the patient. Here may lie the real role of the guardian. As someone close to the patient, someone the patient has chosen to speak for him, he may be testifying that the patient would judge this chance to be worth undergoing all this invasive care. He hasn't put his reasons for his insistence that way, since he talks about what he would want for himself, but it is a reasonable interpretation of what he is saying. We need to remember that the patient chose him as his guardian, presumably because the patient judged that their values were sufficiently similar.

Another aspect of the appeal to consequences needs to be taken into account here.

Those who propose withholding further care against the wishes of the guardian are in effect suggesting an approach to decision making in these cases which might have profound consequences of a negative nature. After all, what is being proposed here is the withdrawal of care from a patient against the wishes of someone the patient has specifically appointed to represent his wishes. Such a policy might well mean a tremendous frustration on the part of the guardian and an uncertainty in the public mind about the extent to which the wishes of those who speak for them will be respected. So there are some real long-range consequences as well.

Two other appeals offer modest arguments for continuing to treat the patient. One is an appeal to respect for persons. The other is an appeal to the patient's nonwaived right to aid against life-threatening illnesses. These arguments are real, but they can offer at best modest support in light of the fact that the probability of success in treating this patient is low.

Mr. O is a patient in the private sector. Moreover, the bed he is occupying in the ICU is not immediately needed by some other patient. Consequently, appeals to cost-effectiveness and justice do not play a role here. We will see other cases in which such appeals are appropriately introduced as arguments against further care.

In short, then, in this case, an appeal to the consequences for the patient, as assessed by the guardian, argues on behalf of continued dialysis and respirator support for Mr. P. This is supported by appeals to consequences for others and by modest appeals to respect for persons and to the right to aid. No other moral appeal seems to present a powerful opposing argument. Any health-care provider whose sense of integrity is offended by his or her perception of the futility of this effort is, of course, free to withdraw from the care of this patient once someone is found to take his or her place. But this case is not like those in which the continued care of the patient is a clear-cut harm to the patient, so this point would probably affect few providers. On the whole, then, it seems that Mr. P should continue to receive the treatment his guardian insists on in the hope that it will reverse his downward course.

## 6.2 Incompetent Patients Whose Families Demand Further Treatment

*CASE NO 17. "How much blood is too much blood?":*
*Counting all the benefits and costs*

FACTS    Mr. Q is a 52-year-old man whose medical history is notable for the fact that he has been a steady drinker (two six-packs a day) since the age of 16, with a 90 pack/year smoking history (three packs a day for the last thirty years). Four weeks before presenting to the hospital, he developed jaundice. He was admitted with an elevated bilirubin of 6 mg/dl, bilateral pneumonia with a white cell count of 25,000mm$^3$, and a hematocrit of 31% with a history suggesting gastrointestinal bleeding. At admission, his mental status was quite obtunded, and he was having some difficulty breathing. A few days after admission, Mr. Q developed massive GI bleeding which required extensive use of blood. His pneumonia did not respond to

antibiotic therapy. Because of progressive respiratory distress, the patient was intubated. As his hospitalization progressed, his mental and respiratory status continued
to deteriorate, and he continued to require extensive amounts of blood to deal with
his GI bleeding. The physicians caring for him became convinced that his condition
was irreversible and that he would die from this constellation of problems ultimately
a result of his liver disease. They are concerned about continuing to provide further
treatment for him in light of his dismal prognosis and the fact that he is making
tremendous demands on a limited blood supply. His family—a wife and two grown
children—is totally unresponsive to any suggestion to limit care. They insist that he
get all the blood he needs. They also insist that he continue to receive respiratory
support and antibiotics for his infections. Their attitude is that he has nothing to lose
and everything to gain from continued aggressive care, and they will not consent to
anything less than maximum efforts to save Mr. Q.

QUESTIONS    Some of the questions here are similar to those about futility raised by
cases 14, 15, and 16. But there are a number of special issues. The first is the
question that will dominate this section of the book. To what extent are physicians
required to continue treating incompetent patients, when they believe that such
treatment is futile, because the family who speaks for the patient insists on continued aggressive treatment? Is the question of futility a purely medical question
which should be settled by physicians? Does it involve other elements? Is family
concurrence required before care can be withheld just because it is futile? The case
of Mr. Q raises still further questions. Mr. Q has a long history of drinking. He was
warned many times of the inevitable outcome, but he paid no attention to these
warnings. Blood products were short during the weeks when Mr. Q was being
treated. Some members of the team, who are usually willing to continue to provide
futile aggressive care at the request of the family, say that the case of Mr. Q is
different. His care demands scarce resources, and his illness is self-induced. They
feel that these two additional factors mandate stopping further care. Other members
of the team cannot agree. They say that if other patients are treated because of
family insistence, Mr. Q should receive treatment as well. Finally, the case of Mr.
Q raises again the very difficult question of what you stop doing if you decide to
stop providing aggressive care. Does that mean not giving Mr. Q blood products
and letting him bleed to death? Does it mean not giving him antibiotics and letting
him die from infection? Does it mean extubating him and letting him die from his
inability to breathe? And if it is decided to discontinue aggressive care against the
wishes of the family, should they at least have a say about this last set of questions?

THEORETICAL ANALYSIS    A number of the points that emerged in section 6.1 need
to be kept in mind as we look at this first case involving an incompetent patient
whose family demands further care. The most crucial are the following. (1) It is
important not to be overwhelmed by the claim of medical futility. It is often
inappropriate to say that further aggressive care for a patient will make absolutely
no difference. Such care usually offers the prospect of at least some modest prolongation of life, even at a very low level of functioning. It sometimes even offers
the prospect of some improvement in functioning for a period of time before death.
In this case, those who are claiming that further care for Mr. Q is futile can at best

mean that the probability of any benefit is very low, and the benefit in question sufficiently modest, so that it is not worth it. This is a value judgment and not a medical judgment, and it ought properly to be made by the patient or by those who best know how the patient would evaluate this situation. (2) The family's right to participate in decision making is limited here. They are no doubt the best source of information about how the patient would have judged the possible benefits of continued aggressive care. They are no doubt the best source of information about whether the consequences for them are worth the costs to them. We need to keep in mind that in this case, as in the previous three, no appeal to their right to participate in decision making is going to have any significant implications. This is because we have distinguished the strong right to refuse care from the nonexistent right to receive the care one insists on receiving. There will be no rights-based arguments for the patient getting the care the family demands, since there is no rights-based moral obligation to provide that care. At most, the family would have an argument for their right to transfer care of the patient to someone else.

Keeping these two points in mind, let us turn to the various arguments for and against providing further care to this patient. First, there is an appeal to the consequences of continuing to provide that care. Are the potential benefits to the patient worth the costs, as the family insists? Are there other beneficial or harmful consequences that we need to take into account?

Let us examine these questions from the perspective of the consequences for the patient. The family says that Mr. Q would judge the consequences (buying him some time with some reasonable quality of life) as worth it, even though their probability of occurrence is not high. We need to be very careful about their testimony. To begin with, it may well be based on a far more optimistic evaluation of the situation than is warranted. Secondly, we need to be sure that they are not simply saying that they would judge the benefits of continued care worth its burdens. So some work must be done to find out what the family is really telling us. If we do conclude that the family is really giving us reliable testimony about Mr. Q's values, then we will have one consequence-based argument for continued treatment of Mr. Q.

Another consequence argues for the continued care of this patient. This argument examines the consequences of continued care for the family. We saw in chapter 2 that an appeal to the consequences for the family is also part of a legitimate appeal to consequences. The family clearly has a strong desire for this patient to receive aggressive care. If the patient continues to receive that care, then there is an immediate benefit to them in that their desires have been respected. Moreover, if, as is likely, the patient dies in spite of the aggressive care, then the family will have the consolation of knowing that they made sure that everything possible was done for Mr. Q. Suppose, however, that their wishes are not respected and care is withheld from Mr. Q. Then they will suffer just because their wishes were not respected. Moreover, they will have to live with continued feelings of grief and perhaps even guilt, based on the idea that if only they had been more effective advocates for Mr. Q he might have received aggressive care and survived for a while. So, from the perspective of an appeal to the consequences for the family, there is much to be said for continued aggressive care given the family's wishes and desires.

Are there any appeals to consequences which argue the other way? In chapter 2, we noted that there were three appeals to consequences: the consequences for the patient, the consequences for the family, and the consequences for all those affected. Are there any others affected? How do the consequences look from their point of view? One relevant group is the health-care providers. Given that the care is not likely to be of benefit, continuing the care produces an undesirable sense of frustration on their part. But it is unlikely to be as bad as the consequences of stopping the care for those most involved, particularly since the team's frustration is limited by the patient's limited life expectancy. There is, however, another consequence which some members of the team have alluded to and which may be very significant. This is the consequence of the continued use of blood products for this patient. This patient has already required extensive use of blood for his GI bleeding, and blood products are in short supply. How serious an argument is this for not giving aggressive therapy to Mr. Q? A lot depends on just how short the blood supply is at the particular moment. Would continued aggressive care for Mr. Q really mean that other patients who would benefit more from receiving the blood products would not receive them? Although the team has talked about blood being in short supply, it is not generally true that the provision of blood to one patient actually means that someone else will not receive the blood they need. So, in the usual circumstances, this appeal to dire consequences will not hold. But suppose that we are in one of those unusual circumstances in which others who can benefit more will not get the blood they need if Mr. Q gets the blood he requires. Then there will be an important appeal to consequences arguing against aggressive care for Mr. Q. How significant it will be depends on how much the other patients need that blood, how much they will suffer from the failure to get it, and how those bad consequences stand in comparison to the bad consequences of not providing care for Mr. Q. Also, if blood is that short, there will be considerations of justice which argue against continuing to supply Mr. Q with the blood he requires, even though Mr. Q is a patient in the private sector. Some just decision will have to be adopted about the allocation of blood to Mr. Q and to others claiming it.

One other relevant moral appeal that might be invoked is Mr. Q's right to aid in life-threatening situations. Here, the self-induced nature of Mr. Q's illness is relevant. As we saw in chapters 2 and 4, the right to be aided certainly has far less significance when the threat against which one will be aided is self-induced. This is the extent to which members of the team are right when they argue that the cause of Mr. Q's illness is relevant. But it is only relevant to this argument and has no relevance to the appeal to consequences, which is in any case the major argument for continued care. It also has no relevance to the appeal to respect for persons, which argues (with modest significance, give the low probabilities of a favorable outcome) for continued care as the only chance for restoring this patient for a short period of time to the capacity to perform those activities whose performance we value so much.

What about the appeal to integrity? Once more, any health-care provider whose sense of integrity is offended by the provision of this care is free to withdraw from the care of this patient once he or she can find someone to take his or her place. As in the case of Mr. P, however, the continued care of Mr. Q is not a harm to this patient, so this point will probably involve few providers. It might, however, involve more than in the case of Mr. P, since the sense of futility is surely greater in this case.

The appeal to consequences, particularly if we clarify the basis of the family's wishes, will support the claim that the patient should continue to receive the care the family requests. This appeal is strengthened by an appeal to respect for persons. However, it is important to keep in mind that this conclusion is based on the factual assumption that blood is not in such short supply that others will be significantly harmed by Mr. Q's continuing to receive the aggressive care the family demands. Given this assumption, it would seem that the family's wishes ought to be respected and that Mr. Q should continue to receive aggressive care.

CASE NO 18. *"Why should we consider the wishes of the husband?"* : *Carefully examining the motives of the family*

FACTS Mrs. R is a 72-year-old woman who worked for years as a cleaning lady in a very dusty warehouse. She has a long history of chronic bronchitis. In recent years, she has had difficulty breathing and has been admitted to the hospital on several occasions. On some of those occasions, when her condition was very bad, she was intubated and put in the ICU. She never expressed any feelings about this care. On this particular admission, she has been intubated once more, has developed progressive pneumonia in the face of antibiotic therapy, and has also become hypotensive. She is febrile and completely disoriented. Although people in the unit see her case as hopeless, they are willing to keep her on a respirator to help her breathe, but they don't want to treat her hypotension. They feel that it is silly to continue to try to pull her through. Mrs. R's husband has been approached for his permission to institute a "do not resuscitate" order and to not treat her current infection and hypotension. He insists that she be treated for the hypotension and that she be resuscitated if her heart stops beating. He says that he cannot live without her, because she has always taken care of him, even when she has been ill, and he wants her back.

QUESTIONS The case of Mrs. R raises many of the same questions as the case of Mr. Q. But a crucial difference between the two cases has attracted attention. Mr. Q's family insisted on further aggressive treatment because they believed that it was in the best interest of Mr. Q as Mr. Q would judge it. While recognizing Mr. Q's dim prognosis, they felt that he had nothing to lose and everything to gain from further aggressive treatment. These are not the considerations that are motivating Mrs. R's husband. He has never expressed any concern except that she get better so that she can take care of his needs. Should this make a difference? Some members of the staff feel that it should. They think that his failure to attend to the best interests of his wife disqualifies him as a surrogate decision maker. Others believe that this is too harsh a judgment. They suspect that he finds it easier to say what he is saying than to articulate his concern for her, so they are not prepared to accept his remarks at face value. Moreover, they feel that whatever the basis for his decision, he is the closest family member, and it is his wishes that count. Still others think that the question of his motives is irrelevant because families have no role to play in the decision to withhold further aggressive care when that decision is a purely medical judgment based on futility. The case of Mrs. R also raises many familiar questions about what forms of care should be withheld if care is to be withheld. But those are not the issues that have attracted most of the attention of the staff; they have focused on the question of whether the expressed reasons of Mr. R should disqualify him from playing any role in decision making.

THEORETICAL ANALYSIS    The first thing we need to note is that this case should remind us of the importance of talking to chronically ill patients whose condition is deteriorating about the level of aggressiveness with which they wish to be treated as their condition worsens. Mrs. R has been admitted to the ICU because of her chronic bronchitis and associated pulmonary problems on several occasions, and one could easily have predicted a continued downward course for her, a course that has now resulted in her being very ill. The staff notes that she never really expressed any feelings about her previous admissions, but no one ever asked her how she felt about them. We have all the ambiguities in this case about what to make of her husband's wishes for further aggressive care just because no one ever took the opportunity to explore her wishes with her.

The second thing we need to note is the familiar point that many members of the staff have misanalyzed this case because they have seen it as being settled by a medical judgment that further aggressive care for this patient is futile. In fact, while her progressive pneumonia and hypotension in the face of antibody therapy are certainly ominous, particularly in a patient with a long history of pulmonary problems, it is hardly clear that she has no chance of being pulled through this current crisis and returning to the baseline condition she was in before her current hospitalization, where she functioned at a reasonably normal level. Keep in mind that she has been pulled through several earlier similar crises and has been restored to that baseline level. Here, even more than in the earlier cases in this chapter, the claim of pure medical futility seems inappropriate. The question of whether all she is being put through is worth it to her is a value question to be settled (if possible) in light of her values; it is not a medical question.

We know that further aggressive care for this patient carries with it some possibility of substantial benefits and that we have no way of finding out from the best possible source—the patient herself—whether that possibility justifies her being put through all that she is currently being put through. The crucial question is whether the husband's expressed wishes constitute any evidence of whether the benefits are worth it to her. It seems that they do not, for all of his comments concern what her survival or demise means for him. His demands for further care can hardly be taken as evidence that she would have judged the benefits as worth it. So, if we appeal to the consequences to the patient in trying to determine what ought to be done in this case, we really are in no position to decide since we have no way of finding out whether the patient would have judged the benefits worth the highly aggressive and highly invasive therapy she is currently receiving.

Some members of the staff have suggested that the husband may be talking the way he is because he has difficulty verbalizing his true feelings, which are that he believes that she would have judged the chance of survival as sufficient to justify continued aggressive care. That hypothesis is no doubt possible but hard for us to rely on. It would even be hard to accept what he would say if we were to put to him directly the question of whether he can tell us how she would have judged the benefits and losses to her from continued aggressive care. Even if he were to say in response to direct questioning that she would surely have judged the possibility of success as worth what she is undergoing, we could not have very much confidence in his testimony. We would have to be suspicious that his answer reflects his perception of what he wants for himself rather than his perception of how she would have judged the benefits and losses. So we are not going to be in a position to decide what to do in this case by any appeal to the consequences for her. One suggestion that has been made is that we seek other possible sources of information about how Mrs. R would have judged the benefits and losses. That is a useful general suggestion. When the role of the immediate family is that of testifying to the values of the patient, alternatives sources of reliable testimony can be of equal value. Unfortunately, in this case, such alternative sources are not available.

What about the appeal to the consequences for the husband? One thing is certain: he certainly believes that the consequences of continued aggressive care are extremely valuable for him. That is what he has been telling us again and again. Moreover, if we did not attend to his wishes and simply kept this patient comfortable until she died, he would not only suffer the loss of his wife but would also undergo a tremendous feeling of anguish from knowing that the physicians made decisions about the care of his wife which conflicted with what he wished. So this aspect of the appeal to consequences seems to argue for continued aggressive care for this patient. The husband's aggressiveness in demanding continued care for his wife, coupled with his constant references to how much he needs her to take care of him, seems to have provoked a fair amount of hostility on the part of many members of the team caring for this patient. That's understandable but not necessarily justified. After all, he is an elderly person who is confronting the loss of his spouse of many years and the need to live on his own, and he is understandably scared and frightened. Perhaps we would think more kindly of husbands who, while feeling all of these feelings, would focus a bit more on what all this current illness and care mean for their wives. But we need to be careful not to be harshly judgmental in our feelings about this individual. We also need to be careful to remember that his behavior does not change the fact that it is appropriate to consider the consequences of the various courses of action for this husband. So the appeal to consequences does provide us with a substantial argument for continued care for Mrs. R.

There is also an argument from respect for persons. Of all the patients we have looked at so far in this chapter, Mrs. R may have the highest probability of pulling through her crisis and being restored to normal functioning for a considerable period of time. This is because her pneumonia and her hypotension might yet be overcome by aggressive therapy, and success in treatment means that she will be capable of living a life full of those activities whose performance we value so greatly for some substantial but undetermined period of time. So an argument from respect for persons joins together with an argument from consequences—considering the consequences to her spouse—in supporting the claim that she should continue to receive aggressive care.

There is a residual sense of unease about this case, based on the fact that we can't take into account the consequences for the patient. If we had evidence of the patient's wishes, we might well treat this case very differently. But we don't, and we are forced to settle the case without considering any appeal to the consequences for the patient. We need to do the best we can with the information available to us. This feeling of unease should at least produce a firm intention to ensure that Mrs. R is given the opportunity to express her feelings about both her current care and any future care if she is successfully pulled through the current acute crisis.

*CASES NO 19, 20. Pulling a vegetable through:*
*How much is a long-term vegetative patient worth?*

FACTS    Mr. S is a 62-year-old man whose previous medical history is nearly nonexistent. His family reports that he has never seen a physician as an adult. They also report that he has always been childlike in nature but has managed to hold a series of odd jobs and to function in his home environment, where he lives with his three unmarried brothers and sisters. Mr. S was brought to the emergency room by his family because he had not gotten out of bed for two days and because they had noted slurred speech. His blood pressure on admission was 250 over 130, and he was lethargic, with evidence of considerable right hemiparesis. His CAT scan showed a very edemous left hemisphere and a large left-hemisphere infarct. His neurological status worsened quite rapidly after hospitalization, and he became comatose. In addition, he required intubation. After a week of no improvement, the physicians treating Mr. S had a long talk with his family. They explained that his death was by no means imminent and that they probably could extubate him in time, but there would always be considerable destruction of brain functioning. They also explained that he might survive for a long time but with only minimal neurological functioning. They asked the family whether they want Mr. S to receive further respiratory support to save his life if the best outcome is that he would survive as a near vegetable. The family say that they understand what that means, but they insist that he still be treated.

QUESTIONS    What is the role of family wishes in this case? Some argue that the final decision is clearly the family's. After all, the question presented here (unlike in cases 17 and 18) is not the medical question of whether there is any hope that this man can survive but the value question of whether his survival with severely diminished neurological functioning is of sufficient value to justify continued care. Such a value decision can only be made by the family. Other members of the team see it differently. To begin with, they are not sure that the family really understands what the patient will be like if he survives. They suspect that the family thinks that the patient will just be a little worse than he has always been. Although considerable efforts have been made to explain to the family what he will be like, this group believes that the family doesn't fully comprehend (perhaps because they don't want to face reality), and it would be inappropriate to allow them to make the decision based on a misunderstanding. In addition, this group argues that the family in question has limited financial means. The continued treatment of the patient would require extensive social and medical services that the family cannot afford. The cost will have to be borne by society. Why should the family be allowed to make this type of decision and impose heavy costs on the rest of society? There is, however, a conflicting set of considerations that trouble many members of the team. The major health care that the patient is currently receiving, besides supportive nursing care, is respiratory support. He probably can be weaned from this eventually, but any current attempt to discontinue support would probably result in his imminent death. This leads some members of the team to conclude that there is no choice but to continue treating the patient.

FACTS    The story of Ms. T is a very sad one. She is 28 years old and has been a patient either in the hospital in question or in an affiliated nursing home for the last two and a half years. When she was 25 she sustained extensive head injuries in a motorcycle accident. Since then she has been totally comatose and unresponsive. She has been able to breathe on her own, and she shows evidence of some brain-stem reflexes, so we know that she is not brain dead.[6] In the last two and a half years, however, she has shown no evidence of higher brain functioning. Most of the time she receives only nursing care. She needs to have her airway suctioned to prevent secretions from blocking it, and she is regularly turned in bed to avoid bed sores. She is fed through a tube. Her major medical needs arise from intermittent infections that require careful workups and extensive antibiotic treatment. In severe episodes she is transferred from the nursing home, where she normally lives, to the hospital. That happened two days ago. The family of Ms. T has been heartbroken since her accident. She is her parents' only child, they took great pride in all of her achievements, and they cannot bring themselves to accept the fact that she will never again be able to function normally. They know that if she is treated carefully she can survive for a long time. They hope for a miracle or for some medical advance that can cure her. Many unsuccessful attempts have been made to explain the futility of this. The team treating her has spoken to the family again, now that she has been transferred back to the hospital, and the parents have reiterated their desire that her infection be treated.

QUESTIONS    Many members of the team don't wish to treat Ms. T's infection. One reason is a feeling of compassion for the family. In the two and a half years since Ms. T's accident, her family's life has centered around their regular daily visit to the hospital or the nursing home. They sit with her for hours. Their normal life has come to a stop. Continued treatment for Ms. T, these people argue, means a continued living hell for the family. Her death would lead to grief but also, it is hoped, to a renewal of their life after a period of time. A second reason is based on cost considerations. Ms. T's family cannot pay for her nursing home or hospital care, and her continued treatment is a real cost to society. There is no reason why she cannot live on for many years. Mrs. T's family has no right, this argument runs, to impose these costs on society given her condition, and this is a reason for disregarding the family's wishes. A third reason, offered by many of the nurses who have had to provide most of the treatment for Ms. T over the years, is that the staff is frustrated by the tremendous efforts required to maintain her. They want to use their professional time and talents in more constructive ways.

The major question raised by all of these points is whether they are relevant. Are they of greater significance than the family's wishes in this matter? After all, don't we have here a fundamental ethical and even metaphysical judgment about the value of life per se, no matter what its quality, a judgment that can only be made by the patient's immediate family? Those who believe this are not arguing against taking quality-of-life considerations into account; all they are arguing is that these are issues which the family needs to consider, and it is their wishes that need to be followed.

THEORETICAL ANALYSIS    The cases of Mr. S and Ms. T are strikingly different from the other cases we have examined in this chapter for two major reasons which are absolutely central to our examination. The first difference is that neither Mr. S. nor Ms. T is suffering from a terminal illness that will definitely result in their death in the reasonably near future. Patients such as Mr. S and Ms. T have been known to live on in their sad condition for many years.[7] The second and related difference is that the emotional and financial burden of caring for these patients is far more significant than the burden of caring for any other patient whose case we have examined in this chapter, primarily because their need for care can continue for so long.

It is helpful to begin by reminding ourselves that no appeal to procedural or substantive rights is going to play a major role in the resolution of these cases. Withholding and withdrawing care from these patients (respirator support from Mr. S and antibiotics from Ms. T) would not be violating either their substantive right not to be killed or their substantive right not to be harmed, since, as I have already pointed out many times, doing so would simply mean letting the disease process take its natural course. The procedural right of the patient and/or the procedural right of the family to be decision makers is also not going to be relevant to either case. The patient's procedural right is totally irrelevant because the patient is incapable of participating in the decisional process. The family's procedural right is going to be mostly irrelevant because this is not a case of the family's exercising the right to refuse care but rather the family's demanding care. There is no right to the care that one demands for family members. At most, they have the right to transfer the patient's care to some other set of providers.

The second point is that no appeal to respect for persons is going to play any role in the resolution of these cases. Neither patient is currently capable of performing any of those activities whose performance we value so much. Despite the hopes and dreams of their families, the probability of either patient ever being able to resume any of those activities is near zero. This differentiates these cases from the cases of Mr. Q and Mrs. R. These cases clearly illustrate how the appeal to respect for persons differs from the appeal to the sanctity of life, which would make a difference to the resolution of these cases. Both patients can be kept alive by aggressive nursing and medical care for considerable periods of time, and an appeal to the sanctity of life would strongly urge continued medical and nursing care for them. The incapacity of these two patients to perform any of those activities whose performance we value so much would not in any way diminish the significance of the argument from the sanctity of human life for continued treatment. An appeal to respect for persons is very different. Given the inability of these patients to perform any of the relevant activities, it would present no argument for continued care.

This way of objectively looking at quality-of-life considerations is built into the appeal to the respect for persons. The question of whether the patient is capable of performing those activities whose performance we value so greatly (e.g., thinking, feeling, interacting) is an objective medical question. The quality-of-life judgment that the patient is incapable of engaging in those activities is an objective judgment which can be made on purely medical grounds. None of this is to say that all quality-of-life considerations are objective medical judgments. We will look at another such judgment shortly, namely whether the patient's continued existence in this low quality of life is a desirable or undesirable consequence for him or her. That type of subjective quality-of-life judgment will, of course, be treated very differently.

It looks as though the major moral appeals that we will need to examine are the appeal to consequences and the appeal to cost-effectiveness.

We need to look at the consequences for these patients, for their families, and for the rest of society. Is their continued existence in their current state a benefit to these patients, a loss to them, or something of no value either way? In certain frameworks for evaluating consequences (for example, the hedonist framework discussed in chapter 2), the answer is clear. It is of no value to them either way, since they are incapable of experiencing pleasure or pain, and only those experiences determine value. However, we have adopted the preference-satisfaction approach, and this means that it is possible to evaluate continued existence from the perspective of the patients' preferences when they were still competent, to see whether this continued existence might be a gain or loss to them.[8] Here, unfortunately, we have no information about whether or not these patients would have preferred this type of continued existence.[9] It is unlikely that there could be such information about a patient like Mr. S. Given his limited mental functioning in the early parts of his life, it is unclear whether he could have ever understood, much less formed a preference about, the question of whether continued existence without mental functioning is of value to him. So there seems little point to trying to ascertain from the family of Mr. S what his preference would have been. The case of Ms. T is different. Before her accident, she certainly was capable of having preferences on that topic. But there is nothing the family has said in all of the discussions with them that indicates that she ever expressed any preferences on this matter. Direct questioning at this point might elicit from them some claims about what her wishes would have been, but these claims could not be taken very seriously as evidence. They would be tainted by the fact that the family has been fighting for continued care for their daughter for so long. We will just not be able to tell whether or not the consequences of care (continued existence without significant mental functioning) would be of any value to these patients. This is a subjective value-of-life consideration which only the person in question could decide. Since we have no evidence for how they would have decided, we cannot legitimately invoke this type of value-of-life consideration in deciding whether the consequences for the patient are worth it or not.

Initially, it looks as though a consideration of the consequences for the family argues for continued treatment for both of these patients, much as it argued for continued treatment for Mr. Q and Mrs. R. After all, the clear preference of both families is that these patients continue to be treated, so continued treatment will definitely satisfy their preferences. Stopping treatment will go against their preferences. Therefore, from a straightforward appeal to the consequences for the family, there is a major argument for continued treatment. This argument has particular significance in the case of Ms. T, since the preferences in question are long-term intensively held preferences. However, matters are not that simple. Members of the staff have correctly pointed out that continued care for Ms. T is actually imposing tremendous costs on her family. They have not gotten on with their lives, because they have devoted themselves to hanging around their daughter's hospital. Her continued existence is a tremendous loss for them, as well as a source of much frustration. One might say that this is their choice, but I think that is too simple-minded. It confuses the correct claim that the individuals affected are the ones whose preferences must determine the value of the consequences with the incorrect claim that these individuals are always the best judges of which course of action will lead to the satisfaction of most of their preferences. Ms. T's family has no prefer-ence for living the way they are living. They only hope that it will ultimately result in a favorable outcome—the recovery of their daughter. They are wrong about this. She will never recover the functioning they wish to see her recover. Continued aggressive care will produce a set of consequences (a continuation of the way they live) which they themselves judge not to be of value without the compensating consequences (her improvement) which they would judge as being of value. So we can say quite correctly that the consequences for this family of continued care for Ms. T are unfortunate even from their own perspective. The case of Mr. S is much more recent. Nevertheless, similar points must be made about the consequences of continued aggressive care for Mr. S. Over a period of time, the family will get the benefit of having their wishes respected and will pay the price of coming to live the way Ms. T's family lives. There is, however, one notable difference between these two cases. Ms. T's family has lived with her condition for a number of years, has developed their pattern of life, and is not likely to change. However, the relatives of Mr. S might well change their desires about his continued care after some further period of time when they come to see more realistically what his condition is and what his prospects are. So continued aggressive care for Mr. S, for at least some short period of time, might preserve the good consequences for the family of having their wishes respected while not necessarily leading to bad long-term consequences for them. This difference will be of great significance in our final resolution of this case.

What about the consequences of continued care for these patients from the per-spective of the rest of society? Here there are two obvious points that need to be made. The first is that continued care poses a great burden of frustration on the health-care providers, which is particularly significant in these cases because this frustration is ongoing and will continue over a long period of time. Secondly, and perhaps even more importantly, the continued aggressive care of these patients poses considerable financial costs to society. Again, because these patients are not confronting death in the reasonably near future, these costs will mount over a period of time.[10]

Putting all of these appeals to consequences together, we seem to be led to the conclusion that these patients should not be maintained indefinitely. This is rein-forced by another appeal which certainly must be invoked. As was pointed out in the initial description of these cases, the heavy financial burden of caring for these patients requires a considerable expenditure of public funds. As was argued in early chapters, an appeal to cost-effectiveness is certainly appropriate in treating public patients. Lacking a full-fledged theory of cost-effectiveness, it is difficult to come to any definitive conclusion about the cost-effectiveness of care in these particular cases. However, in light of the heavy expenditures over a long period of time and the fact that it is hard (but not impossible) to see how, even from the perspective of these patients, their continued existence could be of great value to them, it would not be implausible to suppose that the appeal to cost-effectiveness would also argue against continued aggressive care.

One additional issue is the question raised by members of the staff about what forms of care ought to be withdrawn and/or withheld from these patients. It is clear in the case of Ms. T that the crucial question is that of withholding antibiotic therapy when she develops her next infection. That would impose the least psychological stress on those involved, since it would be a nondramatic withholding of care leading to a peaceful death and would therefore be supported by an appeal both to consequences and to the virtue of compassion. A similar approach might well be adopted in the case of Mr. S, particularly if we are going to take up the earlier suggestion of giving the family a bit more time in the hope that they will come to agree with the decision. Given that time, he might be weaned from his respirator, and the crucial question will be antibiotic therapy.

Another issue has to do with honesty. Some might be tempted, either by prudence or by a sense of compassion for the family, to withhold antibiotic therapy from these patients without telling the family what they are doing. We need to remember, however, the great significance of the virtue of honesty in the patient-physician relationship. Moreover, the strategy of not telling the family is of dubious value from the point of view of compassion, since it will stop being a compassionate act if the family discovers what has happened. It will not be easy to deal with the family; it will not be easy to get them to come to grips with the fact that the time for continued aggressive care is over, whatever their wishes may be. Here is where a recognition of the virtue of courage in the health-care setting is vital.

One final complication: the families of both of these patients do have a right to transfer care of these patients to another physician. They may be tempted to do so if they realize that the current physicians are planning to discontinue aggressive therapy. Being honest with them involves the risk of this. One can only hope that they will listen to what the physicians are saying to them and/or that they will find that other physicians say the same thing and refuse to take the case given the family's insistence on continued aggressive care.

We are led to the conclusion that, despite the family's wishes, these two patients should not continue to be treated just to preserve their mere biological existence. In the case of Mr. S, it would be appropriate to continue to treat him for some period of time to give the family an opportunity to adjust to what has happened to him, in the hope that they will come to agree to no further therapeutic measures. In the case of Ms. T, the time to stop has certainly been reached. In both cases, the best approach is to not treat further infections with antibiotics.[11]

This analysis seems morally sound. However, it is not clear that current American law would allow such a decision to be carried out. The problem is not with the withholding of antibiotics from patients who are permanently comatose and/or vegetative. It is rather that our analysis indicates that this ought to be done regardless of the family's wishes, and current law seems to require family approval. Our analysis argues that they are entitled to an honest account of what is happening but not to continued deference to their wishes. One of the crucial legal issues in the area of death and dying in the next few years will be whether or not society is prepared to forthrightly confront the question of the benefits and costs of continued therapeutic measures for this very sad class of patients or whether it would prefer, for one reason or another, to continue its policy of deferring to the wishes of their families.

In this section, we have seen four patients who are no longer competent to participate in decision making about their own medical care. Their families are present, however, and this is what distinguishes them from the patients in cases 14, 15, and 16. In all four cases, the family insists on further health care against the recommendation either that such care is futile (cases 17, 18) or that the resulting quality of life makes it pointless (cases 19, 20). These are merely a sampling of a large number of cases of this sort. In the next section, we will look at a few cases in which family members wish to stop treatment and physicians wish to continue treatment.

## 6.3   Incompetent Patients Whose Families Wish Treatment Discontinued

*CASE NO 21. "Dad had planned to sign a living will":*
*Many reasons for respecting a refusal of care*

FACTS    Mr. U is a 66-year-old widower with a history of congestive heart failure and chronic obstructive pulmonary disease. He has been admitted to the ICU and has required respirator support several times in the past. On this particular occasion, Mr. U's son called an ambulance to take his father to the hospital because Mr. U was having difficulty breathing. On the way to the hospital, he arrested. He was resuscitated by the ambulance staff, intubated on arrival in the emergency center, and transferred to the medical ICU. A CAT scan revealed a right brain infarct. It is difficult at this point to say how severe his neurological deficits will be. Attempts have been made to wean him from the respirator, but they have not been successful. The son who called the ambulance and his two brothers have asked the physicians to extubate their father and simply keep him comfortable until he dies. They all believe that this is what their father would wish. When asked why, they say that their father had read in the newspaper about the local natural-death act (which allows individuals to prepare a living will asking that aggressive health care be withheld or withdrawn when their death is imminent) and had asked them to make an appointment with his attorney to fill out such a document. Unfortunately, say the sons, they were unable to make the appointment before the father's latest attack.

QUESTIONS    The case of Mr. U has caused much controversy among those caring for him. Some members of the team say that his death, while not necessarily imminent, is not too far away, and they see no point in pulling him through this particular crisis so that he can live in a diminished neurological state until he dies from his chronic problems. Others agree that this is a patient with severe medical problems, but they do not see his further care as futile. It may be able to buy him some time, and they are not convinced by the evidence that his neurological deficits will be so great that the time is worthless. So there are questions both about the futility of this care and about the quality of life of this patient if he is pulled through. This debate has occupied many members of the team. Others, however, view it as irrelevant. They feel that this is a choice for the family to make, and the family has made it in light of their understanding of what the patient would have wished. They are, moreover, impressed by the fact that the family is appealing to the patient's expressed desire to fill out a living will. Others are less persuaded. They see Mr. U's announcement that he wished to fill out a living will as the family's only evidence, and they wonder how much credence should be given to this evidence. After all, they argue, Mr. U never had a living will explained to him, and, had it been explained to him, he might not have filled it out. Moreover, the local living will, like most living wills,[12] refers only to the withholding and/or withdrawing of care when the patient is terminally ill and his or her death reasonably imminent, and they remind us that this patient's death is not necessarily imminent. Still one more set of issues is raised by many members of the team. Previous attempts to wean this patient from his respirator have failed. If he is extubated at this point, he is likely to die very quickly. Some find this objectionable because they view withdrawing the respirator at this point as killing the patient. Others find it objectionable because they think that it would be cruel to withdraw this care from the patient and allow him to die short of breath and gasping for air. While it is true that the gasping reflex might be stilled by the use of morphine, they are concerned that this would be actively killing the patient. So the difficult case of Mr. U raises many questions about the meaning of futility and the quality of life, about the role of the family and possible advance wishes of the patient, and about the borderline between letting a patient die and killing a patient.

THEORETICAL ANALYSIS The family of Mr. U is requesting that he be discon- nected from his respirator and sedated with morphine to keep him comfortable until he dies. The first question we need to consider is whether this is a request that can be honored. Many members of the team feel that it cannot be, because it would constitute killing the patient. Some feel that the killing would be performed by withdrawing the respirator; others feel that it would be done by sedating him with morphine which would depress his respiratory functioning. In any case, the patient's right not to be killed would be violated, and these members of the team feel that this right is of sufficiently great significance so that avoiding its violation should take precedence over any other considerations. The family's request must therefore be denied.

It might be suggested in response that this is no problem, because the patient has waived his right not to be killed. He did that when he indicated that he wished to fill out a living will. This is incorrect. Whatever the implications of that wish for other questions, it certainly does not constitute a waiver of the right not to be killed. Even if the patient had actually filled out a living will, that is a request to be allowed to die and not a request to be killed.[13] So even if one agrees with the theoretical claim of chapter 2 that the right not to be killed is a waivable right, one cannot use that to resolve the problem posed by those members of the team who see deferring to the family's wishes as actually murdering the patient.

There is reason, however, to reject their claim. To begin with, as already argued, the withdrawal of a respirator, even when the patient is incapable of breathing on his or her own, is at most a case of allowing the patient's underlying illness to cause death; despite the fact that one physically does something, the withdrawal of the respirator is not the cause of death. So if this is a case of killing, it must be because of the decision to provide the patient with morphine. This is a much more difficult issue. Some would claim[14] that as long as our intention is just to keep the patient comfortable, we would not be killing the patient by providing the morphine, no matter how much morphine is provided to keep him comfortable. That claim rests on the presupposition that it is our intentions which determine whether we have engaged in an illicit act of killing. I have argued in chapter 2, however, that we will have killed the patient if our action causes the patient's death, whatever our intentions. There is, therefore, one crucial restriction on the family's wish that must be understood and accepted by the physicians and the family if respecting their wish is to be an option. This is that the provision of morphine must be limited by our ability to do so without actively causing the death of the patient. More precisely, the dosages must not be so high as to make it likely that the patient's death will result from the depression of respiratory activity. When that limitation is pointed out to the family, they may change their minds about the request. But they may not, because they may hope that the amount of relief given Mr. U within the limits of not actually killing him would be sufficient. They may feel that the small temporal duration of discomfort from gasping is justified in order to avoid the longer suffering of this patient. The question we face is whether the wishes of the family should be respected, given that this limitation is understood.

The first crucial argument for respecting those wishes is that the patient has in advance refused the form of care in question by expressing his intention to sign a living will, and he has a right to have his refusal respected. Looked at this way, the family is providing evidence of Mr. U's wish to refuse care. This can be at best a modest argument for discontinuing care for Mr. U. To begin with, there is the question of how seriously we should take the patient's wishes to have an appointment made with an attorney as evidence of an advance refusal of care in such circumstances. As has been pointed out by many members of the team, the patient may not have fully realized what is involved in a living will and the circumstances under which it might be employed, so a mere expression of a wish to make an appointment is not overwhelming evidence of a refusal of care. Moreover, even if he had signed the living will, we would have no evidence that he would want to refuse care when his death is not imminent. Finally, any advance wish to refuse care, just because it does not involve knowledge of the exact circumstances in which the decision will be made, must have less significance than a wish to refuse care at the time in question.[15] So if the family's decision is simply testimony about the patient's wish to refuse care under these circumstances, it provides only a modest argument from the patient's right to refuse care on behalf of withdrawing respiratory support.

There is, however, a second way of looking at the family's request. It may well be that they are not simply testifying about what the patient would have wished; they may also be expressing their wish on behalf of this no longer competent patient to refuse care. Keep in mind that families do have the right to refuse care for incompetent family members. It is crucial, of course, that we clarify that the family is both testifying about what they think the patient would have wished and also expressing their own wishes. But if they are saying both of these things, as seems to be the case here, then there is a second argument for withdrawing respiratory support from this patient and providing morphine subject to the above-mentioned restriction. This would be acting in accordance with the family's refusal of care, and they have a right to have that refusal respected, given the patient's incompetence and the lack of firm knowledge about his wishes. Moreover, in light of the fact that this refusal is a strongly requested refusal and seems to be rooted in some centrally held beliefs about how bad continued care would be for Mr. U, this right to refuse care seems to have particular significance in this case.

There is also a significant argument from an appeal to consequences on behalf of respecting the family's wishes in this case. If care is provided for Mr. U so that he pulls through the current crisis, he will live for a modest but unknown period of time with an unclear neurological status. Even before the neurological problems, the fact that he expressed a wish to see his attorney provides us with some reason (even if not overwhelming evidence) for thinking that he would view continued survival as not worth the price of the aggressive therapy required. Keep in mind that he has experienced intubation and ICU care several times in the past. So an appeal to consequences, evaluating the consequences from the perspective of Mr. U's evaluation of them, seems to argue against treating this patient. A similar point can be made about the appeal to consequences for the family. A failure to respect their wishes would produce the consequences of a tremendous sense of frustration on their part.

What are the arguments against respecting the family's wishes even when we keep in mind the limitation on the amount of morphine that can be used? An appeal to the respect for persons might provide some reasons for continuing to treat this patient. With luck, Mr. U can be pulled through and go on for at least some period of time to perform at least some of those activities whose performance we value so greatly. But because of his multiple medical problems, the period of time is not likely to be very long. With his neurological deficits, he will be able to perform fewer of those activities than the ordinary person. So the appeal to the respect for persons does not have tremendous significance in a case like this. Similar considerations make the appeal to the right to be aided, even if we agree that the patient has not waived that right, of modest significance here. It appears then, that the many reasons for respecting the family's wishes settle the case by favoring the withdrawal of Mr. U's respirator and the provision of such symptom relief as is required, so long as that provision doesn't cause the patient's death.

*CASE NO 22. "How can we listen to what he tells us?"* :
*The need to carefully examine family motives*

FACTS    Mrs. V is a 73-year-old woman who was widowed eight years ago. She has
no immediate family except for her second husband, whom she married seven
months ago. Her physician, who has know her for many years, describes this
relationship as being a matter of two old, lonely people thinking they would be
better off living together. Last week, Mrs. V had a stroke. It is clear that her
permanent capacities will be diminished by the stroke, but it is not clear at this point
just how badly. For the moment, she is not very responsive and has developed a
host of management problems, including a serious infection and some difficulties
with breathing. Her husband has expressed the wish that the doctors not treat these
conditions. He wants them to just keep her comfortable until she dies. He claims
that they often talked about the great difficulty with functioning after serious illnesses and that his wife said she did not want to live that way. However, on more
than one occasion, he has also told a nurse that he just cannot see spending the rest
of his life caring for an invalid. These remarks have led people to wonder about his
motives. However, her physician does agree that Mrs. V has been a very independent lady and that she would probably not like to live as a dependent invalid. The
physician is just not sure what conclusions can be drawn about what she would have
wished in such a case.

QUESTIONS    Perhaps the most crucial question here is how we should view the role
of the family in decision making in such cases. Some of the people caring for Mrs.
V say that the decision to continue to provide care belongs to the family (in this
case, the husband) unless there is strong evidence of an inappropriate decision.
There is no doubt that the husband is concerned about what it will mean for him to
care for this woman whom he married more out of convenience than anything else,
but the evidence is not sufficient, this group feels, to disqualify him as the decision
maker. Others feel that decisions to withhold care on the basis of the family's claim
about a poor quality of life are always tenuous and can only be justified when there
is overwhelming evidence that the family truly understands what the patient would
have wished and is making the decision based on that perception. This group
concludes that they cannot make any decision based on this husband's expressed
wishes. There is still another issue bothering everyone. Many feel that it would be
inappropriate to make a decision to withhold care at this point. They just don't see
enough evidence about permanent disability on which to base an appropriate decision. Others are less convinced. They have seen too many previously proud and
independent stroke victims leading a dependent existence. If they could only be
convinced that the husband's judgment was appropriate, they would be prepared to
support his decision that aggressive medical measures should not be initiated.

THEORETICAL ANALYSIS    The case of Mrs. V needs to be contrasted with the case
of Mrs. R. In both cases, there are family members whose reasons for their wishes
concerning treatment for the patient raise doubts about their ability to serve as
appropriate surrogate decision makers. There are, however, two crucial differences
between the two cases. First, in the case of Mrs. R, the husband is insisting on

further care. Mrs. V's husband, on the other hand, is demanding that further therapeutic care be discontinued. This distinction is important when we examine the appeal to the right of the family to make decisions. After all, Mrs. R's husband has no right to have his request for treatment respected, but Mrs. V's husband, as the closest family member of a currently incompetent patient, has a right to have his refusal of care respected. Unless there are reasons for disregarding the husband's wishes because of his motives, that refusal will have considerable significance. Second, Mrs. V's prognosis is considerably better than that of Mrs. R. Mrs. R has a progressive deteriorating illness, and her current condition is relatively dismal. Mrs. V's condition, on the contrary, does not involve a necessarily progressive illness. Moreover, Mrs. R's baseline functioning was already limited because of her difficulties. Mrs. V's condition, if she is pulled through her current problems, will involve some deficits, but their extent is as yet unknown, and there exists a real possibility that they will be quite limited.

Keeping these differences in mind, we begin with the major argument for discontinuing care for Mrs. V: her husband, who is the closest family member, has requested that her care be discontinued. Note that there are really two arguments being offered by the husband. The first is that the care should be discontinued because his wife has in advance refused aggressive medical care if she is ever in these circumstances. On this argument, the husband is simply testifying to his wife's earlier refusal of care, and it is her right to have her refusal of care respected which grounds the argument against continued aggressive care. The second argument is that he is the closest family member, and, as such, he has a right to have his refusal of further care respected. So there are two rights-based arguments for withholding and/or withdrawing care, and these arguments must be separately examined in light of the suspicions about the husband's motives.

The most serious reason for suspicion is that Mrs. V's husband has on more than one occasion said to members of the team that he cannot see spending the rest of his life caring for an invalid. This has led some to feel that his testimony cannot be trusted, thereby undercutting the argument for not treating her because she has refused care in advance. Moreover, they suspect that he is making decisions in light of his own interests rather than her interests, thereby undercutting the argument that he has a right to refuse care on her behalf. Some would add to this the fact that they are a recently married couple whose marriage seems to be based more on convenience than on any deep affection. It is extremely difficult for outsiders to assess all of this in any definite fashion. The least that can be said is that these considerations weaken the significance of any appeal to the procedural rights of the patient and/or the family as a basis for decision making in this case. So we need to look at other considerations that argue against continued care.

Could we argue that the consequences for the patient would be best if she did not survive this illness? There is evidence over and above the husband's testimony that suggests that she would find dependence unsatisfactory. Her physician, who has known her for a long time, says that she is a proud and independent woman who would find the limitations from her stroke unacceptable. The physician cannot testify, as the husband is doing, to any advance refusal of care by the patient in such circumstances, because he was not present during any discussion with her about these matters, but he can at least testify to her general values. This independent testimony, combined with the husband's testimony, might be sufficient to ground an appeal-to-consequences argument against further care. The trouble is that his testimony is also flawed. He is telling us—and we have no reason to doubt his testimony—that she would find dependency troubling. But given that even he doesn't know at this point the exact extent to her permanent dependencies given her stroke, he is hardly in a position to testify about how she would evaluate the consequences of living with this stroke. His knowledge is just too general to help us in this case. So we have no firm basis for an argument against treating her.

One argument on the other side is an appeal to respect for persons. While we cannot at this point tell the extent of Mrs. V's limitations if she is pulled through the current crisis, we do have reasonably good reasons for believing that she will be able to perform at least many of those activities whose performance we value so greatly. The trouble is that our inability to say what will be her resulting condition makes it difficult to assess the significance of that appeal.

We seem to be in one of those difficult situations in which none of the appeals speaks strongly on behalf of any conclusion. Suppose we consider an alternative compromise strategy that has been suggested by some members of the team: attempting to treat the patient's current acute problems—her difficulty with breathing and her infection—in the hope that as these conditions improve she will become sufficiently clear-minded and responsive so that she can become involved in decision making about her future care. There is certainly a risk in doing this. If these current crises are resolved, the major decisions may have been made before she becomes capable of participating in decision making. If in fact her husband's claim is correct, we may have condemned her against her wishes to existence as an invalid. But it is important to keep in mind that seriously disabled stroke victims often have further medical problems, and she will have the opportunity to make explicit and definite arrangements for refusal of future care if that is what she wants. It is also important to keep in mind that if we don't pull her through the current crisis, there is also the risk that her husband's views are not a correct expression of her wishes and she will die unnecessarily and against her wishes. That is a risk we cannot correct later.

Buying time to get further information is never a very comfortable strategy because it seems to be based on ignorance rather than knowledge and because it carries with it the risk of being wrong. But there are times when we just don't have enough information to feel confident about any decision, and there are risks either way. In such cases, buying time may be our best bet. If we firmly resolve to clarify Mrs. V's wishes as soon as she has improved sufficiently, and if we firmly resolve to follow those wishes even if it means withholding care for easily correctable residual problems, buying time appears to be the best way to deal with the case.

CASE NO 23. *"The family is just too pessimistic"*:
*Trying to be fair both to patients and to their families*
FACTS    Mr. W is a 69-year-old patient who presented six weeks ago with squamous cell carcinoma of the lung and demonstrated metastatic disease in his brain. He received X-ray therapy for the brain metastases but no treatment for his primary carcinoma in the lung. Three days ago, he became acutely short of breath and

arrested just after arriving in the hospital. He was intubated in the emergency room and transferred to the ICU. His respiratory function has started to improve, and the unit staff feels confident that they can pull him through the current crisis and buy him some months of reasonable life at home. Since the patient's admission to the unit, however, his entire family has been extremely upset about seeing him in this condition. Again and again, they have said that they don't want their father to die a slow, agonizing death connected to tubes. They admit that they never talked about such issues in the past, so they don't know what he would have wanted, but they all feel strongly that he should be taken off his respirator and allowed to die now. They keep saying that a quick death is better than a long, lingering death.

QUESTIONS   This case has troubled the entire staff. Many feel that the family is being excessively pessimistic. The patient has suffered an acute crisis, but he's coming out of it, and with proper care he can live for some months in a reasonable state of comfort. Why should that be denied to him? Moreover, they are impressed by the family's admission that they really don't know what the patient would have wished. All of this leads them to feel that continued aggressive care for Mr. W is justified. As others see it, while this patient's death is not imminent, it certainly is not that far in the future. They see a compassionate family making a judgment that it would be best for the patient to allow him to die now, and they think it would be cruel to violate the wishes of the family. The first group concedes this last point, but they feel that the way to deal with the family's agony is by proper counseling, not by accepting their wishes. Still another viewpoint has emerged: the patient should be pulled through this crisis and after proper counseling should be asked to express his wishes about what should be done in a similar situation if, as is quite likely, it arises again.

THEORETICAL ANALYSIS   The case of Mr. W is in many ways closer to the case of Mr. U than to that of Mrs. V. Mr. W, like Mr. U, has a family that is concerned with his best interests. However, unlike the case of Mr. U, the family of Mr. W has very little information relevant to the question of what he would have wished.

We have distinguished three ways in which families of patients can play a role in decision making when the patient is incompetent. They may testify about the patient's previous wishes, thereby giving us a basis for withholding care on the grounds that the patient has refused it at an earlier time. They may testify to the patient's values, thereby giving us an appropriate basis for evaluating the consequences of further care. Or, finally, they may exercise their own right to refuse care for the patient in light of such considerations as they find relevant. It is clear that in this case, unlike the case of Mr. U, the family is capable of playing only the third role, since they explicitly say that they never discussed such issues with the patient in the past. So we first need to examine the significance of the argument that the patient's aggressive care should be terminated on the grounds that his family, who is speaking on his behalf, wishes this care to be terminated.

Obviously, the significance of the appeal to the right to refuse care is greater here than in the case of Mrs. V; there is no question here of the suspect motives that were present in the case of Mrs. V's husband. I think, however, that there are several reasons why this appeal is less significant than the appeal to the same right in the case of Mr. U. To begin with, the family of Mr. W is less competent to make a decision because they have had no experience with what is involved in the care in question and because they are far more agitated than Mr. U's family, which is much more experienced with these crises. This readily apparent agitation, combined with the lack of full knowledge of acute crises and the ways in which they can be reversed, certainly casts some doubts on the full competency of the family and must weaken to some degree the significance of their right to refuse care for Mr. W. Moreover, this decision of the family is a relatively new one, brought on by the sudden onset of a crisis. It cannot compare to the more long-standing decision of Mr. U's family, which really grows out of their willingness to support him when he originally decided to see his attorney about the living will. None of this is to say that the family's right to refuse care for Mr. W is of no significance at all, just that it fails to have the significance that it has in other cases.

Two other arguments might be advanced on behalf of withdrawing care from this patient. First, the family clearly wishes that care be withdrawn, and refusing to do so would clearly produce a tremendous sense of frustration and unhappiness. This is an undesirable consequence and offers an argument, based on an appeal to the consequences for the family, for withdrawing care. Second, it would certainly be compassionate to not impose on this family, struggling as they are with the illness of their father, an extra judgment that they have been precipitous and have acted wrongly in demanding that care be withdrawn from this patient. So an appeal to the virtue of compassion also argues on behalf of withdrawing care.

On the other side, the first argument is the argument from respect for persons. As has been pointed out by many members of the team, Mr. W's current crisis seems to be reversing, and there is a good probability that he will be able to go home and live for some period of time performing all of those activities whose performances we value so much. To be sure, the patient's life expectancy is not great, and that means that the appeal to respect for persons does not have its full significance in this case; it would certainly have more significance in a case where the patient had a greater life expectancy. But, unlike Mr. U, this patient, if pulled through the current crisis, will be able to resume normal functioning for some period of time; that gives the appeal to respect for persons greater strength.

What about the appeal to the consequences for the patient? This is an important issue and one that is difficult for us to evaluate at this point because we just don't have any information about the patient's values. On the one hand, allowing Mr. W to die now might help him avoid much further suffering that he would undergo from further acute crises, and this consequence speaks on behalf of withholding care. It is, in fact, the very consequence that the family is invoking. On the other hand, pulling this patient through would buy him some very good months, and that is certainly a consequence worth taking into account. The crucial question is which of these two consequences is more important according to the values of the patient. We do not have an answer at this point.

We will have great difficulties resolving this case because crucial information about the patient's values is missing and because the various relevant appeals on both sides have less than their full significance. The third option suggested by members of the team seems promising. It suggests that we continue the course of care to enable the patient to surmount the current crisis and then get a firm reading from the patient on what his wishes would be for the next crisis and how he would value a chance at some further months versus having to go through another period of aggressive care. The best method would be to convince the family of the merits of this approach. Should the family agree, then there would be little doubt about the moral superiority of the approach. It would then be in accord with the family's wishes, it would involve full respect for the personhood of the patient, it would avoid the lack of compassion in totally disregarding the family's wishes, and it might well produce the consequences that would be best given the patient's own evaluation. The much harder question is what to do if the family adamantly refuses to accept this compromise suggestion. Absent the crucial information about how the patient would evaluate the consequences of dying quickly now without further suffering versus a good chance of some good months plus another acute crisis (even with the clear promise that no aggressive therapy would then be provided), it is impossible to form any clear-cut judgment. We have a reasonably significant but not overwhelming appeal to respect for persons as the main argument on the one side and a very significant appeal to the consequences for the family and a modest appeal to respect for their right to refuse care for the patient as the primary arguments on the other side. Reasonable clinicians might have different judgments about how such a case should be managed if the family doesn't agree with this compromise.

This leads to one final reflection about this case. The compromise strategy is a way of obtaining information now that could have been obtained earlier on. A patient presenting with squamous cell carcinoma of the lungs and metastatic disease in the brain will shortly face acute crises and doesn't have a very long life expectancy no matter what is done. This is one of those patients with whom discussions about levels of care should have taken place earlier on. The fault, if we wish to talk about fault, lies both with the family and with the physician who neglected the opportunities before this crisis to determine the patient's wishes. Having such discussions with family members and/or patients is not an easy matter, as anyone who has ever been part of such discussions knows, although it often turns out to be not as difficult as expected.[16] In any case, we need to be reminded here of the virtue of courage and its implications for the idea that those who deal with the terminally ill, whether as physicians or as family members, need to find the courage to talk to them about their wishes so that we have the relevant information in cases like this.

We've seen patients without a family, patients whose families wish further care, and patients whose families wish aggressive care to be stopped. But we have not exhausted all of the possibilities. In the final section of this chapter, we will look at three additional cases, cases in which the patient is incompetent and in which the family and providers are both present and divided. This total division and ambiguity among all of the parties will make these last three cases so difficult.

## 6.4   Incompetent Patients Whose Families Are in Disagreement or Unsure

*CASE NO 24. "Can't you see that she's changed her mind?":*
*Dealing with conflicting wishes*

FACTS   Ms. X is a 57-year-old woman with a long history of medical problems for which she has refused care. She has a documented history of aortic valve disease, for which she has refused surgery, and a ten-year history of COPD which has become progressively worse. She presented a few days ago after suffering several episodes of blacking out. These were shown to be caused by intermittent third-degree heart block. The normal treatment would be to insert a pacemaker. In accordance with her usual approach, Ms. X initially refused permission. However, when her brother and sister realized that she could die without the insertion of the pacemaker, they talked her into signing a form consenting to surgery. Her pulmonary problems required prior treatment, so she was being treated with medications and pulmonary toilet in preparation for eventual surgery. However, it became increasingly clear that this was inadequate, and the suggestion was made that she be intubated. Despite her agreement to have the surgery and her agreement with the medical management of the pulmonary problems, she absolutely refused to be intubated, although it was not clear that she fully understood what was at stake. She is now severely hypoxemic ($PaO_2 = 30$) and disoriented. In accordance with her wishes, the physicians do not want to intubate her. In the meantime, her brother, who was sitting with her, heard her saying, "Help, breathe," which he interpreted as her saying that she wished to be helped to breathe. He insists, therefore, that she be intubated. The sister sees it differently. She wants the doctors to do something to relieve the discomfort caused by Ms. X's gasping for breath, but she believes that it would be wrong to intubate her because of her long history of refusing medical care and her specific decision to refuse intubation.

QUESTIONS    Everyone has a profound sense of uncertainty about what to do here. To begin with, there is the question of how binding should be Ms. X's previous refusal of intubation. Her brother insists that it must be overruled by her current desire for help to breathe, even if that desire is not that of a competent patient. He insists that she didn't understand what it would be like to die gasping for breath, and he urges that her earlier wishes be disregarded. He says, moreover, that Ms. X's agreement to surgery shows that she really wants to live. The sister, on the other hand, believes that the patient's firmly expressed wishes when she was competent must take precedence. She agrees that the patient wants some help, but she interprets the patient's wishes as a desire for relief from gasping for breath, and she raises the question of sedation by morphine. This conflict between brother and sister is shared by most of the team caring for the patient. They also don't know what weight should be given to Ms. X's earlier expressed wishes and what weight should be given to her current desire for relief. Some, however, don't see the issue that way. They feel that the patient's previously expressed wishes are too confused to be taken seriously and that this should be treated as a case of family decision making. They have pushed the brother and sister to say what they would want done for the patient if the decision were up to them. Unfortunately, even when the question is put to them that way, the brother and sister disagree. The brother says that if it were up to him, he would urge intubation, continued attempts to reverse the pulmonary problems, and the insertion of a pacemaker, hoping that this would buy Ms. X some good years. The sister is impressed by the fact that Ms. X has been so sick for so long and by the fact that her long-term outlook is just not that good. If it were up to her, she would just let Ms. X die. Whose wishes should take precedence when family members disagree? There is still a third set of questions raised by this case, having to do with the sedation of patients gasping for breath. Some view this as a perfectly appropriate act of compassion when the decision is made not to intubate the patient. Others wonder whether this isn't active euthanasia. They feel that the patient should be either intubated or left to die without any use of morphine. Ethical, legal, and medical questions are involved here. There are substantial clinical questions about how much morphine can be given to relieve distress without compromising respiratory functioning, as well as substantial ethical and legal questions about whether compromising respiratory functioning would constitute an illegitimate crossing of the borderline between passive and active euthanasia.

THEORETICAL ANALYSIS    The case of Ms. X is very perplexing because we have too much information about patient and family wishes, and this information leads to conflicting conclusions. Our problem is how to sort out this conflicting information to help resolve the issues raised by the case.

One thing seems clear. The choice we face at this point is between intubating the patient and providing her with simple relief for her gasping for breath by use of morphine, subject to the upper limitations on the use of morphine noted in section 6.3. Judicious use of morphine is morally licit, so there is no reason to withhold the compassionate aid Ms. X needs if we don't intubate her. In other words, the choice facing us is whether to simply relieve her current suffering or to attempt to save her life through aggressive management of her current pulmonary problems followed by surgery.

It becomes clear that there is at least one significant moral appeal which unequivocally argues for aggressive management of the patient's current pulmonary problems and for surgery. This is the appeal to respect for persons. Ms. X, if she is aggressively managed during her current crisis, has a good chance of being able to go home and resume for a substantial period of time her normal life activities, which have included until now a great many of those activities whose performance we value so greatly. The appeal to respect for persons is far more significant here than it was in many of the earlier cases (e.g., Mr. W) because she has the prospect of normal functioning for a considerable period of time, something which has not been true for many of our previous patients in whom we have invoked this appeal. It would be even more significant if we could be sure that our aggressive efforts would succeed. The chances seem good enough, however, to give this appeal considerable significance. So we begin with a strong argument for trying to pull this lady through.

What about the appeal to consequences for this patient and for her family? Here we begin to encounter ambiguities. Is Ms. X's continued existence for a lengthy period of time with normal functioning something she desires? Does she see it as a positive result? We cannot ask her. All we can look at are her previous decisions. But shall we look at the decisions she made in past years not to be treated and her decision just before she became incompetent not to be intubated? Or should we look at the fact that she did agree to the insertion of the pacemaker when she recognized that she would otherwise die? The answer, I believe, is that we need to look to both; each teaches something different about her values. Her many refusals, both in the past and just before she became incompetent, testify to her negative evaluation of undergoing health care. Her willingness to undergo pacemaker installation testifies to her desire to live and her view that continued existence is a positive value for her. Having both of these desires is a perfectly possible, even if frustrating, desire structure. Which of these values is more important to her? There is a modest argument that suggests that continued existence is a greater positive value for her. On the one occasion when she clearly confronted the question of dying or allowing herself to be treated, she agreed to be operated on so as to avoid dying. Her refusals before the current hospitalization did not involve confronting this question in a direct fashion. Her refusal of intubation just before she became incompetent did not necessarily raise this question to her, since we have no clear evidence that she understood when she refused intubation that this would mean she would die. The evidence we have, as conflicting as it is, does suggest on the whole that in her estimation survival is a greater gain than the loss of undergoing medical therapy. If this argument is correct, then we have an appeal to the consequences for her (as judged by her) which argues on behalf of continued care.

What about the consequences for the rest of her family? The two most relevant family members seem to be her brother and sister. Each strongly desires that we follow a different option, and so one would benefit and the other would lose whichever option we adopt, and there is no reason to think that the gain to one would be greater than the loss to the other. The appeal to the consequence for the family does not lead to any conclusions.

We come now to the procedural right to refuse care. Two such rights might be invoked in this case: the right of the patient to refuse care and the right of the family of the incompetent patient to refuse care.

How significant is the appeal to the patient's refusal of intubation? Many factors speak on both sides of this question. On the one hand, her refusal of intubation, while itself a relatively new refusal, is part of a long-standing pattern of refusal of medical care and therefore seems to carry the greater significance of a long-standing refusal. Moreover, it seems to be rooted in some central beliefs and values of this patient. Exactly what these values and/or beliefs are remains a mystery (and it is unfortunate that this issue has never been explored with the patient in the past), but it remains a fact that her refusal of intubation just before she became incompetent carries with it considerable significance because of what it is rooted in. But that is not the full story. On the other side, probably the most significant factor is the question of the patient's competency to refuse care. There are significant reasons for doubting Ms. X's full competency. One is the fact that the patient was already hypoxemic at the time in question, although certainly not as badly as she is now. That automatically entails certain hesitations about the complete competency of the patient. But perhaps even more significant is the fact that the immediate life-threatening nature of her problem was not made sufficiently clear to her, and she was operating with less than the full information required to be a fully competent decision maker. This might explain her refusal of intubation just shortly after her acceptance of the idea of surgery. In short, then, we have a definite refusal of care of mixed significance. Some would add that her current confused remarks are testimony to her desire to be helped to breathe and therefore a reversal of her refusal of intubation. However, we shouldn't be moved by that argument. To begin with, she is now clearly incompetent, so any reversal of her earlier decision made at a time when she was more competent, even though not fully competent, should hardly count. Moreover, it is not clear that she is doing anything more than expressing great discomfort at her inability to breathe. The evidence of a reversal of her refusal is just too marginal, if present at all, to weigh in our deliberations.[17]

What about the right of the family to refuse care for Ms. X? The trouble is that the argument is blocked by the fact that the family is split. We have no evidence that either of these siblings was closer to the patient or that the patient would have preferred one to speak for her rather than the other. It was argued in chapters 2 and 4 that the right of the family to refuse care for the patient is in fact a delegated authority of the patient to the family to exercise the patient's right to refuse care. It was also argued that it is a right had by the family member who is closest to the patient (where, in the case of the previously competent adult patient, that it is to be understood as the right of the person who is most likely to be the one the patient would have chosen). When family members are in disagreement about what ought to be done for a no longer competent patient and where there is a family member who is more likely to be the person the patient would have chosen, then we have a basis for following the wishes of that particular family member. When there is no such individual who is clearly the one the patient would have chosen, but when all of the prime candidates are in agreement about what should be done, then we have a basis for following their agreed-upon decision. When there is no such person and no such consensus, but there is a clear majority of the relevant candidates wishing a particular approach, then perhaps we have a basis for following their wishes on the grounds that it is more likely[18] that they include among them the person the patient would have chosen. But in our case, none of these reasons applies, we have no basis for determining whose wishes should be followed, and we have no basis for invoking the right of the closest family member to refuse treatment.

Our analysis seems to lead to the conclusion that this patient ought to be intubated, pulled through the current crisis, and prepared for the insertion of a pacemaker. The major hesitation arises from the conflicting evidence about the patient's values. Should we be totally wrong about all of this, and should it turn out that the patient really prefers to die, then she will have another chance no matter what we have done. She still faces the life-threatening heart block and will have another opportunity when she is clearly competent to refuse life-saving therapy and to choose to die. That is, of course, not the major argument that we have offered for treating her aggressively at this point, but it should serve to console us with the thought that we have a way of avoiding permanently imposing an unwanted life on this patient if we have misunderstood her wishes and values.

*CASE NO 25. "Who is the patient, anyway?":*
*The difficulties of compassion*

FACTS   Mr. Y is a 48-year-old man with a long history of diabetes and serious kidney problems. About a year ago, he required a left nephrectomy. A week ago, he was admitted to the hospital in a coma. His neurological status improved slightly after admission so that he was responsive to pain but to little else. As his treatment continued, his respiratory status worsened. He required intubation and mechanical ventilation. Moreover, he became hypotensive and required dopamine. At that point, his only relative in the community, a cousin with whom he lived, agreed to a "do not resuscitate" order, saying that the man's situation looked hopeless and he saw no point in prolonging the agony. In fact, the cousin challenged the continued use of the dopamine and the ventilator in light of the patient's dim prognosis. That issue was being actively discussed by the staff when a further complication arose. The cousin contacted Mr. Y's son, from whom Mr. Y had been alienated for many years, and the son spoke to the physician of record and demanded that everything be done to keep his father alive, including resuscitating him if he arrested. The son wanted to have a last chance to see his father and make his peace with him. The physician explained that the father's mental status made a reconciliation impossible, but Mr. Y's son responded by saying that even if his father couldn't understand, he had expressions of regret that he had to say to his father. The cousin is furious about this. He claims that the only thing the doctor should worry about is not prolonging Mr. Y's agony. In addition, the staff is acutely aware of the fact that Mr. Y's continued support in the ICU, which is very crowded, means that there are other potential patients who could benefit more from its services who might not be admitted to the ICU and that actual patients already in the unit are not getting everything from which they could benefit.

QUESTIONS    Some staff members feel that the whole issue should be settled by considering the patient's dim prognosis and the crowded conditions in the ICU. They feel that it is inappropriate to lower the level of care for everyone in the unit in order to keep Mr. Y alive for a short period of time. Others feel that even a DNR order, and certainly a discontinuation of dopamine or of the ventilator, requires the consent of the family appropriately (even if not entirely) considering what is in the best interests of the patient and cannot be settled simply on the basis of the unit's problems. This latter group, however, is severely divided over which family member should make the decision. Some argue that it ought to be the cousin, the only member of the family who has lived near the patient and who has been close to the patient in recent years. Others argue that the choice belongs to the son, because the son is, after all, the closest relation. There is still a third group who sees this case entirely differently. Their view is that it would be an act of compassion to allow his son his chance to express his final farewells to his father, even if (or perhaps precisely because) they have been alienated for all these years. They feel that this compassionate act justifies maintaining Mr. Y for a day or two until the son can come to see his father. Others sharply disagree. They feel that the patient's interests are what have to be considered and not the needs of the son. As one of them put it, who is the patient?

THEORETICAL ANALYSIS    The case of Mr. Y is particularly interesting because it reminds us once more that, in making difficult life-and-death decisions, we are making decisions that affect the family as well as the patient and that we need to consider the needs of the family.

Two moral appeals argue for continued aggressive care for Mr. Y, including resuscitating him if necessary. One is the appeal to the consequences for Mr. Y's son; the other is an appeal to the virtue of compassion. Both of these appeals are rooted in the fact that Mr. Y's son, who has been estranged from him for many years, has a very strong need to see his father alive for a short period of time before the father dies and can do so only if the patient is aggressively managed for the next day or two until the son arrives. Some people have difficulty understanding the son's request because they point out that Mr. Y's mental status will not allow the son to successfully communicate with Mr. Y. This is true. The son may well be talking to a father who cannot hear what he has to say. None of this takes away from the fact that the son feels this great need to say what he has to say to his father while the father is still alive, and an approach that will enable the son to do this has consequences for the son which the son evaluates as very important. Moreover, if he is denied this opportunity (especially if he knows that he could have had the opportunity if only people had managed his father's care a bit more aggressively), the son is likely to feel a great sense of loss and suffering. The virtue of compassion calls us to help the son avoid this suffering, if possible. Moreover, both of these appeals have considerable force in this case, because the son's desire is very strong and because the sense of suffering he is likely to feel if he does not have this opportunity is likely to be great.

There are several arguments against following the request of the son, and each needs to be looked at carefully. They include the right of the truly closest family member—the cousin—to refuse further care for this patient, possible detrimental consequences to the patient, and the allocations of resources within the ICU.

The cousin is refusing further care for this patient. While it is true that the son is the legally closest family member, it is also true that the cousin has actually been the closest person to the patient for many years. In light of the analysis of closeness in chapters 2 and 4, the cousin is likely to be the closest family member, the one entitled to exercise the right of decision making for this patient, because the cousin is most likely to be the person Mr. Y would have chosen to make decisions for him. It is understandable why the law has its rule about the closest family member. It is also understandable why that rule does not correspond in cases like this to moral reality. So there is a moral argument against further aggressive care for this patient, including an argument against resuscitating this patient: the closest family member has refused that care. How significant is that appeal in this case? This is not a long-standing refusal, even if it is a perfectly reasonable and appropriate reaction to the sudden crisis the patient is in. Moreover, even if we aggressively maintain this patient, we would not be totally disregarding the wishes of the cousin but simply postponing following those wishes for a day or two to allow the son to get here. When this is explained to the cousin, so that it is clear that we are not going to be imposing on this patient any long-term aggressive management, the cousin might agree to this short-term aggressive management. But even if the cousin does not agree and exercises his right to refuse further care for the patient, there are still factors that give our short-term disregarding of that refusal less than its usual significance.

The second appeal is to the consequences for the patient. But there is a grave difficulty in ascertaining what such an appeal implies in a case like this. How would the patient assess the consequence of being kept alive for a day or two with a certain amount of pain and discomfort so as to allow his son to come and say what he has to say? We really have no way of knowing how the patient would have assessed these consequences. So, contrary to what was said by some members of the team, we have no way of knowing what an appeal to the consequences for the patient says about this case, and this is not a clear-cut case of a conflict between what is best for the patient and what is best for the family.

We turn to the third and perhaps most important argument against the aggressive management of this patient, the question of its implications for other actual and potential patients in the ICU. One way of looking at this argument is as an appeal to the consequence for others. Another way sees it as an appeal to the injustice of this allocation of scarce resources. These are significant considerations, but the case description does not enable us to ascertain just how significant they are. We are just not given enough information to know whether or not the continued aggressive management of this patient for only a day or two is going to impose a grave burden on actual or potential patients in this ICU. Naturally, the more claimants for a place in the unit and the more crowded the unit, the more these considerations will count against the son's request. Again, in thinking about these issues, it is important to keep in mind that we are only contemplating a short-term aggressive management of this case, just long enough to allow the son to come and say his farewells to his father.

All of this seems to lead to the following conclusions. First, the cousin should be approached with the suggestion that he concur with the son's request for short-term aggressive management (including resuscitation) for Mr. Y with a clear understanding that this aggressive management will come to an end as soon as the son arrives and says his farewells to his father. Second, if the cousin agrees, but perhaps even if he doesn't agree, this option should be adopted as a compassionate act aimed at relieving the suffering of the son. Third, none of this should be done, however, if the consequences for other actual or potential patients of the short-term aggressive extension of this patient's life become seriously detrimental. The appeal to compassion is an important moral appeal which calls on us to make extra efforts to alleviate the suffering of the families of the dying. It is not important enough, however, to call on other sick patients to suffer severe losses.

*CASE 26. "What do you do when nobody has any strong feelings?":
A look at total ambiguity*

FACTS   Mr. Z is a 72-year-old man with a long history of snoring and coughing. A recent chest X-ray showed an infiltrate near the hylum, and a bronchoscopy confirmed the diagnosis of oat-cell carcinoma of the lung. There is no evidence of metastatic disease. The decision was made to put him on radiation therapy and chemotherapy in light of their demonstrated success in prolonging life in such cases. Just before treatment was begun, he became acutely short of breath, was moved into the ICU, and was intubated. In the next few days, his condition deteriorated rapidly. He went into renal failure, and it was impossible to wean him from his ventilator. At that point, the question arose about what to do for this patient. His family had been very supportive of the earlier decisions made by the physicians with the patient's strong concurrence to treat him aggressively. They felt that he wanted to survive and that they would be there with him, for better or for worse. Now, with his rapidly deteriorating condition, they are not so sure. They wish they could ask him, but his neurological status has deteriorated sufficiently so that one can't have any real conversations with him, although he is by no means fully comatose. They just don't know what to do, and neither does the staff.

QUESTIONS   Many members of the staff feel that this issue should be settled solely on the basis of the patient's medical prognosis. Although Mr. Z's rapid decline has been surprising, it inspires little optimism. In any case, in light of his underlying carcinoma, the patient does not have a long life expectancy. They conclude, therefore, that the best thing to do is to just keep the patient comfortable and let him die. Most members of the staff cannot agree. They find it hard to accept the claim that this patient will not survive the present crisis, in large measure because they do not understand why the crisis has developed but also because they suspect that it might be reversible with aggressive treatment. They concede that the patient's long-term prognosis is not good, but they argue that if he can be pulled through the current crisis he can have some good time. They are unwilling to stop aggressive care unless the family insists; they feel there is no clear medical basis for such a decision. Unfortunately, the family is unwilling to make that decision. Some members of this group argue that the benefit of the doubt should be given to aggressive treatment. Other do not see the justification for this presumption. They are unclear about what ought to be done, but they feel that any decision needs to be justified and that the presumption appealed to is illegitimate.

THEORETICAL ANALYSIS   The case of Mr. Z is very troubling, as is evidenced by the total lack of firm conviction on the part of either the family or the care providers. Let us begin by examining this case from the perspective of the appeal to consequences.

If Mr. Z is not managed aggressively at this point, with the hope of pulling him through the current crisis so that he can receive the originally planned chemotherapy and radiation therapy, then he will die in the very near future. If he is managed aggressively, then there certainly is some chance that therapy can succeed in buying him some good time. Is this chance worth all the burdens to Mr. Z of the care in question? We do know that he chose to undergo radiation therapy and chemotherapy in the hope it would buy him some good months. His cancer is very responsive, at least in the short run, to the aggressive use of these modalities of care. So we know that he values prolongation of life sufficiently to undergo very rigorous radiation therapy and chemotherapy. That is some indication of how he might evaluate the consequences of the current choice, but it cannot be taken as conclusive evidence. The probability of a successful outcome is now much lower in light of the current crisis, and what he must undergo at this point is even more invasive than the initial therapy for his cancer. So, while we have some indication that he might see the favorable consequences of aggressive therapy at this point as worth the effort, we cannot take his earlier agreement to undergo therapy as anything like definitive evidence. At most, the appeal to consequences for the patient, as evaluated by the patient, might give rise to a modest argument for continued aggressive therapy.

Several crucial points which emerged in the discussion of earlier cases are relevant here. First, the decision in this case, as in many others, cannot be settled by some appeal to total futility. We can rarely say that continued aggressive care is futile in the sense that there is no chance that it will in any way affect the outcome for the patient. In this case, claims of futility (as opposed to improbability of success) of the current aggressive care are particularly suspect in light of a lack of knowledge about the etiology of the current crisis. The real question is whether or not the burdens of the care in question are worth the possible successful outcome in light of the values of the patient. That is why an appeal to consequence always is an appeal to consequences as evaluated by the patient. Second, figuring out whether it is worth it to the patient, particularly when the patient cannot help us at the current moment, is very tricky. We have to fall back on such expressions of the patient's values as we have available to us and try to infer how much the patient would value various outcomes. That is particularly difficult when, as in cases like this, the attitudes were those the patient expressed when facing one set of circumstances, but the patient is now facing a different set of circumstances. These two points undercut the arguments offered by various members of the team in this case. Those who argue that there is no point to continued care for Mr. Z because such care is futile have failed to take into account the first point. Those who argue that Mr. Z's earlier choice for chemotherapy and radiation therapy is an indication of how he would value possible outcomes of the current choice have failed to take into account the second point. Properly taking both of these points into account results in a better evaluation of the appeal to consequences for the patient, and that evaluation tells us that we have at most a modest argument from the appeal to consequences for continued aggressive care.

What other arguments are there for continued care? Can one, for example, appeal to the respect for persons to provide such an argument? If Mr. Z can be pulled through the current crisis, and if the resulting chemotherapy and radiation therapy are successful, then he will be able to resume for some period of time those activities whose performance we value so greatly. So perhaps the appeal to respect for persons argues for continued care in this case. If it does, and I believe it does, it offers only a modest argument for continued care. As we saw in chapter 4, the appeal to respect for persons will have less significance as an argument for a particular course of action when, as in this case, the likelihood of the patient being restored to an appropriate level of functioning is relatively low.

What arguments are there against continued treatment? If the family was opposed to continued treatment, then we would have an argument from their right to refuse treatment for this patient, a right whose significance we would have to evaluate carefully. In fact, however, the best way to describe the condition of the family is that they are confused. They are not insisting on further care, but they are also not demanding that care be stopped. There is no question here of choosing the family member who is closest to the patient, since these members are not in conflict with each other but rather are jointly unsure about what they want done. The right to refuse care, either as exercised by the patient or as exercised by the family, offers no argument in this case against continued therapy. And it is not clear what are the other arguments against continued care.

Some members of the team have talked about the presumption in favor of continued care; others have challenged the existence of such a presumption. The challengers are right in insisting that there should not be a general presumption in favor of continued care. None of the moral appeals discussed in this book justifies such a general presumption. However, those who argue for it in this case have a point. The patient's own expressed values provide a very modest continued presumption on behalf of continued care. Moreover, the appeal to respect for persons in cases like this provides a modest presumption in favor of continued aggressive care. So we need to accept that presumption in this case while recognizing that it is not a valid general presumption in favor of continued aggressive therapy in all cases.

There is something very unsatisfactory about the resolution of this case. We move forward without any overwhelming confidence that we are acting rightly. Still, there is some basis for moving forward and no principled basis for not doing so. It is perhaps fitting that we end our examination of cases involving adult patients with this recognition that however sophisticated the conceptual machinery we bring to bear on these difficult cases, there will be cases (like that of Mr. Z) in which our analysis leads us in a direction we ultimately follow while simultaneously recognizing that there is no reason for tremendous confidence in the rightness of what we are doing. Perhaps we can be consoled by the thought that this recognition is a sign of increased sophistication about the ambiguities and difficulties of the moral life rather than a sign of intellectual failure.

## Notes

1. The policy options are to have the family concur or to insist that a guardian be appointed. *Superintendent* v. *Saikewicz* 370 N.E. 2d 417 (1977) was widely read as a decision saying that a formal guardian always needs to be appointed. In the Matter of *Dinnerstein* 380 N.E. 2d 124 (1978) helped clarify that the courts would be satisfied with the concurrence of the family in deciding to forego care when the patient was irreversibly ill and death was imminent. Besides being more practical, this policy can be justified by an appeal to the consequences for the family, who might feel very hurt by the need to involve a stranger in their affairs. There has been much less litigation on what to do if there is no family present, as in our case. A Meisel et al., "Hospital Guidelines for Deciding about Life-Sustaining Treatment," *Critical Care Medicine* 14, no. 3 (March 1986): 239–46, offer the following: "In the case of intractable conflict among family members or when there is no appropriate person to serve as surrogate and the patient has not previously designated a surrogate, the judicial appointment of a surrogate must be sought" (p. 245). They fail to say, however, what these surrogates, who are strangers, are supposed to do.

2. This suggestion needs amplification. We have here a case of a surrogate who is a stranger to the patient and who has no testimony about the patient's probable views about the value of her life and/or the patient's wishes about what should be done. So what can the surrogate do? One thing is to review the evidence to see whether there isn't some neglected source of information. A second thing is to review the evidence to see whether the medical conclusions are firmly held by all involved. This could, of course, be done by the team as well. But since they have become advocates of a certain approach, and as their advocacy is

seen to be related to their own (appropriate) frustration, there is something to be said for appointing an outsider. It could be an outsider from the hospital, someone not part of the team, but the appearance of propriety argues for a total outsider, a court-appointed guardian.

3. This likelihood will be reinforced if we remember to explain to Mr. O that one of the reasons for treating his infection was to enable him to recover sufficiently so that we could determine his wishes. If we assume, as was suggested in chapter 2, that many people have an independent desire to be decision makers for themselves, then this increases the probability that he will see the treatment of his infection as having satisfied his relevant desires.

4. My experience with the appointment of guardians is that they are usually lawyers known to the probate judge who are total strangers to the patient. Such guardians can, even with the best of intentions, serve only the limited roles indicated above in note 2. The appointment of close friends of the patient as guardians would be a much better approach, since there is much more they can do.

5. More recent legal developments could have helped Mr. P effectuate his wishes. In the common law, powers of attorney created before a person became incompetent lapsed at the time of incompetency. Hence, Mr. P needed to ask his friend to be appointed guardian if and when Mr. P became incompetent. Newer legal doctrines allow for "durable powers of attorney," which come into effect at the time of incompetency and remain in effect through that incompetency. Those in Mr. P's situation are well advised to consider creating such a durable power of attorney. On these recent developments, see President's Commission for the Study of Ethical Problems in Medicine, *Deciding to Forego Life-Sustaining Treatment* (Washington, D.C.: Government Printing Office, 1983), pp. 145–47. Recent natural-death-act statutes, such as the Texas Natural Death Act of 1985, make provisions (sections 3c and 4b) for issuing a durable power of attorney for the limited purpose of refusing life-sustaining care when death is imminent.

6. That such a patient is not dead is clear from the language of all current brain-death statutes. The clearest is the Uniform Determination of Death Act 12 *U.L.A.* 271 (Supp. 1985), which says: "An individual who has sustained either (1) irreversible cessation of circulatory and respiratory functions or (2) irreversible cessation of all functions of the entire brain, including the brainstem, is dead." Ms. T satisfies neither criterion. Some would redefine death so as to cover cases like that of Ms. T. They include: R. Veatch, "The Definition of Death: Ethical, Philosophical, and Policy Confusion," 315 *Annals of N.Y. Academy of Science* 307 (1978); Youngner and Bartlett, "Human Death and High Technology: The Failure of Whole Brain Formulations," 99 *Annals of Internal Medicine* 252 (1983); and, most recently, D. Smith, "Legal Recognition of Neocortical Death," 71 *Cornell Law Review* 850 (1986). My criticism of their suggestions will be found in B. Brody, "Ethical Questions Raised by the Persistent Vegetative Patient," *Hastings Center Report* 17 (December 1987).

7. The longest cases are described in note 16 to p. 177 of President's Commission, *Deciding to Forego Life-Sustaining Treatment* (Washington, D.C.: Government Printing Office, 1983).

8. For further discussion of this point, see note 52 in chapter 2.

9. This differentiates our case from the much discussed recent cases of *Brophy* (Massachusetts) and *Jobes* (New Jersey). In both of those cases, there was considerable evidence that the patient would *not* have wanted to survive this way and that the patient's survival would actually be a *loss* for the patient. In the *Jobes* case, there even was evidence that the patient had waived her right not to be killed if she was ever in a comatose state.

10. In one such case that I followed closely for a period of time, the best estimate for the annual cost of keeping the patient alive was in the range of one hundred thousand to one hundred fifty thousand dollars (1984 dollars).

11. An alternative suggestion would be to stop feeding and/or providing fluids for this patient. That suggestion has recently (March 15, 1986) been defended by the AMA's Council on Ethical and Judicial Affairs, and by the Massachusett court, with considerable dissent, in *Patrica E. Brophy* vs. *New England Sinai Hospital* (Supreme Judicial Council of Mass., September 11, 1986). My argument for agreeing with the dissenting judges will be found in Brody, "Ethical Questions."

12. A review of the various statutes collected and/or described in Society for the Right to Die, *Handbook of 1985 Living Will Laws* (New York: Society for the Right to Die, 1986), indicates that some requirement that the death is "imminent" or "will occur in a short time" is nearly universal in all of these statutes. It is even found in the more permissive recommendation of the Uniform Rights of the Terminally Ill Act adopted by the National Conference of Commissioners on August 2–9, 1985, and reprinted in the *Handbook* on pp. 35–47.

13. To quote as representative the Texas Natural Death Act of 1985: "Nothing in this act shall be construed to condone, authorize, or approve mercy killing, or to permit any affirmation or deliberate act or omission to end life other than to permit the natural process of dying as provided in this act" (sec. 10).

14. This could be based on an intentional rather than a causal analysis of killing. That intentional analysis is challenged in chapter 2. It might also be based on an appeal to the principle of double effect. See my discussion of that doctrine in note 18 of chapter 5.

15. This is the basis of a powerful argument for preferring durable powers of attorney over living wills.

16. It often turns out that the patient has just been waiting for an opportunity to talk about fears of death, concerns about the dying process, and his or her wishes. The loneliness of the patient who has no opportunity to have these discussions was best portrayed by Leo Tolstoy in his classic work, *The Death of Ivan Illich*. Recent scholarship has simply confirmed Tolstoy's insights. For pediatric patients, see M. Bluebond-Langner, *The Private Worlds of Dying Children* (Princeton: Princeton Univ. Press, 1978). For all patients, see B. Schoenberg et al., *Anticipatory Grief* (New York: Columbia Univ. Press, 1974).

17. All of this suggests that the revocation clauses in natural-death acts may be in trouble in real cases. Moreover, some of them explicitly allow, for reasons that are unclear, revocations by incompetent patients. Section 4(a) of the Texas Natural Death Act, says, for example: "A directive may be revoked at any time by the declarant, without regard to his mental state or competency . . ."

18. I say "perhaps" because this argument invokes a version of the principle of indifference (if we have no evidence, then each possibility is equally likely), which needs justification.

# 7

## Cases Involving Children

In chapters 5 and 6, we were introduced to twenty-six patients whose management posed significant ethical issues. Those cases involved adult patients. In this final chapter, we will look at an additional fourteen patients about whom serious life-and-death decisions need to be made. All of these cases involve children. Some are newborns; others are older children. We will begin with decision making for newborns in cases where the parents insist on further care for their newborn while the caregivers are not sure whether that is appropriate and the opposite type of cases in which the parents want to stop care while the caregivers are not sure of the appropriateness of decision.[1] Finally, we will look at a set of cases involving older children.

### 7.1 Parents Who Want Continued Care for Their Newborn Children

*CASE NO 27. "Save my child and my marriage":*
*Distinguishing motives from decisions*

FACTS    Baby A was born to a 23-year old woman who arrived at the hospital just a few minutes before actual delivery. The baby suffered some perinatal asphyxia and displayed symptoms at birth compatible with respiratory distress syndrome. Because of his difficulties in breathing, Baby A required placement on a respirator. In addition, the baby had an esophageal atresia and a tracheoesophageal fistula. Unfortunately, four days after birth, the stomach perforated and this required emergency surgery. He then developed seizures and was diagnosed as having very significant intraventricular bleeding (bilateral grade three). The chances of this child's survival, in light of all of these worsening problems, is not high. But even if he does survive, the outlook for normal neurologic functioning is problematic.

194

The social history surrounding Baby A complicates matters further. The mother and father have had a stormy marriage, and they separated during the pregnancy. They reunited shortly before the birth, but the relationship is still very troubled. The father blames the mother for all of Baby A's problems, claiming that the baby would have been well if she had gone to the hospital earlier. Attempts to explain to him that this was at most a small contributory factor have failed. He wants nothing more to do with her. She, however, very much hopes that he will return to her if she can take the child home. Moreover, she has tremendous guilt feelings about the child, despite the many attempts to explain to her that his problems are not her fault, and these feelings lead her to insist on full aggressive care.

QUESTIONS    The staff taking care of Baby A finds this case very troubling. Some see aggressive therapy as contraindicated in this case. The child's stormy course suggests a dim prognosis. They feel that this child is doomed to die no matter what is done, and they cannot see the point of continued aggressive care and prolongation of his agony. Other members of the team see this case differently. They admit that the child has many serious problems, but they argue that each of these problems is manageable, and there exists a real, even if not very high, probability that the child will survive. How futile must care be before we judge that it should be discontinued? Then there is the question of the quality of the child's life. In light of the asphyxia and the intraventricular bleeding, the likelihood of normal neurologic functioning if the child survives is dim. But it is very difficult to say how badly retarded the child will be. Some see little point in imposing a child with severe neurologic deficits on a family like this. Such a child, they argue, can have a decent chance only if there is a strong supportive family prepared to do the most for him. That isn't present in this case. Other members of the team find it hard to accept this claim. There is too much uncertainty about the quality of life, they argue, to use that as a basis for withholding further aggressive care. Moreover, they challenge the legitimacy of using social factors (such as family stability) as a basis for making medical decisions.

These debates have seriously split the team. But there are still further issues. The director of the neonatal ICU thinks that his entire staff has incorrectly analyzed this case. As far as he is concerned, the choice about further aggressive care for this child is to be made by the mother and the father. He thinks that all of these issues and arguments should be put before them and that they should decide whether the child should be aggressively managed. Other members of the team strongly disagree. Some claim that no parents facing the sudden crisis of a newborn with severe problems are in a position to make these difficult decisions. Others think that some parents might be able to make these decisions, but they don't think that this particular mother is qualified to do so. They feel that she is too influenced by her guilt and her desire to use the child to save her marriage. Why, they ask, should a person who is not focusing on the interests of the child make crucial decisions for that child?

THEORETICAL ANALYSIS    It is clear that the personal problems of this mother have troubled those who have to deal with Baby A. They understand and sympathize with her problems, but they would prefer that she focus on the child's welfare rather than her plan to use the baby as a way of reuniting her family. But it is important to analyze this case impartially, examining what each moral appeal has to say about it, and attending to the mother's motives only when they turn out to be relevant to assessing the significance of a particular appeal.

Let us begin by examining the appeal to the consequences of our actions for the patient. The issue before the team is how aggressively they should manage Baby A. One thing is reasonably clear: without aggressive management of all of his problems, Baby A will die in a relatively short period of time. Even with aggressive management of these problems, there is a very substantial probability that the baby will die anyway. But there is a real probability of survival with aggressive management, since, as some members of the team have pointed out, none of Baby A's problems is inherently unresolvable.[2] Is that survival a beneficial consequence for the child? Some have argued that it is not, since Baby A may suffer long-term disabilities and retardation because of the extensive damage to his brain. That claim is much too strong for two reasons. First, it is difficult to say at this point how extensive the retardation will be if he survives. And, second, even if there is a significant degree of neurologic damage, with resulting extensive disabilities, it is hard to say with any confidence that the resulting life will not be worth living and that Baby A would be better off dead than alive. Others have argued that it is a beneficial consequence for Baby A since his life would be a life worth living. But that claim is also too strong for two reasons. Given all the neurologic damage, with the resulting extensive disabilities, it is equally hard to say that his life will be worth living. And even if it is, it might be at such a low level of functioning that his survival would be at best a modest benefit, outweighed by the discomfort of all of the necessary invasive treatments. It is hard to draw a conclusion about what the appeal to the consequences for Baby A would imply for this case, because we just don't know what the consequences will be.[3]

What about the consequences for the family? One immediate beneficial consequence for the mother of aggressive treatment is the satisfaction of having her wishes for her child respected. Perhaps, more speculatively, it might also lead to the desirable consequence (in her estimation) of reuniting her family. These favorable consequences for the mother have to be weighed against the possibility that aggressive management of the child might eventually produce a real loss for her, even when the consequences are evaluated from her perspective, if she has to take home a badly retarded child and raise him without the help of his father. Further speculations arise. The mother has the option, if the child survives and the father doesn't return, of putting Baby A up for adoption. In the current climate, where there are many desperate childless families chasing few available children, this may be a realistic possibility. The further speculative consequences for the mother are therefore quite difficult to assess. The one consequence that we can feel confident about is that aggressive treatment will give the mother the satisfaction of having her wishes respected. This offers an argument with some significance for continued aggressive management of this child. What about the consequences for others? Here things are less speculative. Continued aggressive management of this child, particularly by a staff that has real doubt about its value, produces the unfavorable consequence of considerable staff unease, a problem that is particularly significant in a neonatal ICU where staff stress is always a major problem. In short, the appeal to consequences leads to very mixed results in this case.

We turn then to the question of the right of the parents (in this case, the mother) to make health-care decisions for the child. Some members of the team, particularly the director of the unit, think that it leads to a significant argument for continued aggressive care of the child, namely that the mother has a right to have her decision for aggressive care respected. This is wrong. To begin with, the mother is demanding care rather than refusing care. We have already seen that the right to refuse care is a real right; the right to get the care one demands is not a real right. So the physicians in question are not bound by any of the mother's procedural rights to provide the care she requests, although she is, of course, free to seek other physicians who will follow her wishes. Moreover, the question of the mother's motives is relevant here. Even if the mother were refusing care, her right to be a decision maker would lose much of its significance since her refusal is heavily influenced by concerns other than the well-being of the patient.

Another argument for continued aggressive care of this child is based on respect for persons. There is a real possibility of this child surviving and being able to engage in some (it's hard to say how much) of those activities whose performance we value so much. That argues for continued aggressive care. But this is obviously only a modest argument, because of the significant probability that Baby A will die or will be so retarded that he will not be able to engage in most of those valuable activities.

It is important to note that the neonatal ICU is not full at the time when these decisions have to be made and that this patient is in the private sector. No questions of cost-effectiveness and justice can be relevant unless this is a case of a fully occupied medical resource, and it is not. Should that issue have arisen, we would have had to compare Baby A and other potential beneficiaries and determine who should get aggressive care of the type that can only be provided in a neonatal ICU. Fortunately, however, that issue does not confront us in this case.

There seems to be an argument from the real immediate beneficial consequences for the mother for continued aggressive care. This argument is modestly reinforced by a consideration of an appeal to respect for persons. On the other hand, there are some real possibilities of bad consequences for the mother from further aggressive care, and further aggressive care would impose some costs on the caregivers. Is there perhaps some compromise strategy which would capture the benefits for both sides? I believe there is such a strategy, one that allows us at an appropriate time to use data then available about the likely outcome for the child. Suppose that the physicians and the mother could agree to continue aggressive care until such time, if ever, that the child's condition deteriorated in a way that made his survival much less likely and/or made the prospect of substantial functioning if the child survived much dimmer. Suppose they agreed that at that point no further aggressive measures would be employed and that some currently employed measures would be withdrawn. That would succeed in giving the mother the satisfaction of having her desires followed and would give the child some chance for survival with decent functioning. On the other hand, it would limit the potential of bad consequences for the child if he is not going to survive and/or if his prospect of substantial functioning becomes dimmer. It would put some limit on the frustrations of the providers. It would also decrease the likelihood of the mother's having to cope with a baby who survived with an extremely low level of functioning. It seems best, therefore, that the mother and those caring for Baby A should come to some such agreement.

What if they can't? What if the mother insists on every aggressive measure until the child dies, no matter how much Baby A's condition deteriorates? At that point, I am inclined to believe that the team could unilaterally impose such a decision to limit care if Baby A's condition deteriorates, because the arguments for continued aggressive care even after further deterioration would be very weak, and the arguments against that continued aggressive care would be much stronger. Then the virtues of honesty and courage would come into play. These virtues call on the physicians to at least make it clear to the mother that they will impose a limit upon the aggressive care they will give the child, leaving the mother free to seek alternative caregivers who would follow her wishes.[4] Moreover, the virtue of compassion comes into play even now, arguing for compassionate counseling to help the mother work through her feelings and problems. This case illustrates once more the importance of keeping an eye on the virtues as we think about these difficult questions.

CASE NO 28. *"God will save my child":*
*Understandable reasons for bad decisions*

FACTS   Baby B was born at 28 weeks gestational age weighing slightly more than 1000 grams. He was diagnosed shortly after birth as having respiratory distress syndrome. On day four, he suffered a cardiac arrest and was resuscitated, placed on a ventilator with 100% oxygen, and given medications to support his cardiac functioning. He subsequently suffered three more cardiac arrests; in each case, he was successfully resuscitated. An ultrasound revealed very severe bilateral intraventricular hemorrhages (grades three and four). Moreover, he has developed hydrocephalus. His prognosis is truly dim.

The child's mother is a 37-year-old woman who is married for the third time. Her first two marriages ended in divorce, and she describes her earlier self as "a wild woman." Some years ago, she says, she found God and has since been at peace with herself. She married someone who shares her religious beliefs. They were told that they were unlikely to have a child, but they prayed for one, and they now have the child for whom they prayed. They really want this child, and they believe that the pregnancy was an indication that God wanted them to have this child. They insist that if the physicians continue to resuscitate Baby B, no matter how often he arrests, he will eventually survive and become the healthy baby that they want.

QUESTIONS   In some ways, the case of Baby B is easier than that of Baby A. Baby B's chance of survival, while not nonexistent, is clearly worse. It is really a miracle that he has survived this long. In other ways, however, this is a harder case. Baby B's parents clearly believe that it is in the child's best interest that aggressive medical therapy be continued. They also believe that if they show sufficient faith, God will pull the child through. No doubt, deep psychological needs underlie these beliefs. Nevertheless, the parents of Baby B (unlike Baby A's mother) are not making decisions based on ulterior motives. That makes it harder to disregard their wishes. Many members of the team see this second factor as settling the case. From their point of view, the decision of whether or not to continue resuscitation every time the baby arrests should be a parental decision. These parents have made their decision, even if it's not necessarily the decision that the treating team would make, and it ought to be respected. Other members of the team view this as a straightforward case of medical futility. They argue that while the child can be resuscitated again and again, he will die sooner or later. They believe that if the child is not resuscitated the next time he arrests, this would save the family, the child, and the staff considerable further pain and anguish. They argue that what the parents need is compassionate counseling to accept the inevitable death of their child rather than continued deference to their unrealistic wishes.

THEORETICAL ANALYSIS    The parents of Baby B have had an easier time with the staff than the mother of Baby A. People are moved by the fact that the parents are focusing on what they perceive as best for their child, by the fact that this may be their only chance for having a child, and by the way in which they use their deep religious faith to support themselves through this crisis. But it is as important in this case as it was in the last case to differentiate our feelings about the family and their motives from the question of what we ought to do. It is vital that we analyze this case carefully, examining what each moral appeal has to say about it, and that we attend to these facts about the parents only to the extent that they are relevant in evaluating the significance of our appeals for the management of this case.

The analysis of this case must take into account that the probability of Baby B's surviving to leave the hospital is far less than the probability for Baby A. Moreover, the even greater seriousness of the bilateral intraventricular hemorrhages and the development of hydrocephalus make the prospects of Baby B's having even a modest amount of normal functioning, if he should survive, lower than the prospects for Baby A. Continued aggressive management (as the parents have pointed out) is Baby B's only chance, but the probability of a favorable outcome is extremely low, and that means that the appeal to what is best for the child cannot provide much support for continued aggressive care.[5] In fact, given that continued aggressive care imposes substantial burdens on the child as he is subjected to many invasive procedures, the appeal to the consequences for the child argues far more significantly against aggressive care. For the very same reasons, the appeal to respect for persons offers little support for continued aggressive care in the case of Baby B. In the case of Baby A, where there was a better (although not very good) probability that the child could survive and function in some of those ways we value so much, that appeal added an argument of some significance for continued care. Here, the probabilities of survival and of being able to perform substantial activities is just so low that the appeal to respect for persons can offer at most a minimal argument for continued aggressive care.

Are there any arguments for continued aggressive care which have more significance in this case? We have seen in the case of Baby A that it cannot be an argument from an appeal to the parental right to be a decision maker. One possibility is the appeal to consequences for the parents. Stopping aggressive care for Baby B, just like stopping aggressive care for Baby A, would certainly produce the undesirable consequence of parental frustration because their wishes are not being respected. In this case, as in the last, the probability of that consequence's being serious is heightened by the fact that these wishes are connected to many other important feelings and hopes. So the argument from the appeal to the consequences for the family, which was significant in the case of Baby A, is equally significant here.

What about the arguments against continued aggressive care? We have already seen that the appeal to the consequences for the patient argues against aggressive care in this case. Moreover, the appeal to the consequences for the providers, as they have to deal with their frustrations in providing aggressive care when they feel that this care is inappropriate and harmful, also speaks against aggressive care. Finally, providers whose sense of integrity is offended by care which they think is needlessly harming the baby will appeal to the virtue of integrity as an argument against further aggressive care.

In a way, Baby B's current condition resembles the condition in which Baby A's continued aggressive care would be stopped if the compromise proposal advocated in the previous case were adopted. So there is little room left here for negotiations between the physicians and the parents. Short of actually dying, despite resuscitative efforts, there is little room for further deterioration in Baby B's condition, and so there is little room for agreeing that aggressive care would be stopped if there were further deterioration. This leads to the conclusion that continued aggressive care should be stopped in this case, where that means among other things withdrawing some of the support systems that are now keeping the child going. Honesty and courage, as in the previous case, call for making clear to the parents what is being done, thereby allowing them to seek out other caregivers whose values allow them to follow the parental wishes. But the virtue of compassion needs to be mentioned here as well. It calls on the medical staff to ensure that the parents are offered counseling help by hospital chaplains and/or other clergymen from their faith to help them analyze whether their faith that God will produce a miracle for their child is the only appropriate religious response to this tragedy.

*CASE NO 29. Parents who wish to keep their dead baby intubated:*
*Forcing people to accept reality*

FACTS   Baby C's mother suffered from severe medical problems during her pregnancy. Several weeks before the birth, she was admitted to the hospital with low cardiac output and renal failure. When increased fetal distress was noted, Baby C was delivered immediately by cesarean section. The baby did not breathe at birth, and resuscitative efforts began. In the midst of these resuscitative efforts, a very acidotic cord pH of 6.73 was reported, which was consistent with the fact that there had been a 60% abruptio placenta. Resuscitation was continued despite this information, and the child was eventually successfully resuscitated and intubated. Later that day, seizures were noted. They were treated with phenobarbital. Shortly afterward, Baby C stopped showing any signs of spontaneous functioning. The staff began to suspect that the baby was clinically dead. An EEG was ordered. It was flat, but no final determination of brain death could be made because of the high phenobarbital levels. Throughout this time, the mother was unavailable for any consultation because of her own medical problems. The father was clearly in a terrible emotional state, but he insisted that everything be done to save his child. The staff was initially quite willing to do this, primarily because they thought it would be pyschologically helpful for the parents to see that every effort had been made for their child but also because they weren't sure the baby was really dead. However, from the very beginning, the neonatal ICU was crowded, and other patients who might have been helped by care in the unit had been denied transfer from outlying hospitals. Now, in light of Baby C's clinical condition, the staff is beginning to reconsider its initial willingness to go along with the father's request.

QUESTIONS    The case of Baby C, even more than those of Baby A and Baby B, forces us to confront the very difficult question of the limits of respecting parental decision making. Some members of the team remain convinced that care cannot be withheld from a baby until death is definitely determined so long as the parents wish care to be provided. Other members of the team see things differently. To begin with, they question the competency of this father to participate in decision making. He is in the midst of a terrible crisis, involving a very sick wife and a probably dead child, and he is in a state of shock and confusion. They do not see how he can function as a decision maker. Moreover, there is the question of the allocation of resources. The director of this overcrowded unit argues that whatever the father may want, it is inappropriate to deprive other neonates in the unit of adequate care because of a child who is probably dead. And what, the director asks, has happened to the newborns who were not admitted to the unit from other hospitals because of the crowded conditions in the unit? Other members of the staff find this view unacceptable. They feel that their responsibility is to the newborns currently in the ICU, and they think it is inappropriate even to consider the question of possible transfers. Finally, a third question is raised by the consultants from Neurology. They agree that it is standard medical practice to obtain flat EEGs without the presence of phenobarbital before a neonate is declared dead. But they see this case as involving all the clinical indications of death. They wonder whether or not it wouldn't be appropriate to just declare this baby dead and then terminate care.[6] Other members of the team think that it would be wrong to modify a standard procedure for determining death in a case like this. They see that as a way of hiding what would really be done: withdrawing care from a baby who is not definitely dead against the wishes of the father.

THEORETICAL ANALYSIS    The mother of Baby A wanted continued aggressive care for her baby, who had a real, even if not very high, probability of surviving and attaining some substantial amount of normal functioning. Baby B's parents wanted continued aggressive care for a child with nearly no possibility of surviving with significant functioning. Baby C's father wants continued care for a child who is probably dead but for whom the standard tests of death are not yet definitive.

The major argument for continuing to provide aggressive care for Baby B was the psychological benefit for the parents of feeling that their wishes were being respected. This was also an argument for providing continued aggressive care for Baby A, although, because of his better prognosis, there were other arguments as well. This argument continues to be present in the case of Baby C, whose father is just as insistent on further care as were the parents of Baby B and the mother of Baby A. But that argument from parental benefit was not significant enough to justify continued aggressive care in the case of Baby B, and we must now consider whether it is sufficient in the case of Baby C.

The policy of continued aggressive care for Baby C has a shorter time limit built into it than the policy for Baby B. The high levels of phenobarbital will shortly drop, and then, if the staff's clinical judgment about the baby's being dead is correct, a flat EEG will confirm death, and the baby can be declared dead. All of this means that one of the arguments used against aggressive management for Baby A and Baby B—the imposition on the caregivers—is going to have less significance here because the imposition is only very temporary. Moreover, given that the staff is convinced that the child is dead and therefore cannot suffer any pain or discomfort from continued invasive management, there can hardly be an argument against continued aggressive care for the child either on the grounds that it is imposing unjustified suffering on Baby C or on the grounds that it challenges the integrity of the caregivers who are opposed to harming patients. All of this suggests that a continued policy of aggressive management for a very short period of time until a flat EEG is obtained with an appropriately low phenobarbital level is reasonable, subject to the condition that it be clearly explained to the father that once the child is definitively ascertained to be dead, all support will be discontinued.[7] If the situation is properly handled, the psychological benefits to the father of continued care can be reaped with only modest cost to the caregivers and with no cost to the almost certainly dead baby.

There is, however, one complicating feature: the question of the justice of continuing to use a limited resource in heavy demand to support some of the physiological processes of a probably dead child rather than to aid other children who need transfer to the ICU. The question of justice can be raised here, even though this child is being cared for in the private sector, because, as we saw in chapter 4, questions of justice do arise even in the private sector when the physical resources for providing care are limited. I have deliberately shied away in this book from an attempt to develop a theory of justice in the allocation of limited health-care resources. I have tried to deal with our cases, to the extent that they raise questions of justice, without having to enter into the development of a full-scale theory of justice. In particular, I have tried to avoid the conflict between those who argue for a first-come, first-served squatter's-right approach to justice in the allocation of limited health resources versus those who advocate a triage approach.[8] I hope to be able to continue to avoid that very difficult question with regard to this case. If Baby C is dead, the child is not a claimant for neonatal intensive care. The father might derive some psychological benefit from the child's being maintained in the neonatal unit, even if dead, but it would be hard to think of a theory of justice in which Baby C's father would have a higher claim on the resources of the neonatal care unit than a neonate in need of transfer to that unit. So, unless a living neonate who could seriously benefit from neonatal intensive care presents in the short period of time before the phenobarbital level drops sufficiently, we will not have to confront the question of who has a greater claim to the place currently occupied by Baby C.

I conclude (1) that the father needs to be told that the child is almost certainly dead at this point but that the unit is prepared, if the father wishes, to continue to maintain some of the body's physiological functioning until the last definitive test is performed so long as some live neonate claimee who needs the bed doesn't present and (2) that the father needs to expect that this definitive test will be conclusive in the very near future and that, at that point, the child will be declared dead, and further support of physiological functioning will be withdrawn.

*CASE NO 30. Saving a baby with no brain:*
*Dealing with the right decision maker*

FACTS    Baby D was born to a 16-year-old woman who is unsure of the father's identity. None of the more likely candidates has expressed any interest in the baby. The course of the pregnancy was normal, and the infant seemed normal at birth. However, it was noted by the nurses that the baby was excessively sleepy, cried continuously when awake, and fed poorly because of poor sucking ability. A neurology consult revealed that the child suffered from hydranencephaly, a congenital anomaly in which nearly all of the cerebral hemispheres and the corpus striatum are reduced to a sac covered by intact meninges but filled with clear fluid. This condition is easily detectable; a high-intensity light held up to the skull on one side transilluminates the entire upper skull (since all that is present in the skull is fluid). All of this has been explained to the mother and the maternal grandmother. In order to be sure that they understand the baby's condition, the staff showed them the transilluminated skull. The staff would simply like to keep Baby D comfortable, not ever providing any nourishment, until the baby dies. They feel that if they use more aggressive treatment there is a chance that the infant will survive for some time and that these poor people will be required to take home a child who has no chance for any neurological functioning. The maternal grandmother, who would probably have the responsibility for providing most of the infant's care, totally agrees. Baby D's mother does not. She insists that the baby is alive, and she wants to take Baby D home and give the child as much love as she can.

QUESTIONS    The first question raised by this very troubling case is about who in the family is the relevant person to be involved in decision making. Some members of the treating team believe it is Baby D's mother. Most, however, do not agree. They see this mother as a 16-year-old child whose social history indicates that she is irresponsible, and they conclude that the relevant person to be involved in decision making is the maternal grandmother. They also say that the grandmother should be the one involved because she will have responsibility for the care of the child if the baby goes home.

A second very difficult question is just how far one can go when one makes a decision not to treat a newborn. Some members of the staff feel that it would be morally wrong to fail to provide food and fluids to Baby D. Any child, they argue, is at least entitled to food and fluids. They agree that it would be appropriate to withhold medical care, but they cannot see withholding food or fluids. Other members of the staff disagree. Their view is that once the judgment has been made by the medical staff and the maternal grandmother that this child would be better off dead, we should find that form of withholding care that provides the least painful and degrading death for the child. They see withholding food and fluids as serving that role. A further disagreement about this issue should be noted. One of the problems of such neonates is that they often manifest wide swings in body temperature, as they have difficulty controlling their body temperature. Thorough management of this child requires careful attention to thermal control. Some of those who insist on feeding Baby D would extend this view to keeping the child warm. Others would distinguish between these forms of medical intervention, arguing that aggressive thermal control (anything beyond simply keeping the child properly clothed and wrapped) is not required. What are the boundaries of "mere supportive care"?

THEORETICAL ANALYSIS   The case of Baby D is included in our discussion of parents who wish treatment to be continued because Baby D's mother is asking for further aggressive management of her child's many problems. Nevertheless, it is important to go beyond that fact and ask the question, raised by many members of the team, of exactly who it is that the physicians should be dealing with.

There are difficult legal questions about who should be the decision maker in this case.[9] But the moral situation seems clear. There is little reason to suppose that the teenage mother of Baby D is competent to make decisions for herself or for Baby D. Her general behavior does not suggest any maturity of understanding and reasoning. The argument she gives for wanting to take the child home, namely that she can show the baby love and affection, suggests that she has not really understood the fact that Baby D will never be capable of recognizing love and affection because Baby D lacks those portions of the brain required to do so. Moreover, the mother of Baby D has in no way emancipated herself. She still lives at home and is still supported by her mother. She intends to take the baby home to her mother's house. Since she will not bear the burdens of the decision, why should she be making the decision?

Who should be making decisions for Baby D? We can only rely on the notion of biological closeness. This makes it plausible to suggest that the maternal grandmother should occupy that role. A second argument also supports this conclusion. One can argue that the right to make decisions for this baby is a right of the minor mother which she is not yet capable of exercising and which must therefore be exercised for her by her legal guardian (the maternal grandmother). There are therefore two arguments on behalf of allowing the maternal grandmother to play the role of decision maker.

What we really have here is a case in which the surrogate decision maker for the patient is refusing further health care. The right of this closest family member to refuse care seems to be reasonably significant in this case, since the grandmother has shown throughout the discussion a full understanding of the situation, and her wishes that the child not be treated are strong wishes which have been held steadfastly ever since the child's condition was clarified. So we have a strong argument from the right to refuse care on behalf of the claim that Baby D should not be treated.

There are additional arguments against aggressive management of Baby D. Given the neurological status, continued existence would be neither a gain or loss to Baby D. But aggressive efforts to keep the baby going would impose unnecessary strains on the providers of care and might lead to the unfortunate consequence of the grandmother having to take responsibility for the child until such time as the child dies, a responsibility that would weigh heavily on the grandmother, who already has many other problems. Several appeals to consequences join with an appeal to the right to refuse care in arguing against aggressive management for Baby D.

A believer in the sanctity-of-life position might hold the view that since life must be preserved at any cost, Baby D should be managed aggressively.[10] Our analysis is based, however, on a belief in respect for persons, a respect that makes fewer and fewer demands on us as the person in question becomes less and less capable of engaging in those human activities whose performance we value so much. Baby D is incapable of engaging in any of those activities, and we must therefore conclude that respect for persons offers no reason in this case for further aggressive care.

It is clear then that we should allow Baby D to die. There remains, however, a subtle question raised by various members of the treating team. What should we do about feeding, hydration, and aggressive control of body temperature? Many feel that these forms of support should be treated no differently from any other form of medical care and that they may be withheld in cases like this.[11] I am troubled by that claim. I have maintained throughout this book a distinction between passive and active euthanasia which I have explicated in terms of causality. I have claimed that, absent a waiver by the party in question of the right not to be killed, one violates a fundamental right if one causes the death of a patient, even if one may allow the patient to die from his or her disease. If we fail to provide these simple supports, what would be the cause of Baby D's death—the underlying disease or our failure to provide that support? We know that courts have held that parents who starve a child to death or expose a child so that death results from hypothermia are guilty of causing that child's death.[12] It seems that we are prepared to treat the failure to provide food, fluids, or body warmth to those incapable of getting them on their own as causing their death. I am inclined, therefore, to conclude that this minimum of care must be provided even for Baby D.

The argument just given presupposes two claims: (1) that the failure to provide basic nutritional support and warmth to an infant is active enthanasia and (2) that it would be wrong to kill the patient, even if the right not to be killed is waivable, because the patient has never waived that right. Could we not challenge the second assumption of this argument? Perhaps the grandmother, acting on behalf of the child, could waive that right. This leads to the general question of whether surrogates can waive fundamental rights of individuals, particularly when the waiver, even if no loss to the individual, is no gain either and is based primarily on the benefit to others. This is a difficult question which needs much further investigation. One way to start thinking about it would be to ask whether we would be prepared, if the grandmother is willing to agree to this idea, to kill Baby D by injection with potassium chloride. If not, we should accept the second claim above.

I conclude that Baby D should receive only the minimal supportive care of fluids, food (via an NG tube if necessary), and help in maintaining body temperature. If possible, plans should be made for placement elsewhere if the child does survive, unless the grandmother changes her mind and decides to take the baby home.

*CASE NO 31. Keeping alive a baby in pain:*
*Recognizing the limits of our abilities to make assessments*

FACTS    Baby E was a term infant born to a 28-year-old woman. It was her first child by her second marriage, although she had several children by her first husband. Upon birth, it was noted that the child had severe dermatological problems which were diagnosed as epidermolysis bullosa, dystrophic type. This skin disease results in painful blisters forming all over the body from minimal trauma, in esophageal constrictions which pose feeding problems, and in an inability to swallow. Infection and fluid management is a major treatment challenge for such children. All of this was explained to the parents. It was also explained that while the child's death was not imminent and while there are some reported cases of such children living to their early teens, the child would always be in considerable pain and discomfort and would eventually succumb to the disease.[13] In fact, Baby E was obviously in considerable pain and discomfort at the very time all of this was being explained to the parents. The baby had developed a serious infection, and it was suggested to the parents that the pain, but not the infection, should be treated and the child allowed to die. The parents vacillated about this issue but eventually concluded that they wanted the child's infection to be treated. They could not find any justification for not treating a readily correctable infection.

QUESTIONS    One set of issues here was raised by the severity of Baby E's problems. Some find it unconscionable to keep this baby alive. Given the nature of the condition, they argue, life would be a real loss rather than a gain for Baby E. Who would want to live in a condition of constant pain, where the simple acts of handling and feeding, which are so important to any infant, are a source of continuous discomfort? Their conclusion is that treating Baby E's infection was immoral. Other members of the treating staff do not see it this way. Some agree with the family members that simple medical management of readily correctable problems is something we are obliged to provide to this infant, whatever judgment we may make about quality of life. Others would have been willing to not treat the infection if the parents would have agreed but cannot see any justification for making a quality-of-life judgment and disregarding the wishes of the parents.

A second set of very difficult issues posed by this case relates to the fact that the parents vacillated many times between the option of treating the child's infection and the option of simply letting the child die. Some members of the team wonder how seriously we should take parental decisions arising out of such clear internal conflict and whether it wouldn't be more appropriate to view this as a case in which the parents could not make up their minds and the treating team needed to guide them to what it viewed as an appropriate decision. Others see the parents as having made a decision, even if it did come after some vacillation.

There is still one final issue which particularly troubles some of the social workers who have been working with the family. This is a family of limited means, and they already have two children to provide for. Taking this child home and providing care is going to be an expensive and time-consuming matter. The continued care of this child until eventual death will be at the cost of a considerable portion of the family's resources and time. The losers, this argument runs, are the other children. It is wrong to save Baby E for a short, painful life at a tremendous cost to the other children. Other members of the team disagree. Some feel that this is an irrelevant issue. We need to do what is right for Baby E. We cannot consider, no matter how much we may be concerned about them, the implications a decision has for Baby E's siblings. Others treat all of these considerations as excessively speculative. Sometimes, they point out, families grow in strength as they care for a very sick child with many problems. How, they argue, can we know what would be the implications to this family of taking Baby E home?

THEORETICAL ANALYSIS    The case of Baby E is radically different from most cases of defective newborns about whom the question of aggressive management is raised in that there is no question here of neurologic impairment. Baby E will undergo normal cognitive development. The problem is that Baby E's life, however, long it lasts, will be filled with considerable pain and suffering. The question that the parents and the team have to confront is whether it is a life worth saving.

One thing can surely be said. Children like Baby E are prone to infection, and that is a very likely pathway to ultimate demise. The failure to treat the current infection with antibiotics would, therefore, be a decision to allow the child to die from the underlying illness and its complications. Such a decision would certainly not constitute a morally illicit killing of the child. In other words, antibiotics are one of those things that may be withheld from patients in cases like this. So those members of the team who feel that we are always required to provide antibiotics are mistaken.

Let us first examine the consequences for Baby E. The question that must be asked is whether or not a life with normal neurologic functioning but with considerable pain and discomfort is worth living. If Baby E were an adult patient with a sense of values of his own, that question could be put to him. But he is not, and there is a significant probability that he will never live long enough to develop a set of values sufficient to answer this question. The parents concluded that Baby E's life will be worth living, even though it will be relatively short and even though it will be filled with considerable pain. Some members of the team think that it will not be a life worth living. Neither side feels any strong confidence in its claim. Moreover, it is hard to see how either evaluation is relevant, from the perspective of the appeal to consequences, given that consequences are supposed to be evaluated in light of the values of the person affected.[14] An appeal to the consequences for Baby E seems to lead to no determinate conclusion.

What about the consequences for the family? Some feel that saving Baby E will in the long run impose an intolerable burden on the family, even if the family thinks at this point that it will not. Others feel that that is inappropriately pessimistic and that the care and upbringing of Baby E may lead to positive outcomes for the family. Either of these claims may be true, but it is hard to be confident about either. One thing certainly can be said. The family, after considerable struggling, believes that Baby E's problems should be treated so that he can have his best chance at life. Following their wishes would at least produce the result of the family's having the satisfaction of knowing that their decisions are being respected. This type of support for the family certainly stands as an argument for continued aggressive care for Baby E, as it did for the first four cases in this chapter.

What other moral appeals might be relevant to this case? The appeal to the procedural rights of decision making will once more play no role here, for this is a case of a family requesting care rather than refusing care for a child. The appeal to respect for persons certainly offers some argument for continued attempts to pull Baby E through his current medical problems. Since Baby E is neurologically intact, he will be capable, for the time that he lives, of engaging in some of those human activities whose performance we value so much. To be sure, those activities, as part of the life of Baby E, will be accompanied by ongoing pain and suffering. But that does not take away from the fact that he has the capacity in question, and respect for persons therefore offers some support for Baby E's being treated at this point.

The argument until now suggests that the best course of action would be to continue to treat Baby E's infection. Take note, however, that the parents have vacillated in the past and may at some later time change their minds. That should lead us to recognize that we may be making a different decision for Baby E at a later stage if the parental attitude changes. As the parents come to better understand the nature of the quality of Baby E's life and its implications for the whole family, they may come to believe that future medical problems should not be treated. If that point is reached, a proper analysis would lead to a very different conclusion. We would then have a family refusing further care for their child, a refusal based on more extensive knowledge of what the child's condition means both for the child and for themselves. That refusal, particularly if maintained over a period of time, would have considerable significance. It would probably make it appropriate at that point to not provide further care to Baby E. This means that the decision at this point to treat the infection is not necessarily a permanent decision about all of Baby E's problems. The family and the providers need to have enough self-honesty and courage to recognize that they are moving forward with a particular decision that makes sense at this point but which they may regret and change in the future. This case reminds us of the limitations in our understanding of the consequences of various decisions and our evaluation of those consequences. It reminds us that we may move forward in one direction now while recognizing that we may move in a very different direction at a later point.

## 7.2   Parents Who Do Not Want Continued Care for Their Newborn Children

We have just examined the cases of five newborn children whose survival was in serious doubt, whose quality of life if they did survive was likely to be very low, but whose parents wanted them to receive continued aggressive care. This type of case is very common. We should not be surprised by this; parental love often makes it hard to accept the idea of letting a newborn child die. There are other cases, however, in which the parental reaction is quite different. The physicians caring for these children recommend continued aggressive medical therapy, but the parents, for a variety of reasons including parental love, do not accept that recommendation.

*CASE NO 32. "Respect our wishes, since you are likely to fail anyway":*
*Probing the limits of parental authority*

FACTS   Baby F was a term infant born to a couple in their mid-thirties with three other children. At birth, Baby F's rapid respirations made it evident that she had major problems. A full evaluation revealed that she was suffering from hypoplastic left-heart syndrome. In this syndrome, there is a severe failure of development of the left ventricle, leaving the right ventricle to do all of the work normally done by both parts of the heart. In the past, such children usually died relatively quickly. In the years just preceding this case, however, some surgeons had developed a very complicated two-stage surgical procedure, the Norwood shunt procedure, which offered some hope of survival for these infants.[15] The quality of their life in the years after the surgery was not clear. One of the physicians in this unit approached the family with the suggestion that they agree to have Baby F undergo this procedure. The physician explained to them that while its results were not very promising, it offered the best hope for their child. The parents were initially very excited about this possibility, even though they had begun to adjust to the idea that their child was likely to die. When they realized, however, that it would be impossible to carry out this procedure without the use of blood products, their whole attitude changed. They explained that as Jehovah's Witnesses they cannot risk their salvation and their child's salvation by agreeing to the surgery. The physician in question explained that it is standard policy in this unit when surgery is indicated but refused by parents who are Jehovah's Witnesses to get a court order taking temporary custody of the child so that surgery can be performed.[16] The parents responded by begging him not to do that in this case. They said that whatever the merits of the policy in other cases, it is very inappropriate in this case where the procedure is highly experimental.

QUESTIONS   The physician who initially approached the parents feels that the experimental nature of the procedure is irrelevant. The child will surely die without the surgery. Why, he argues, should we condemn Baby F to certain death when there is a real, even if unknown, chance of meaningful survival with this procedure? He feels that the religious beliefs of the parents should be disregarded in this case, and a court order should be obtained so that he can do what is best for the child. Other members of the team strongly disagree. A few have doubts about the general policy of getting court orders in such cases. They wonder whether it is ever appropriate for the medical team, with the aid of the court, to overrule the religious values of parents. Most are willing to accept this general policy of overriding parental wishes, with court authorization, in cases where the benefit for the child is well established and clear-cut, but they are less willing to do so in cases like this. To be sure, Baby F has nothing to lose and everything to gain by the attempt, but it will produce tremendous psychological harm and suffering for the parents, and they see no justification for this when the benefits to the child are unknown but not probable. So this case raises questions involving religious freedom, the authority of parents over their children, and the role of compassion for the family in decision making for the child. Not surprisingly, this case has produced tremendous controversy in the unit.

THEORETICAL ANALYSIS    Baby F's parents have refused permission for surgery on their child. That refusal provides one considerably significant reason for not going forward with the surgery. After all, they are competent decision makers with a clear understanding of the implications of their decision, their decision is based on their fundamental values and beliefs about what is best for the child, and it is a decision they have made firmly and repeatedly. In short, all of the factors that need to be present in order for a refusal of treatment, either for oneself or for someone else for whom one is acting as a surrogate, to have maximum significance are present in this case.

There is a second argument, from an appeal to the consequences for the parents, which reinforces this first one. The parents would clearly be immensely frustrated, upset, and angry if their strongly expressed preferences, which mean so much to them, were disregarded. So any decision to go ahead with surgery on Baby F would also produce these very undesirable consequences for the parents.

What are the arguments for proceeding with the surgery? One is an appeal to the consequences for the child. Without this surgery, the child will certainly die very soon. With it, she has some chance, even if not a very high chance, for surviving and being able to live a reasonably normal life. So an appeal to the consequences for the child seems to argue unequivocally for the surgery. But the argument, while unequivocal, is not very significant, primarily because the probability of success with the surgery is not very high. Any appeal to consequences where the consequence only have a modest probability of occurring is not a particularly significant appeal. The very same point needs to be made about another argument for proceeding with the surgery, an appeal to respect for persons. Baby F, if the surgery is successful, may develop into a person who is capable of performing those activities whose performance we value so much. Respect for persons argues for surgery for the child. The argument is not very significant, however, because the probability of Baby F's surviving with the surgery and developing into a person who can perform these activities is not particularly high.

It seems reasonable to judge that we ought to respect the parents' wishes. But this is so only because the treatment in question does not have an established significant probability of success. This helps explain why this case is different from the many other cases in which the courts have mandated care for children of Jehovah's Witnesses against the wishes of the parents when that care involves the use of blood products. In those cases, the treatments in question had much better success rates which had been confirmed over long use. The appeal to the consequences for the child and the appeal to respect for persons then have much greater significance and take precedence over the parental right of refusal.

All of this has significant implications for future Baby F's. When the case of

Baby F arose, heart transplants in newborns were just beginning. That is why the Norwood shunt procedure was the surgery being considered. Since that time, a track record for transplants has come into existence, and it seems to offer a significant chance for such children. If our analysis until now has been correct, the conclusion we need to draw is that parental refusal of surgery should be overridden if a heart becomes available for transplanting a future Baby F.[17]

We need to remember an important point made earlier in connection with adult Jehovah's Witnesses. There are two ways in which a team can move forward with heart-transplant surgery. One would be to talk the parents into agreeing. The other would be to take temporary custody of the child, by virtue of a court order, and then proceed with the surgery. There is more to be said for the latter strategy. To begin with, for the parents to agree with the surgery because of the pressure of the current situation would be for them to act in a way that is not consonant with their principles, showing a lack of integrity. Moreover, if they do agree, then we are laying the foundation for tremendous guilt feelings later on when they have to confront the question of whether or not they have sinned. Wouldn't it be better for both of these reasons simply to take custody of the child?

In conclusion, it was morally appropriate not to press forward with the surgery in the case of Baby F.[18] In the future, however, it seems that getting court orders to take custody for children like Baby F so that heart transplants can be performed (providing that an organ is available) would seem to be the morally appropriate action.

*CASE NO 33. "It's too much of a burden on him and us":*
*The need to clarify what the parents are saying*

FACTS   Baby G was born with spina bifida cystica. Because of the failure of the neural tube to close during the first trimester of pregnancy, this baby developed an opening in the upper lumbar region of the back that left exposed both membrane tissue and nerve tissue (a meningomyelocele). In addition, he had a moderate degree of hydrocephalus. Finally, there were clear indications of significant weakness of the legs and of neurogenic bladder dysfunction. The physicians have explained to the parents the nature of all of these deformities. They have also explained the complicated medical and surgical management currently employed for such cases. This includes closing the opening to prevent infection, shunting the child to lessen the accumulation of fluid in the brain, and then, at a later stage, performing extensive surgery to improve (as much as possible) motor and urinary functioning. They have admitted to the parents that it is difficult to say how successful this complicated set of procedures would be but that their experience indicates a reasonably good chance that this child will have close to normal mental functioning and only some moderate physical dysfunctioning. As the parents began to realize the complexity of the situation, they have begun to have serious doubts about the physicians' recommendations. To some degree, those doubts are based on their concern about whether the physicians are being excessively optimistic concerning the child's resulting quality of life. There are, however, additional factors present in their thinking. The parents have a moderate income, and they already have three other children. They have expressed tremendous concern about the financial implications for long-term care for this child; they are worried about how the tremendous amount of time they would have to give to this child would affect their ability to care for their other children. Having thought about it for a few days, the parents have requested that the child be allowed to die, presumably from the infections that will set in if the open lesion is not closed.

QUESTIONS   The first question here centers around quality-of-life considerations. Some members of the team object to the very introduction of quality-of-life considerations in this case. They believe that aggressive surgical management means that the child will survive, and they believe that it is inappropriate for either staff or parents to make decisions against aggressive management on quality-of-life considerations. Others accept the legitimacy of quality-of-life considerations in at least some cases but believe that they cannot appropriately be invoked in this case. Their argument is that the location of the lesion and the nature of the other problems puts this case on the borderline between those in which the resulting quality of life is likely to be clearly acceptable and those in which the resulting quality of life is clearly unacceptable. In these borderline cases, they argue, it is inappropriate for either physicians or family to decide against surgery on quality-of-life considerations. Other members of the team don't see this issue either way. They feel that quality-of-life judgments may be taken into account and that there is sufficient doubt about the resulting quality of life to allow the medical team to go along with parental wishes to let this child die.

There is also the question of the relevance of the financial and psychosocial implications of the continued existence of this child for the parents and for their other children. Some view these implications as additional reasons why the parental wishes should be respected. Why, they argue, should we impose tremendous additional burdens on this family when the outcome is so unclear? Others see it very differently. They feel that the parents are not attending to what is in the best interests of this child; their concern is primarily with themselves and with their other children. In the minds of these members of the team, this fact makes the parents inappropriate decision makers for Baby G. Members of the medical team, who are concerned with the best interest of this child, should make the decision for surgery.

In a further complication, some members of the team have pointed out that there are good parents willing to adopt such children. Would it not be more appropriate, they argue, to arrange for such an adoption, with the consent of the natural parents, rather than allow this child to die? This would avoid the family's suffering the losses about which they are concerned. Others don't see the question of adoption as relevant. Their view is that the decision has to be made by the physicians and/or the parents of the child, not by outside potential adoptees.

Still one final set of issues complicates this case. Some members of the team think that it is unacceptable to leave the lesion open (exposing the child to infection) and to not treat the infection. They view this as equivalent to killing the child. They feel that even if we respect the parental wishes, we must at least close the lesion and treat the infections. Others think that if we decide to simply let this child die, we should leave the infections alone so that he will die in a reasonably short period of time.

THEORETICAL ANALYSIS    The case of Baby G and those of other babies like him have attracted much attention among neonatologists, bioethicists, and legal scholars in recent years.[19] Spina bifida children have become classic cases around which the discussion of the legitimacy of withdrawing treatment for quality-of-life reasons has centered. Scholars have found this type of case to be one of the most difficult to resolve. Therefore, we need to approach this case with particular care.

The first thing to note is that there is a fundamental ambiguity about the reasoning of the parents. Are they refusing surgery primarily because their judgment is that it would best for the child if he were to die, and is their talk about the burden on the family just an extra consideration, or is the burden on the family an essential part of their decision, and would they make a different decision if it weren't for that problem? Why is it important to resolve this ambiguity? It is not because there would be something wrong with a parental decision for which the burden on the family was one of the essential reasons. We have already argued that it is legitimate for a family to take into account the implications of its decisions for all members of the family, not just for the child in question. It is only when the parents place too much emphasis on the implications for others that their decision comes to have less moral force. The reason why it is important to clarify the parental reasoning is very different. It relates to the possibility of the parents agreeing to the surgery and then giving up their child for adoption, a real option in these days of a very limited supply of children available for adoption. If an essential reason for the parents' decision is the great burden care for this child would impose on their family, then it would seem that they should agree to the adoption option. We would then have a case with a very different moral structure, since we would no longer have to deal with a parental refusal of care. If, however, their judgment about the quality of the child's life is a sufficient reason for their refusing permission for surgery, and if the talk about the burden on the family is simply an extra argument for their decision, then they should refuse the option of giving the child up for adoption postsurgery. The case would then have parental refusal as an essential feature, and any moral analysis would need to take this into account. So it is really very important to settle this question.

For the rest of this discussion, we will assume that the parents of Baby G oppose the adoption option and refuse surgery for the child, insisting that in the end their judgment is based on the belief that the child would be better off if he were not treated and were allowed to die. This is, of course, the harder case.

What are the arguments against surgery? The first and the most important is, of course, the fact that the parents, who are the appropriate surrogate decision makers for Baby G, have refused permission, and they have a right to have that refusal respected. This right is of considerable significance here. After all, this is a refusal made by competent decision makers who have a good understanding of the uncertainties and ambiguities about the outcome if Baby G is aggressively managed and who understand the strong probability that he will die if it is not. Moreover, having arrived at that decision, they have continued to hold it very firmly over a period of days as the discussions between them and the caregivers have continued. While not rooted in some central theological belief of theirs, such as in the previous case of Baby F's parents, their decision is rooted in a general philosophy about what constitutes a life worth living. All in all, then, it is a refusal of treatment which generates a very significant argument against treating the child.

There are substantial consequences for the family that argue against surgical management of this case. To begin with, going ahead with the surgery against the wishes of the family after this whole process of discussion would certainly cause them much distress and frustration; they would feel deprived of the right to make decisions for their child. Moreover, after surgery, there are two options. One is that the child would eventually go home with these parents, and this would result in a great burden on them. Alternatively, they might at that time agree to give up the child for adoption, and they would suffer the extra anguish of knowing that decisions made against their wishes resulted in their being put into a situation where they felt compelled to give up their child. Neither outcome is particularly satisfactory from the perspective of the family. So there are strong considerations from the appeal to the consequences for the family which argue against going ahead with the surgery.

What are the arguments for the surgery? One would be an appeal to the consequences for the child. Surgery gives this child his best chance for surviving with a reasonable quality of life. However, this satisfactory outcome cannot be guaranteed. The child may die anyway as a result of the complications of the disease and/or of the treatment. Alternatively, the child may survive with a significant level of mental and/or physical disability. Any appeal to the good consequences for the child cannot be a very strong moral argument, because the probability of a good outcome is far from certain.

A similar point needs to be made about the argument from respect for persons. Respect for persons comes into play here because we might argue that surgery offers the best chance of continued existence of the child as a person capable of performing those activities whose performance we value so much. All of this is true, but the argument cannot be taken too far since the probability of that favorable outcome is far from certain.

It is important to note, as one immediate corollary, that the situation would be very different if the lesion were lower or if there were no accompanying hydrocephalus. In such cases, where a prognosis for survival with a reasonably good level of functioning would be much better, the arguments for going ahead with the surgery—the favorable consequences for the child and the demands of respect for persons—would be much more significant. This means that the development of well-defined protocols for judging likelihood of success is a valuable help for sound moral decision making in this area.

The arguments for respecting the wishes of the parents, given that those wishes have now been clarified, appear to take precedence over the arguments for going ahead with surgery against their wishes. But it is important to note that the analysis might be quite different[20] if the medical facts of the case were somewhat different.

Many health-care providers might be very uncomfortable with the decision the parents have made. Many would feel that it would be better if surgery were performed. This feeling would be based on a different assessment of the value of Baby G's life even with quite substantial physical and mental disabilities. It would seem perfectly appropriate for such people to withdraw from the case of Baby G, if continuing to care for the baby in a mere supportive fashion without aggressive surgical management sufficiently offends their sense of values and their integrity. The parents need to understand that others may feel just as deeply about this case and that they are not entitled to impose their values on those others by insisting on mere supportive care for the child until he dies. The parents need to seek out health-care providers who feel capable of participating in the choices made by the parents without that participation offending their sense of integrity.

What should be done for the child in the meantime? The parents, if they really mean what they have said, should probably also refuse treatment for Baby G's infections.[21] What would be the point, given their view that the child is better off dead, for treating infections with sac closure and with antibiotics? That would only prolong the child's life and might even result in the child surviving without getting all of the surgery he really needs for survival with good functioning. It seems that consistency calls on the parents to make the decision to simply have the child fed and kept warm and comfortable until he dies, probably from infection. Doing so would not be, as some members of the team have said, killing the child. The cause of the death will be an infection resulting from the underlying medical problems of this child born with a neural tube defect. Not treating infections with antibiotics is simply a way of allowing the child to die from the complications of his underlying disease.

*CASE NO 34. "Why do anything if the baby is going to die anyway?":*
*Facing the ends-means problem*

FACTS At birth, Baby H had severe abnormalities, including low-set ears, an unusually small jaw, rocker-bottom feet, and a clenched hand with tapering fingers and a malformed thumb. In addition, Baby H had difficulty breathing and had clear signs of congenital heart problems. It did not take long to diagnose Baby H as having trisomy 18. The staff met at that point with the parents and explained to them the full extent of Baby H's problems. They told the parents that the chance of the child's surviving for even one year was less than 10%, that even those children who survived that first year had very little chance of surviving childhood, and that the surviving children had extremely severe mental and physical defects. The staff recommended that little be done to treat the medical problems except to feed the baby and keep him comfortable until he died. The parents, a young couple with no other children, were devastated by what had occurred. At the beginning, they simply accepted the staff's recommendations. After about a week, there was a change in their thinking. When they received genetic counseling and came to understand that it was very likely that they could have normal children, their attention turned to the question of having another child. They began to wonder why anything at all was being done for this child. Why not simply stop feeding the child and let him die, they asked? As time has progressed, their insistence has become greater. They want to be done with this terrible situation, to complete their grieving, and to get on with their life. They can't see why the staff insists on doing anything.

QUESTIONS    This heart-rending case has troubled the entire team caring for Baby H. Everyone is comfortable with the decision not to provide this child with any aggressive medical therapy.[22] But the parental reaction has provoked considerable disagreement. Some members of the team agree with the parents. They see the continued existence of this child as a source of suffering. They also see the child as consuming medical resources with no gain for anyone. They see no reason, there-fore, to do anything to keep the child alive, including feeding. Other members of the team cannot agree. Some take the view that failing to feed or provide fluids to a child is always equivalent to killing, and they can see no justification for ever doing that. Some agree that there might be cases in which it would acceptable to neither feed nor provide fluids to a child. These would be cases in which the child's continued existence is a loss because the child is in tremendous pain which cannot be relieved. None of these considerations is present in this case. They recognize that the child's parents would like to have this over with and that there are considerable expenses involved in maintaining the child. But they argue that neither of these is a sufficient reason for accepting the parental wishes, which they feel go too far in this case.

THEORETICAL ANALYSIS    In many ways, the case of Baby H is much clearer than that of Baby G. On the one hand, whatever is done, Baby H's chance of surviving for even one year is very low, and the ability of Baby H to function for however long that survival lasts is extremely limited. So one can hardly argue for keeping Baby H alive on the grounds that it produces desirable consequences for the patient. For similar reasons, there is little, if any, argument for that course of action from an appeal to respect for persons. This case illustrates once more the important dif-ference between an appeal to respect for persons and the more extreme appeal to the sanctity of life, which would support keeping Baby H alive. There is much to be said, on the other hand, against treating any of Baby H's problems aggressively. The parents don't want it, and their refusal certainly is entitled to considerable respect. The consequences for the family and for the staff from prolonging the dying of Baby H are pretty bad, and this provides an additional reason for not going ahead with any aggressive care. The virtue of compassion for all those involved also speaks on behalf of nonaggressive management of Baby H's problems. So there is far less moral ambiguity in this case.

There is, however, one major problem: the parental request that Baby H not be fed so that he will die more quickly. We have already argued that this is morally prohibited, for it would involve killing the baby by causing his death from dehydra-tion and/or starvation. This case illustrates once more the ways in which a complex moral approach, which recognizes the plurality of values, differs from other moral systems. Someone who focused merely on the consequences, on the ends, would find it hard to see any justification for feeding this baby. After all, everyone agrees that the baby's demise would be desirable. So why prolong the time of dying? It is only when we recognize additional moral values, including the constraints imposed by the right not to be killed, that we come to see that we need to focus on the means of obtaining certain ends and not just on the ends themselves.

But haven't we argued that this right not to be killed can be waived? It can certainly be waived by a patient, but can it be waived by a surrogate? That is a different question, which we have already looked at in the case of Baby D. It was argued there that the right cannot be waived by a surrogate in cases where the waiver produces no gains for the patient. We might be prepared to accept the view that surrogates can waive the patient's right not to be killed when the waiver actually produces some benefit for the patient, as in a case where the patient's condition is very painful and agonizing. But we should not extend this point to cases like this one in which that factor is not present. If we did, we would need to accept the idea that the parents could legitimately insist that the child's death should be produced immediately by injecting the child with potassium chloride. And if we are not prepared to accept that conclusion, doesn't that mean that we cannot accept their request not to feed and provide fluids for the child either?

These questions are intellectually difficult and emotionally painful. They would be much easier if we treated the right not to killed as a nonwaivable absolute right. But the right not to be killed can be waived by a patient. We have seen in several cases that this might be extended to a surrogate waiving the right for the patient when the patient cannot waive it for himself or herself and when the continued existence of the patient is actually a loss to the patient because of great pain and suffering. But our thought experiment suggests that we are not prepared to extend the capacity of a surrogate to waive the right not to be killed to a case where the patient's continued existence is not a loss to the patient. And if we are not prepared to go that far, then we need to refuse the parental wish to starve Baby H.

One additional point needs to be made. The parents of Baby H are clearly suffering tremendously as they live through the dying of this child. The virtue of compassion calls on us to extend to these parents all possible support. They need to be helped to understand why their request cannot be accepted. They need help to deal with their frustrations, their anger, and their unhappiness. It is just not enough to say to them that we have gone as far as we can go and that we will go no farther, even if that would be saying the truth.

*CASE NO 35. "I don't want this monster":*
*The importance of body image*

FACTS Baby I represents a truly unusual case, because of both the mother's attitude and the child's medical condition. Baby I's mother is a highly successful businesswoman who in her mid-thirties decided that she wanted to have a child although she had no husband. She was artificially inseminated[23] and had a relatively uncomplicated pregnancy for the first five or six months. Then she started to experience premature labor. Finally, there was a premature rupture of the membranes. She was delivered of Baby I. The baby was normal by physical examination from the umbilicus upward. Below the umbilicus, there was an absence of genitalia,

LIFE-AND-DEATH DECISION MAKING

of an anal opening, and of a urethral opening. There was no evidence of a functioning kidney. There was simply a single lower appendage which contained bone and
tissue and ended with a single toelike structure. In short, Baby I suffered from the
"mermaid syndrome" (sirenomelia anomaled complex). Such children usually die
because of poor lung development, but this was not true in the case of Baby I. The
mother's attitude to her baby is very straightforward. She wanted to have a healthy
child, and she has not gotten it. She has no interest in this child, whom she describes
as a total monster, and she sees no reason why any effort should be made to keep
Baby I alive.

Keeping this child alive would involve extreme surgical measures. To begin
with, immediate surgery would be required to create an opening for the GI tract and
for urine flow. Secondly, peritoneal dialysis would be required until the child was
old enough and big enough to get a kidney transplant. Thirdly, the baby would need
extensive treatment afterward to avoid rejection. Even with all of this, the child
would continue to have no lower limbs and a resulting motor dysfunction. But there
is no reason to believe that the child would suffer from any mental deficiencies. So
we are talking here about a major set of interventions which, if successful, would
preserve a child who was neurologically intact but suffered from motor deficiencies
and a terrible set of deformities.

QUESTIONS    This very difficult and unusual case raises many questions. Some
members of the team find the mother's wishes unacceptable. They recognize that
this child suffers from physical deformities which are not correctable, but they feel
that the child has a real chance for a meaningful life. They point out that the child
has normal mental functioning and that there would also be full use of the upper
extremities. In these ways, the child would be better off than many of the children
regularly saved in neonatal ICUs. To their way of thinking, this child deserves the
best chance of as normal a life as possible. This means surgery now, dialysis for a
few years, and then a kidney transplant. This plan involves many risks, but, they
argue, it is best for the child. They see the mother as concerned only with herself.
She wanted a normal child and has rejected this child because of the deformities.
Other members of the team see this case very differently. Some claim that the
child's quality of life, given the severe physical deformities, would be too questionable to justify intervening against the wishes of the mother. Some point out that this
child would require extensive care, especially during the period of peritoneal dialysis, and they cannot see imposing all of this care on a reluctant mother. Some
argue that the mother is not required to simply consider what is in the best interests
of the child. She should be allowed to make a judgment taking into account all of
the factors in the case, and her judgment should be respected. Some wonder, in
passing, whether some of the conflicts in this case aren't the result of negative
judgments about this woman and her decision as a single woman to be artificially
inseminated.

THEORETICAL ANALYSIS    This case is both interesting and difficult because it raises
fascinating questions about the ways in which we value human beings and human
activities and about the importance we ascribe to bodies and their functioning. We

need to begin by reviewing the usual moral appeals to see what they have to say about this case.

One argument against beginning surgery for Baby I is that the mother, who is the surrogate decision maker, has refused permission for that surgery, and she has a right to have her refusal respected. How significant will that right be in this case? I believe it will not be very significant. The reason for this is relatively straightforward. In all of the discussions with the mother, it has been clear that she is focusing simply on the question of whether or not this is the baby she wants to fulfill her needs. She seems to be paying little, if any, attention to the question of what would be best for Baby I. While it is true that parents acting as surrogate decision makers need not focus entirely on what is best for the child but may take into account the implications of various decisions for all members of the family, it is also true that they can overdo that. They may also focus excessively on the implications for others. To the extent that they do so, their right to have their refusal respected becomes less significant. In this case, where the mother seems to be focusing entirely on the question of what all of this means to her, we can only conclude that little, if any, significance can be given to her right to refuse treatment for this child. It is important to contrast this case with that of Baby F. Both parents are refusing experimental therapies that have a high chance of failing. Baby F's parents are doing so in light of their judgment about what is best for Baby F. Baby I's mother is doing so in light of what she wants for herself. That difference in motives changes the whole case. It would be very different if Baby I's mother was insisting that Baby I would be better off dead.

We need to turn to the other moral appeals. If the complicated course of surgery suggested for Baby I is successful, then the baby will be capable of performing most of those activities whose performance we value so greatly. All of the evidence is that Baby I is neurologically intact and will be able to develop cognitively and affectively in ways that will make those activities possible. Moreover, Baby I's upper extremities seem perfectly normal, and Baby I will be no more limited in physical functioning than many other functional physically disabled individuals. In these respects, Baby I is better off than Baby G. So there is an argument from respect for persons for beginning the surgery in question. It is not, of course, an overwhelming argument, in part because it is quite likely that the proposed dramatic set of operations will not succeed. There is a considerable chance that Baby I will die either from the surgery or from one of the complications of the underlying problems. Still, there is also a significant, although hard to quantify, probability that the surgery will be successful and that Baby I will then be able to function in valuable ways.

What about the appeal to consequences? One thing is certain. If we disregard the mother's wishes and go ahead with surgery for the child, that will immediately produce the bad consequence of her feeling frustrated because her wishes about how her child should be managed are not being followed. There is, of course, the possible additional bad consequence to her, as she evaluates the consequences, of being stuck afterward with this child she doesn't want. Of course, that bad consequence for her can be alleviated if she puts the child up for adoption. So we have some reason from an appeal to the consequences for the mother for not going ahead with treatment for the child. In this connection, it is worth thinking about one further issue. Can we alleviate her feeling of frustration by negotiating with her in advance that she will give up the child for adoption? We know that this option, if carried out, will avoid her being stuck with a child she doesn't want. Knowing this in advance, and agreeing to it, might also lead to her feeling less unhappy about the fact that her decisions are not being followed. It may well be the case that all of her refusals are simply based on the fact that she doesn't want the child and that she may feel no sense (or, in any case, much less of a sense) of frustration about her wishes not being followed if she knows that she will not be stuck with the child. If this speculation turns out to be correct, then that will undercut the argument against treatment from a consideration of the consequences for the mother.

In examining consequences for the child, the question is whether the life that Baby I will lead, if all of the surgery is successful, will be a life that Baby I, at some later stage, will judge as worth living?[24] Or will it be the case that Baby I, at that later stage, will find life so hampered by the major deformities as to be unaccept-able? This is a very hard question to answer. It relates very much to the issue of how important body image is in one's evaluation of one's life. For some people, living with a body as deformed as Baby I's would be so troubling and so disquieting that they would find it unacceptable. Others might see it differently. They certainly would wish that they were not so deformed, but they would still see the many potentialities open to them in their life and would still judge it as worth living. Some evidence on this question might be obtained when we think of the ways in which paraplegics and others who have lost the functioning of the lower portions of their body view their lives as still worth living. I am inclined to judge that the appeal to the consequences for Baby I would imply that we should go ahead with the surgery. Thinking of the case of paraplegics, I am inclined to suppose that the higher probability is that Baby I, at a later stage of life, will find the consequence of being alive desirable. I recognize, of course, that this may be a reflection of my bias as an intellectual which leads me to think that it is more important that Baby I is neu-rologically intact than that Baby I will always suffer from these physical deformities and the corresponding bad body image. So, while I tend to suppose that Baby I will judge life as worth living if that stage in life is reached, I recognize that this judgment might be mistaken.

I believe that the best course of action would be to speak to the mother about the option of surgery plus giving the child up for adoption. This option would avoid the consequences to the mother of having a child she doesn't want while giving the child a real opportunity for a life that may be worth living and a life that we should respect as part of our respect for persons. If we are successful in this discussion with the mother, then we could go ahead with surgery with her consent. If not, we ought to go ahead with the surgery anyway, while continuing to preserve for the mother the right to give up the child if in fact she really doesn't want it.

As things stand currently, going ahead with surgery against the mother's wishes would require obtaining a court order of guardianship over the child. That is proba-bly a good requirement. It is important that someone independent of the treating team be appointed to ensure that the child's best interests are being considered and that the team is not just overreacting to the mother and her motives.

## 7.3   Cases Involving Adolescent and Teenage Patients

*CASE NO 36. "We want the pain to end, but he wants a final chance":*
*Dealing with the agony of hopelessness*

FACTS   J was diagnosed at the age of 11 as having acute lymphoblastic leukemia. He was treated with a three-drug regimen of prednisone, vincristine, and L-asparaginase, and a complete remission was obtained. Unfortunately, about twelve months later, J relapsed, despite central-nervous-system prophylaxis and despite maintenance chemotherapy. Several other remissions were induced, but the time of remission in each case was smaller and smaller. The last induction of a remission was particularly unpleasant. J developed GI toxicity, nonspecific infections, terrible nausea, and respiratory problems. At that point, the physicians met with the parents, and they jointly came to a decision that no further attempts would be made to induce a remission, in part because there were few options open and in part because they saw the resulting pain and suffering as not worth the slight chance of a short remission. When they told this to J, he objected. He says that he can bear the pain and suffering but that he could not bear giving up hope entirely. He insists that he is old enough at 13 to have his wishes respected. Everyone has tried to explain to him that his hopes are unfortunately unrealistic, but he insists that it is his life and that he knows what he wants.

QUESTIONS   The first question raised here has to do with whether anyone, an adolescent or an adult, can legitimately compel his or her health-care provider to provide treatment which the provider sees as both futile and harmful. Some members of the health-care team say no. They feel that it would be wrong for them to put J through another difficult regimen of chemotherapy, no matter what he (or even his parents) want, because it isn't going to do him any good and because it's going to hurt him. Others feel that if the parents had requested further chemotherapy, then it would be appropriate for the physicians to accept that judgment. This group argues against chemotherapy in this case only because the parents don't want it.

Another question is the role of an adolescent patient in decision making. All of those who have met J are impressed by his maturity of manner and his understanding of his medical condition. Many believe that he has demonstrated the type of maturity which gives him, rather than his parents, the right to participate in decision making. They conclude that the providers should negotiate with J regarding the appropriate form of care he should receive. Others don't see it that way. They believe that J is still a 13-year-old, understandably afraid of his imminent death, and that his providers need to be making decisions with J's far more mature parents. Those who take this view face still another difficult question. J's parents have asked for counseling from Social Work and from Liaison Psychiatry. What, they ask, should they do about J's desperate request that he have another chance? Should they reverse what they feel about this case and go along with what he wants, or should they try to get him to accept the inevitability of his death?

Finally, J's parents are reasonably comfortable but by no means affluent, and their out-of-pocket expenses for J's care in the last two years have increased to a point where it is threatening the financial stability of the family.[25] On more than one occasion, they have expressed concern about what these expenses mean for J's 15- and 17-year-old sisters, who will shortly be ready to go to college. They are concerned that any further attempt at chemotherapy will only increase the costs which are already hurting them tremendously. Everyone is sympathetic with this aspect of their problem, but there is considerable disagreement about the implications of it for all of the issues mentioned above. Some people think that this is one more reason why the parents should have decisional authority. At the end, whatever is done, J will be dead, and the parents will be left with a tremendous burden. Others are concerned that these financial issues may be leading the parents to make an inappropriate decision in opposition to the wishes of their child.

THEORETICAL ANALYSIS   J's case is extremely agonizing. Nobody wants to hurt this 13-year-old, but every possible course of action seems to carry with it some terrible consequence for him. Treating him will bring terrible side effects with little or no gain. Not treating him brings the agony of hopelessness and the frustration of not having his wishes followed.

Before analyzing this case, one point must be noted even if it will not affect this particular decision. A boy who develops acute lymphoblastic leukemia at the age of 11 and whose initial remission lasts no more than a year has a very poor prognosis. One wonders whether or not J's inability to deal with the hopelessness of his case at this point is a reflection of his having received too much encouragement during the induction of the last few remissions and whether or not there were sufficiently realistic discussions with him in the past. While none of this can make a difference to the decision that needs to be made now, it should remind those who treat such patients that encouraging hope in cases where the prognosis is very poor may not always be a good idea.[26]

Let us begin analyzing this case by an appeal to consequences. Whether or not J receives further chemotherapy, he will die relatively soon. But if he receives further chemotherapy, he will probably suffer many of the particularly bad side effects that he suffered in the last induction of a remission. If he does not receive chemotherapy, he will be able to avoid those terrible side effects. These consequences for J argue against chemotherapy. But failing to give chemotherapy will produce two very bad consequences for the patient. To begin with, he will feel the frustration of not having his wishes respected. Moreover, he will have to face up to the hopelessness of his situation. He is telling us that he would find the consequences of living without any hope very bad. So an appeal to the consequences for the patient seems to lead in conflicting directions, and it's hard to say which of the approaches would lead to consequences which would be worse for J, as J evaluates them. Some would say that J's wishes indicate that the consequences for him would be worse if he did not get the chemotherapy he wants. This is a mistake. It confuses the truth that we need to evaluate consequences in light of the values placed on them by the affected individual with the falsehood that the individual is always the best judge of which course of action will lead to the best consequences for him or her. In making his decision, for example, J may be underestimating the probability of the side effects of the chemotherapy being very bad. It may be that if J were to properly assess those probabilities, he would judge that the consequences of chemotherapy are worse. Again, J may be assuming that the sense of hopelessness will stay with him and continue to be a source of tremendous suffering. While he certainly is the only one who can assess the agony to him of his current hopelessness, he may be wrong about how long it will remain. The physicians and his parents may understand better than he does the ways in which people adjust to hopelessness and accept their impending doom. So we must conclude that an examination of the appeal to the consequences for the patient will not settle this issue, as we have no reliable way of assessing which approach will lead to the better consequences.

What about the consequences for J's family? Again, it initially seems as though an appeal to these consequences leads to a clear recommendation. After all, if we don't give J chemotherapy, J's parents will at least have the satisfaction of knowing that their wishes and judgments are being respected. Moreover, they will be spared the agony of watching J suffer from the side effects of further chemotherapy. Finally, a decision to forgo very expensive chemotherapy will help alleviate some of the financial pressures on the family, a consequence which is certainly relevant when one is examining this appeal. But it would be wrong to conclude that an appeal to the consequences for the family speaks unequivocally in this case. There is one potential consequence of not providing the chemotherapy which could be devastating. Will the parents be able to handle the anger that J may feel toward them if their wishes are followed and he receives no further chemotherapy? Or will they come to feel both anguish and guilt in response to J's unhappiness? And if they do, will those consequences be worse than the benefits to the parents? It is very hard to answer these questions. It would be a mistake to simply say that the parents' expressed wishes tell us which of the consequences are worse. That would, once more, be confusing the truth that the consequences have to be evaluated in light of the parental values with the falsehood that they are necessarily the best judges of what will lead to the best consequences as they value them.

These reflections suggest, to our considerable dismay, that an appeal to the consequences for those most directly affected by the choice—the patient and his family—is not going to provide tremendous guidance in this case. We need to turn to various other moral appeals, the first one being procedural decision rights.

One thing can be said for sure. If we decide that it is J, and not his parents, who has the relevant procedural right of decision making, that will not lead to an argument for providing further chemotherapy for J. He is, after all, demanding care that the health-care providers do not want to provide, and we have already seen many times that one does not have the right to receive the health care that one wishes, although one certainly has the right to seek out other health-care providers who might provide it. The physicians and nurses who are reluctant to provide the care which they think is futile and will hurt J are not required to provide that care by any procedural right of J, even if he has the procedural right of decision making.

But what about the parents who are refusing care and don't want J to receive any further chemotherapy? Don't they have a right to refuse care? Shouldn't that help settle this case? Perhaps, but there are some difficult questions that need to be considered. J is claiming that he is sufficiently mature so that it is he, and not his parents, who has the right to be a decision maker. Are J's claims well founded? He is certainly not independent of his parents, so that basis for acquiring the right of decision making is not present in this case. But those who have talked to J find that he has a pretty mature grasp of the issues and displays considerable maturity in his discussion of his conflict with his parents. Even those who disagree with J's wishes are not inclined to simply dismiss them. J falls on the borderline of maturity. Perhaps the best we can say is that the significance of the right of J's parents to refuse further care for him is weakened in this case because of J's claim to decisional authority, a claim that cannot be fully dismissed even though it cannot be fully accepted. This means that any argument against chemotherapy on the grounds that the parents have refused it and they have a right to have their refusal accepted is at most a modest argument against further chemotherapy.

What about the appeal to respect for persons? Doesn't that offer an argument for attempting to prolong J's life by further chemotherapy? If it does, it cannot be particularly significant. Further chemotherapy is not likely to work, so there is only a small chance that it will even modestly prolong J's life. Therefore, chemotherapy cannot be argued for on the grounds that it will significantly extend the life of a person capable of performing those actions which we value so greatly.

I see one further moral appeal that has considerable significance in this case: an appeal to the integrity of the health-care professionals. Those involved in the care of J, even though they are sensitive to his claim that he does not want to be left hopeless, feel strongly that providing further chemotherapy would be hurting their patient. This offends their own professional value of not harming patients. Some have suggested that they will also be harming the patient by not providing chemotherapy, because this will produce a psychological sense of hopelessness. Others have responded, I believe quite correctly, by saying that that is something for which they are not responsible, while they would be responsible for inflicting pain on J by further chemotherapy. An appeal to the virtue of integrity argues then against providing further chemotherapy. If J were an adult who could seek out his own health-care providers, this problem of integrity could perhaps be avoided, as in other cases in earlier chapters, by transferring the patient to other providers. But that is not a live option here; it is only J's parents who could seek out other providers for J, and they have no reason to do so given that they oppose further chemotherapy.

All of this seems to suggest that J should receive no further chemotherapy, in part because his parents continue to have a right to refuse that care which they judge to be harmful to him, but primarily because the providers are called on by their values to not provide care that would harm the patient. Other moral appeals that are relevant here, such as an appeal to consequences, seem ambiguous or unclear in their implications.[27]

Much of this argument depends on the fact that the parents are continuing to refuse further chemotherapy for J. But there is another question. Should they refuse that chemotherapy? Shouldn't they be guided by J's wishes? I see no reason why they should be so guided. They should take into account J's evaluations of the consequences. But they are no more bound by J's decision than we are, for they can equally claim that J is making the wrong decision even in light of his evaluation of the various consequences.

All of this does not mean that we should simply not provide J with any further chemotherapy. The virtue of compassion, combined with an appeal to consequences, argues for extensive psychosocial support for J, designed to help him deal with his frustration and rage and to help him make the best of the time that is left to him.

A refusal of further chemotherapy combined with the best efforts possible to provide psychosocial support for J appears to be called for in this case. But this is not an easy decision, and the agony of dealing with this case should remind us of the importance of seeing to it that patients in the future have a more realistic understanding of their prognosis at an earlier stage so that they have time to adjust to it. A policy of being more realistic at an earlier stage is certainly supported by an appeal to the virtue of honesty. A consideration of cases such as this suggests that such a policy is also supported by an appeal to consequences.

*CASE NO 37. "He is tired, but we won't give up":*
*Respecting the wishes of mature minors*

FACTS    K was diagnosed at the age of 12 as having nasopharyngeal carcinoma. He was treated with local radiation and chemotherapy, and he initially responded very well. Within a year, however, his condition worsened, and he required radical neck surgery followed by postsurgical chemotherapy. After surgery he was symptom-free until shortly after his fifteenth birthday, when he presented with headaches and nausea and clear evidence of recurrence of his cancer. At that point the only options left open were several experimental chemotherapy protocols. The physicians explained to the parents that K's long-term prognosis was very poor but that these new protocols could probably buy him some time. K is his parents' only child, the family has been close, and the parents have been very involved at all stages of K's care. They definitely wanted the physicians to make every effort to buy some more time for them with K. When all of this was presented to K, however, he was opposed to being enrolled in any further chemotherapy protocols. He said that he was tired of all he had gone through and that he just wanted to be left alone to die in peace. Several conferences involving the physicians, the entire family, and various counselors have been held, but the conflict has not been resolved. There is real tension in this previously close family.

QUESTIONS    There are obvious parallels between K's case and J's case. Both involve terminally ill young adults who are in conflict with their parents about further chemotherapy versus palliative care. But there are two crucial differences between these cases that need to be noted. To begin with, J is asking for further chemotherapy and does not want palliative care; K, on the other hand, is refusing chemotherapy and is asking that he only receive palliative care. Secondly, in J's case, the chemotherapy he is requesting is unlikely to do him any good, which is why his providers and parents don't want to put him through it. In K's case, the chemotherapy that K is refusing has a real chance of buying him at least some good months.

These differences have been the focus of much attention in the discussions about K. Some members of the team have focused on the first difference. They argue that it is one thing to accept the wishes of an adolescent (J) against the wishes of the parents when the adolescent is requesting one further chance at inducing a remission. They would be willing to consider following the wishes of the adolescent in such a case. It is a different matter, they argue, to accept the wishes of K against the wishes of his parents, for K is requesting that he be allowed to die and not receive any chemotherapy. Others have focused on the second point. They see J's request as totally unrealistic, and they oppose following the unrealistic wishes of an adolescent patient against the wishes of the parents. K's case, according to them, is different. While K is turning down a treatment which could buy him some time, his is not an unrealistic assessment. Many of us could see ourselves making the very same decision. So their comparison of the two cases leads them to be more willing to accept K's wishes than J's wishes.

There are members of the team who are not impressed by any of these differences and who would treat the two cases similarly. Some see K (like J) as a relatively mature minor and believe that we should respect the wishes of both. Others see these two, however mature they may be, as children under the care and responsibility of their parents, and they fail to see any justification for overriding parental authority in either case. Needless to say, everyone is further confused by the fact that K's parents, like J's parents, don't know how to handle this disagreement with their child. Like J's parents, K's parents are unsure whether they should insist on their judgment or whether they should accept their child's wishes.

THEORETICAL ANALYSIS    The case of K needs to be compared with the case of J. The team handling both patients was the same, and many of their arguments were based on such comparisons.

Let us begin by considering the question of the procedural rights of the various parties in this case. Several points emerge immediately. First, the parents have no right to have their wishes respected; they are, after all, requesting further care rather than refusing it. This would be true even if there were no opposition from the patient. It is even more true in light of the opposition from the patient. Second, K is at least as mature as J. In fact, many judge him even more mature. He is moreover older, and that in itself makes an appeal to his mature refusal of treatment more significant. There is, then, an argument against chemotherapy from K's right to have his refusal of chemotherapy respected. This argument, while having some significance, is not overwhelming, however, because K still lives with and is supported by his parents, so he is not yet fully emancipated.

What about arguments that appeal to consequences? Here we are led in a different direction. Consider the appeal to the consequences for the patient. Chemotherapy holds out hope, but no certainty (this is an experimental protocol), of some good months at the price of a variety of side effects. K feels that the consequences are not worth it. It would be hard, in light of the experimental nature of the proposed therapy, for anyone to claim that further chemotherapy is worth it to K in light of his values. Moreover, we know that failing to respect his wishes will certainly produce considerable agony as K undergoes the side effects of a treatment he doesn't want to receive. That suggests that an appeal to the consequences for the patient argues against further therapy.

What about an appeal to the consequences for the family? Here, once more, we see conflicting good and bad consequences. Following the wishes of the family will certainly produce a sense of satisfaction in their control of the decision making. But it also leads to the real possibility of disastrous consequences at a later stage. If the therapy produces no improvement in the patient's condition, as may well happen, and if K suffers from the side effects, then there is the real possibility that the parents will undergo the anguish of seeing their child suffer from a decision they made against his wishes. Perhaps the possibility of the beneficial consequences outweighs the possibility of these disastrous consequences, but perhaps not. At best, we can expect an appeal to the consequences for the family to offer only a very modest argument for chemotherapy for K.

Some might feel that an appeal to respect for persons would offer an argument for chemotherapy. After all, it provides K with a real chance of being able to have more time in which he is capable of performing those activities whose performance we value so much. This is no doubt true. However, it cannot be too significant an appeal, because, at best, we are talking about some months of further existence, and again there is a real possibility that even that will not occur.

Few health-care providers hold the value that one should impose experimental therapy on people who do not want it when that therapy offers only a modest hope of a modest prolongation of life. So one can hardly suggest in this case that the appeal to integrity argues for chemotherapy. If anything, it might argue the other way. There are certainly many providers who hold the belief that experimentation must always involve the agreement of those being experimented on, particularly when there is a potential for considerable suffering from the experimentation. That value is embodied in current federal regulations involving research on such patients which require pediatric assent.[28] If anything, the appeal to integrity argues against chemotherapy for this patient. It is reinforced by an appeal to the virtue of compassion, which calls on one not to inflict suffering on someone against his or her wishes.

The evaluation of this case leads to the conclusion that K, like J, should not receive chemotherapy. But the various appeals play different roles in this case. One final similarity joins these two cases. Here, as in the case of J, substantial psychosocial counseling seems mandated both by the virtue of compassion and by an appeal to its potential beneficial consequences. In this case, however, the counseling has to be directed to the parents, who need help to deal with the fact that their son will die in the relatively near future, no matter what is done, and who need to understand the reasons why the providers are respecting the wishes of their teenage son to simply be kept comfortable until he dies.

*CASE NO 38. "We accept her belief that prayer is her best hope": Confronting the prayer issue*

FACTS   L, a 15-year-old girl, was diagnosed as having Ewing's sarcoma, a small-cell tumor of the bone, localized in her leg without any signs of spread of the tumor. At the time of diagnosis, her main complaints were pain and localized swelling and tenderness. Her physicians recommended surgical resection of as much of the tumor as possible, radiation therapy to the entire bone, and multiple drug chemotherapy.

They pointed out to her parents that this treatment would give a very high chance of short-term control and a very good chance of long-term survival. The parents were initially very receptive to this suggestion, as was L, although they were appropriately concerned with side effects and the possibility of long-term failure. Both the parents and their daughter are Pentacostalists who study the Bible and pray regularly. The night after the conference, L, in her prayers, became convinced that God was testing her faith. She felt that if she put her faith in Him and did not seek any other therapy, He would cure her. The next morning, L told both her parents and the physicians that she did not want any surgery, radiation therapy, or chemotherapy. Initially, her parents were strongly opposed to her wishes. After a long discussion with their minister and after much praying, the parents agreed to support their daughter's wishes. They withdrew their consent to all of the recommended treatments and made it clear that they wished to take their daughter home as soon as possible. The physicians involved have suggested a combination of prayer and medical therapy, but L has explained that God wants her to place her total faith in Him, and that is incompatible in her mind with using medical therapy. The parents, with some obvious reluctance, seem resigned to going along with their daughter's wishes.

QUESTIONS    This case is radically different from the two previous cases. Here, there is no longer a conflict between the parents and the teenage patient. They have all agreed to rely solely on prayer. This leads some members of the team to the conclusion that their refusal must be respected. By what rights, they ask, can we violate the deeply held religious beliefs of the entire family? This is not, however, the only crucial difference. It is also important to keep in mind that Ewing's sarcoma, diagnosed at such an early stage, has a very considerable cure rate, so the therapy in question is not a desperate final chance designed to buy some time but rather a good chance at a cure. Many members of the treatment team see this difference as settling the issue. They believe that no teenager, even with the concurrence of her parents, should be allowed to refuse a therapy which offers such a good chance of saving her life. They believe that the team should seek a court order getting custody of this teenager so that the appropriate therapy can be carried out.

Another question about this case troubles many people. They wonder whether the superficial appearance of parental agreement represents reality. Is this really a case of parents in agreement with their teenage child, or is it rather a case of parents too tired and troubled to resist their child's unreasonable request? They wonder whether the more appropriate thing would be to push the parents to insist on appropriate medical care for L.

THEORETICAL ANALYSIS    This is the third case we have examined in which health care is being refused on religious grounds. The first was the case of Mrs. I, the adult Jehovah's Witness who refused blood after unexpected GI bleeding postsurgery. The second involved Baby F, the newborn whose parents refused a Norwood shunt procedure because it might require the use of blood. Both of those cases involved Jehovah's Witnesses. This case does not.

Refusing blood transfusions when they are indicated is an essential part of the religious practices of a Jehovah's Witness. There is no way one can continue to be a sincere Jehovah's Witness while accepting blood products. But there is nothing in the Pentacostalist religious beliefs of this family that requires a refusal of therapy for L.[29] It is just that L feels that God wants her to refuse therapy and rely solely on faith. Why is this difference important? It suggests a possible way of avoiding a very difficult decision. Perhaps, after further religious counseling and prayer, the patient and her family may change their minds and accept medical treatment while continuing to pray to God. This would be compatible with their religious beliefs. In no way, then, will we be calling on them to compromise their integrity if we ask them to seek further religious counseling and to engage in further prayer. So in this case, unlike the cases involving the Jehovah's Witnesses, there is much to be said for trying to help the patient and her family accept the physicians' recommendations.

The harder question arises, of course, if the family and the patient refuse care even after additional prayer and counseling. What are the arguments against seeking a court order so as to be able to provide therapy for this patient? At least the following come to mind: an argument from the right to refuse care, an argument from consequences, and an argument from integrity.

Both L and her parents are refusing care in this case. This distinguishes it from our previous two cases in which there was considerably ambiguity about who had the right to refuse care, and that was important because only the patient or only the parents were refusing further chemotherapy. In this case, however, both the patient and her family are refusing therapy. So it seems to make no difference who has how much of the procedural right to refuse therapy. Moreover, the refusal of therapy after further prayer and religious counseling would be a firmly held, repeated refusal based on, even if not necessarily entailed by, fundamental religious beliefs. All of this seems to give the right to refuse care considerable significance. This analysis, while initially promising, has not been accepted by many courts.[30] They would see this as a case of parental refusal of life-saving therapy and would argue, as we argued in the case of Baby F, that a refusal of life-saving treatment by a surrogate should not be respected. But I think that this legal analysis misses the crucial fact that L has a considerable claim to the right to be a decision maker in light of her age and the maturity she has shown in all discussions with her. When her refusal is supported by her parents, it seems to acquire as much significance as the refusal of an adult.

Two other arguments reinforce this argument from the right to refuse care. One appeals to the consequences for the patient and her family of their refusal's being overridden. Both the patient and her parents will see this as a sin, a violation of God's will. They will have to live with the idea that L is alive only because of her sin. This is certainly a bad consequence of further treatment. Moreover, an appeal to integrity calls on this patient and her family to refuse therapy, and not providing her with therapy is a way of supporting the integrity of the people involved.

It is important to note a difference between this case and the case of Mrs. I, the adult Jehovah's Witness who refused blood products after she started bleeding. In that case, we were able to dismiss these appeals to consequences and to the virtue of integrity by noting that it was not she but the physicians who would sin. This was true because Mrs. I only required a one-time transfusion of blood products, something that could be done without her cooperation. That is not true here. Even if we got a court order mandating the parents to bring the child in for regular therapy, L will not receive the therapy she needs (surgery, radiation therapy, and chemotherapy) without the active participation of the entire family. They would rightfully feel the anguish of a sense of sin, and their participation would, in fact, be in violation of their fundamental values and would compromise their integrity. So we have here two additional arguments, combined with the argument from the right to refuse care, which argue in favor of allowing L to refuse treatment.

There are, however, significant arguments on the other side. The first is a different appeal to the consequences for the patient. There is no doubt that this patient assigns great value to surviving. She very much wants to live. Treating her gives her a high probability of survival, whereas allowing her to refuse therapy almost certainly means that she will die. There is a significant argument from an appeal to consequences for providing the needed therapy. This is reinforced by an appeal to respect for persons. There is no reason why this patient, if she survives as a result of her therapy, cannot go on to live a life full of those many activities whose performance we value so much. There is no guarantee of success, of course, but there is a very good probability for long-term survival that will allow the patient to fully involve herself in those activities. So this argument from the appeal to respect for persons is very significant.

This looks like one of those cases in which no clear judgment emerges and in which good individuals who have carefully analyzed the case may come to conflicting conclusions. My own judgment, as in the case of Mrs. I, is that the arguments from respect for persons and from the favorable consequences are sufficiently significant so that they should be followed. But I recognize that others may judge this difficult case differently. This case, like the case of Mrs. I, illustrates the point of our initial theoretical presentation: that moral systems with many independent appeals result in cases where no decision emerges as a clear-cut best decision, even after one has carefully analyzed the case.

*CASE NO 39. "Pay no attention to him; he is selfish":*
*Looking behind the signature*

FACTS  This case involves a 16-year-old, M, who is a potential donor of bone marrow to a younger sibling who suffers from acute lymphoblastic leukemia and is now in a second remission. The parents and the sibling have agreed to the bone-marrow transplant, despite their awareness of the risks involved in the procedure. They feel that the risks to the sibling are justified in light of his poor prognosis without the transplant and his much better prognosis with it. The problem is that the potential donor, M, is not willing to make the donation. He understands the need for the marrow and the minimal nature of the risks to him, but this makes no difference. The parents say that M has been a serious problem for years. He has run away from home on several occasions, has been a terrible truant at school, and has been in constant minor trouble with the police. They feel that they can get him to agree to donate the bone marrow by threatening to withdraw all types of privileges from him. They are willing to do so, in part because they are angry about his unwillingness to help his younger sibling and in part because they are primarily concerned about saving the life of their younger child. Many members of the treating team wonder whether it would be appropriate to accept such a coerced donation from M. The parents insist that the team should disregard these qualms and go ahead with the planned transplant. They are not prepared to see their other child die.

QUESTIONS    This case raises issues that are radically different from those raised by the previous cases. In cases 36, 37, and 38, the conflicts were among the patients, their parents, and the health-care providers. In this case, the conflict is between the parents, the patient, and the health-care providers on the one hand and a teenage potential donor on the other hand. Some members of the team see this difference as settling the issue. They feel that there is no justification for accepting a coerced donation of bone marrow from a teenager even if he is displaying considerable moral failings. Absent a truly voluntary consent from him, these members of the team oppose the bone-marrow transplant. Other don't see it this way. They raise a number of considerations. One is the straightforward legalistic point that M is a minor whose parents have consented to his being a bone-marrow donor and will obtain his consent in writing. In light of that, they see no need for further inquiry about the legitimacy of the donation.[31] Others who agree with this conclusion argue that the risks to M are minimal and the need for the bone-marrow very great. This leads them to the conclusion that the donation should be accepted, regardless of whether formal consent can be obtained from M, as long as real consent can be obtained from M's parents.

THEORETICAL ANALYSIS    This case is very troubling because the team is clearly involved in a conflict between the feeling that it's wrong to take bone marrow from a donor who is coerced into consenting and the feeling that it would be a great shame for the sibling to die just because M is a nasty person.

We shall begin by a consideration of the appeal to consequences. One consequence argues strongly on behalf of accepting the donation from M. With a bone-marrow transplant, the sibling has a good chance of survival. Without it, the sibling will almost certainly die.[32] So an appeal to the consequences for M's sibling certainly argues on behalf of accepting the donation. This argument is reinforced by a consideration of the consequences for the parents. They are desperate to give the younger sibling his best chance of survival. The satisfaction they will feel if the donation is accepted constitutes an additional favorable consequence that argues significantly on behalf of accepting the bone marrow.

There are other arguments for accepting the coerced donation of the bone marrow. The most important is the appeal to respect for persons. By accepting the donation, the sibling is given a good chance of surviving to lead a life full of all of those activities whose performance we value so much. Without it, the sibling will die relatively soon. So an appeal to respect for persons also argues on behalf of accepting the donation. Still another appeal is the right to be aided against life-threatening situations, a right possessed by M's sibling. Given the seriousness of the threat and the good chance that the aid will work, that appeal also argues on behalf of accepting the donation.

What are the arguments against accepting the donation of the bone marrow? One is an appeal to the consequences for M if the donation is accepted. M will certainly feel very upset about the fact that he has been coerced into donating the bone marrow that he did not wish to donate. The acceptance of the coerced donation has that bad consequence. If this were the only moral consideration that we had to take into account, then it would be simple to claim that the arguments on behalf of accepting the donation are more significant. But there is an additional moral appeal arguing against accepting the coerced donation. It is not based on the right to refuse treatment, since what is being proposed is not treatment for M. It is an appeal to the more general right to refuse to allow something to be done to one's body. The right to refuse treatment is, of course, just an instance of this more general right. M can claim that an acceptance of this coerced donation is an action that violates one of his fundamental rights. That appeal might have tremendous significance, so we need to look at it very carefully.

There are two reasons for thinking that that appeal has less significance than it usually has. One has to do with the fact that M is still a minor. We need to be careful about this point. M is a relatively mature, even if not a very nice, minor. So the fact of his age only modestly diminishes the significance of his appeal to his rights in this case. There is, however, another factor that diminishes the significance of that appeal in this case. M's refusal is not grounded in any deep and fundamental value. His refusal seems to be based on nothing more than a desire to frustrate his family. It is the type of refusal which he might rescind without any fundamental change of values. In light of the general criteria we use to evaluate the significance of this appeal in particular cases, it seems that M's refusal to donate has less significance than it would have in other cases.

I conclude therefore that the treating team may in this case accept the coerced bone-marrow donation from M. But they need to understand that the moral permissibility of doing so is not based on M's agreement. That agreement, resulting from parental coercion, is of no moral significance. They need to understand that the moral permissibility is based on the overwhelming need for the donation combined with the fact that M is a minor refusing permission for less than fundamental reasons. These factors give the right to refuse participation less significance in this case than it would normally have. The case would be very different if M were an adult who had strong and deeply rooted reasons for refusing but was coerced by his family into agreeing to donate bone marrow. Accepting such a coerced donation might not be justified in this sort of case.[33]

It would certainly be much better if M could be brought to agree freely to the donation. The parental strategy of coercing him by threatening to withhold all sorts of privileges, even if it does succeed in getting M's signature on a morally meaningless consent form, is not helpful in accomplishing this goal. Before accepting such a coerced donation, we would do better to see if outsiders, who are not in such an antagonistic relationship with M, could work with M to get him to voluntarily agree to donate the bone marrow. This course of action would clearly be morally preferable, since it would eliminate the objections to M's donation. But if it fails, it would be morally justifiable to go ahead with the bone-marrow donation.

*CASE NO 40. "Let my brother kill me":*
*Dealing with tragic responses to tragic cases*

FACTS    The patient in this case, N, is a 16-year-old junior at a local high school. Before her accident, she was an outstanding student. Her grades were at the top of the class, she represented the school in swimming and in track and field, and she was an outstanding folk dancer. Three months ago, N was in a serious automobile accident that left her paralyzed from the neck down. For the first week or two, there was serious doubt about whether she would survive. Now her medical condition has stabilized. She has a good understanding of her condition and what she must face for the rest of her life. She is totally unwilling to accept what fate has dealt her. When people talk to her about rehabilitative therapy, she expresses absolutely no interest in what they have to say. Her standard response is to ask to be left alone. She expresses great regrets that her physicians pulled her through her immediate crisis after the accident, and she believes that she would be better off had she been allowed to die. She has been living with her older brother since both of her parents died some years ago. She wants to go home to his house, and he is willing to take her home as soon as possible. One of the nurses heard them talking and heard the older brother promise that he would follow her wishes and shoot her when they got home. The nurse reported this to the attending physician, who believes that this conversation best explains why N wants to go home now and why the brother wants to take her home.

QUESTIONS    This case is radically different from any that have preceded it. The question is not that of providing or withholding certain forms of medical care. The question is the legitimacy of discharging a patient, knowing that the patient has arranged for someone else to kill her because she no longer wants to live. Many members of the team believe that this fact settles the case. They argue that this form of active euthanasia is morally wrong. They feel, moreover, that it is the responsibility of the staff to intervene to prevent this from happening and that the best intervention is to refuse to discharge N at this time. In fact, they would want convincing evidence that this is not N's intention before they would discharge her. Others hold a somewhat weaker position. Their main point is that N, however mature she may be, is still just a teenager, has undergone a crisis that would try the understanding and competency of anyone, and can hardly be treated as a competent adult whose wishes should be respected at this point. They feel that the least that is required is that the team confront N and her brother and explain (1) that what N is going through is a standard reaction of many who have suffered such a terrible tragedy, (2) that most patients eventually come to peace with their new condition, and (3) that at least a significant amount of time should elapse before N and her brother consider the extreme measures they now have planned. Still a third group sees the issues very differently. There is no doubt, they argue, that N is very depressed at this point, but she has every right to be depressed. They claim that her achievements, despite the difficult circumstance of growing up with the loss of two parents, is an indication of considerable independence of mind and maturity. They find in talking to her that she has a full grasp of the issues, including the fact that many patients do eventually adjust to the type of circumstances in which she finds herself. They find that she has made a judgment that she doesn't want to become that type of person. They see no reason to impose any other views on her. In short, they are willing to allow her to go home to her brother's house, even though they know what this might mean for her and for him.

THEORETICAL ANALYSIS    Few cases have created as much disagreement among the treating team as this one. Opinions range all the way from the view that there is a moral obligation to prevent this brother and sister from carrying out their plan to the view that we ought to accept their decision and let him carry out their plan. I think it is easy to understand why this case has provoked such diverse but strongly held feelings. What has happened to N is truly tragic. What she and her brother are planning to do is troubling. It is precisely in cases like this, where we are pulled in so many different directions, that we hope that a moral theory can provide the basis for a reasonable decision.

We shall begin with the position of those members of the team who say that what the brother proposes to do is a morally unacceptable act of killing his sister and that we are obliged to prevent this by refusing to discharge her until such time as we can be sure that the plan for the murder has been dropped. There are two parts to this position: the claim that what the brother proposes to do is a morally wrong act of killing and the claim that we are obliged to prevent it.

There is no doubt that what the brother proposes to do is illegal. Is it, however, immoral? As we saw in chapter 2, killing someone is immoral in large measure because it deprives that person of his or her life, something to which he or she has a right. But that cannot be the basis for the claim that what is being proposed here is morally wrong. After all, N, by requesting that her brother shoot her, has clearly waived her right not to be killed. We saw in chapter 2 that that right is waivable. So why should we suppose that the brother's action is immoral?

One might claim that N is not competent to waive her rights. Why? Because she is a minor? But she is more likely to fall under the mature-minor rule than any of the other patients we have discussed so far. She has been independent of her parents since their death. She has shown tremendous maturity, strength of character, and intelligence. Everyone who discusses the case with her is impressed by how much careful thought she has given to her situation. It is hard to see, then, why she should not be able to waive that right despite the fact that she is still only 16. Is she not competent to waive that right because she is depressed? We need to be very careful about that claim. There is no doubt that she is very saddened by her circumstances. In fact, they are terrible circumstances. The mere fact that she evaluates them so negatively cannot, therefore, serve as the basis for claiming that she is incompetent because of depression. There is, moreover, no further clinical evidence of depression. Her affect is far from flat. She has very strong feelings about herself, her circumstances, and her life. Nor are there any other signs of clinical depression. In short, then, there seems to be no reason why she should not be able to waive the right not to be killed.

It is also worth noting that the second assumption of this approach—the claim that we are required to intervene to prevent the brother from shooting her—also raises many important questions. Even if it were true that the brother would wrongfully be taking her life and depriving her of her right to live, we would still need additional arguments to show that there is a moral obligation on the part of the team to prevent that from happening. Given that he is not wrongfully depriving her of her right, however, that question is moot in this case.

This is not to say that there are no moral problems raised by this case. There are a great many, and we need to examine them carefully. All that has been argued so far is that the right not to be killed is not relevant here. Whatever we decide about this case, we cannot decide it on the basis of the simplistic claim that what the brother is willing to do is to wrongfully deprive his sister of that life to which she has a right and that we must therefore stop him.

Let us examine this case from the perspective of our other moral appeals. One which is certainly relevant here is the appeal to respect for persons. Despite the overwhelming physical limitations, N's abilities to think, to feel, and to orally express those thoughts and feelings are not impaired. She is capable of performing a wide variety of those activities whose performance we value so much, since so many of them have to do with thinking, feeling, and communicating. An argument from the sanctity of human life would certainly be for preserving N's life. Even an argument from respect for persons, however, is for preserving N's life. We have, then, one reasonably significant argument for preventing N's brother from killing her. However, it is not as strong as it would be in cases where the patient is less handicapped physically.

There is another argument for preventing the murder. Whatever the morality of the situation, what N's brother proposes doing is clearly illegal. While we cannot be sure what will be the consequences of his killing his sister, there is at least a strong probability that he will be arrested, convicted, and punished. It is certainly the case that none of those things is a consequence that he desires, even if he is prepared to put up with them to help his sister. These bad consequences certainly are an argument for preventing him from doing what he proposes to do.

There is a significant argument on the other side. N has as much right to refuse care as any other patient. That right includes the right to refuse further hospitalization. It is, moreover, a right which has considerable significance in this case because her refusal has been held for quite a long period of time and because it is rooted in her fundamental conception of what she values and how she sees herself as a person. All of this argues with some significance for allowing her to go home.

We have left, then, the appeal to the consequences for the patient. Here we come to what is in many ways the hardest and yet the most crucial issue. Is N better off alive or dead? She clearly thinks that she is better off dead. Having now lived for some months with her tremendous physical disabilities, she is in a better position than most to evaluate whether her continued living is a gain or a loss to her. Keep in mind, however, that we need to distinguish between her evaluation of the various outcomes, which is definitive, and her judgment about which action will lead to the best results, which may be mistaken. What sort of mistake could she be making here? Members of the team suggest that she is not taking into account the possibility that she will acquire a variety of interests which might lead her to say later on that her life is worth living. She has, in effect, dismissed that possibility, saying that that is not the type of person she wants to be. The crucial point that lies behind that remark is that given her current values, not the values she may come to acquire if she is forced to go on living, she believes that she would find the life she is living unacceptable. But our assumption is that the preferences of the patient at the time of the outcome (and not at the time of the decision) are the ones which determine the value of the outcome. Giving that assumption, the nature of the values she will acquire later on is very important but hard to predict. So we cannot say with any confidence what action will lead to the best consequences for the patient; we can say, however, that the question is not settled by any claim she is making in terms of her current values.

What about the suggestion made by members of the team that N and her brother be urged to postpone their plans at least for a while until N can see whether or not her values will change? This argument, as initially formulated, is problematic because it refers to new values which may or may not be adopted. There is, however, another way of putting that point which is more straightforward and provides a different account of the mistake she may be making. N may simply be overlooking at this point the various possibilities (as limited as they are) which are open to her and would be valuable for her even given her current values. So there is the possibility of N's being wrong, even using her values at this point. This possibility needs to be urged upon N.

All of this seems to suggest that the appropriate thing is to keep N in the hospital for a period of time in the hope that she will see things differently. At the end, she must be discharged, and we cannot permanently prevent N and her brother from carrying out their plan. But if it persists, that may tell us that the consequences for N of continued existence are truly undesirable, and that may justify the killing.

## 7.4   Conclusion

We have analyzed forty difficult cases employing the model of conflicting values. None of these has been easy, and some of them remain puzzling even after our analysis. I do feel, however, that the model has helped resolve many and has at least shed light on the rest. That is the argument for the model.

There is, however, one point which I made earlier and which needs to be repeated. Casuistry using the model of conflicting values is a new approach. I would be very surprised if this first attempt was completely successful. It is far more likely that many of the analyses offered can be improved on. Such an improvement would not be an argument against the model. It would only show its ability to be used more and more successfully as time goes along. I therefore welcome collaborative extensions of this model both to the forty cases I have presented and to other cases as well. This book is intended to be the first word in pluralistic casuistry, not the last word.

### Notes

1. The analysis in this chapter, as in the previous chapters, is meant to be an analysis of the moral issues, not the legal issues. Nevertheless, neonatal cases are special in that a definite prolife moral structure has been legislated into the child abuse laws in the United

States by Public Law 98-457 (October 9, 1984). That statute treats a failure to provide medical care in response to a child's life-threatening condition as a form of child abuse unless the infant is chronically and irreversibly comatose, the provision of such treatment would be futile in terms of the survival of the infant, or the provision would be virtually futile in terms of the survival of the infant and the treatment itself would be inhumane in such circumstances. It seems appropriate, therefore, to analyze what that law would say about each of our cases, and I will do so in a footnote to each case. There has been a tremendous literature surrounding these issues. An excellent summary of the prelegislation literature is R. Weir, *Selective Nontreatment of Handicapped Newborns* (New York: Oxford Univ. Press, 1984). More recent books include E. Shelp, *Born to Die* (New York: Free Press, 1986); H. Kuhse and P. Singer, *Should the Baby Live* (Oxford: Oxford Univ. Press, 1985); R. Gustaitis and E. W. D. Young, *A Time to Be Born, A Time to Die* (Reading, Mass.: Addison Wesley, 1986); and F. M. Frohock, *Special Care* (Chicago: Univ. of Chicago Press, 1986).

2. It seems, then, that aggressive management of Baby A is mandated by PL 98-457, since we cannot say that the provision of that care would be virtually futile in terms of the survival of the infant, and one certainly cannot say that Baby A is comatose.

3. Even if we could get some better indications of that, we would still have the problem, mentioned in the text, of deciding how to assess the value of such a life for a patient who has never had any relevant preferences. We will return to this issue in later cases. For now, the uncertainty of the actual consequences for Baby A makes it unnecessary for us to consider the question of how such consequences should be evaluated.

4. Should the mother be allowed to transfer the child to other physicians in order to get further aggressive care even after Baby A's condition deteriorates? She should, unless we are prepared to treat her demand for further care at that point as child abuse. We badly need a theory of this form of child abuse.

5. It also makes the case one in which the provision of further care is at least virtually futile in terms of the survival of the infant and in which the treatment would be inhumane. Withholding further care from Baby B seems to be legally allowable under PL 98-457.

6. It is certainly true that initial protocols for determining brain death, such as the classic statement found in Ad Hoc Committee of the Harvard Medical School, "A Definition of Irreversible Coma," *JAMA* 205, no. 6 (August 1968): 337–40, stressed the importance of a confirmatory EEG. This emphasis on the EEG has rightfully diminished. See, for example, "Guidelines for the Determination of Death," which is Appendix F to President's Commission for the Study of Ethical Problems in Medicine, *Defining Death* (Washington, D.C.: Government Printing Office, 1981). Neonatal cases are, however, notoriously difficult, and there is much to be said for waiting for the confirmatory EEG.

7. A fine point here is worth noting. In a world in which the physical-resources problem is not present, one could argue for continued support even after a patient is dead for a short period of time until the family accepts what has happened. Compassion and an appeal to consequences would be the basis for doing so. But that is only a fallback response to a family which insists on continued support. There seems to be nothing wrong with starting off with a firm statement that support *will* be stopped.

8. See, for example, H. T. Engelhardt and M. Rie, "Intensive Care Units, Scarce Resources, and Conflicting Principles of Justice," *JAMA* 255, no. 9 (March 1986): 1159–64.

9. Many states have passed statutes authorizing minor parents to make decisions for their minor children and/or emancipating minor parents. The details of the current legal situation are summarized in J. Morrissey, A. Hofmann, and J. Thrope, *Consent and Confidentiality in the Health Care of Children and Adolescents* (New York: Free Press, 1986). The argument in the text should be taken as an argument against that development and for the alternative of seeing on a case-by-case basis whether the minor parent is covered by the emancipated-minor rule or the mature-minor rule discussed in section 5.1.

10. PL 98-457 would not, however, require that aggressive care. It is not, therefore, based on a sanctity-of-life position. It is probably best understood as a respect-for-person approach which simply gives very high significance to any capacity to perform any of the relevant activities. Such an approach would authorize withholding care only if the child is irreversibly comatose.

11. See, for example, the statement of March 15, 1986, of the AMA's Council on Ethical and Judicial Affairs. Interestingly enough, PL 98-457 is ambiguous in this matter, requiring only the provision of *"appropriate* nutrition, hydration or medication" (italics added).

12. Such cases are discussed in R. Perkins, *Perkins on Criminal Law,* 2nd ed. (Mineola: The Foundation Press, 1969).

13. Would this be a case of the third exception to PL 98-457 that care need not be provided if its provision would be virtually futile and the treatment itself inhumane in such circumstances? Or would the chance of survival for some time and the noninvasive nature of the treatment require that treatment be provided? Such are the "joys" of "Baby Doe jurisprudence."

14. The careful reader will note that the only case in which we appealed to the consequences to the child was that of Baby B. There we could do so because nearly all who have values seem to desire the cessation of pain, and we only needed to appeal to this simple evaluation. Here we would need to appeal to a much more complex set of evaluations, and they are unavailable. The careful reader will also note that this last point only deals with evaluating consequences for the sake of the appeal to consequences.

15. The classic paper describing this procedure is W. J. Norwood, et al., "Physiologic Repair of Aortic Atheria Hypoplastic Left Heart Syndrome," *NEJM* 308, no. 23 (1983).

16. Many court cases have clarified that this standard procedure is the law in the United States in connection with life-threatening illnesses that have standard therapies with well-established significant success rates. For the details of these cases, see A. Holder, *Legal Issues in Pediatrics and Adolescent Medicine,* 2nd edition (New Haven: Yale Univ. Press, 1985).

17. I am referring, of course, to human transplants, not transplants of hearts from other species.

18. PL 98-457 does not, as far as I can see, distinguish between experimental and nonexperimental therapies, mandating simply that the physicians use the approach most likely to succeed. One might have been able to argue, however, that the Norwood shunt, in light of its experimental nature and its modest success rate, still left this case as one in which treatment was "virtually futile."

19. Attention was first focused on these cases by the writings of John Lorber. See, for example, J. Lorber, "Results of Treatment of Myelomeningocele," *Dev Med Child Neurology* 13 (1971): 279–303. See also R. Duff and A. G. M. Campbell, "Moral and Ethical Dilemmas in the Special Care Nursery," *NEJM* 289 (October 1973): 890–94. A recent example of this approach is found in R. Gross et al., "Early Management and Decision Making for the Treatment of Myelomeningocele," *Pediatrics* 72 (October 1983): 450–58. Weir, *Selective Nontreatment,* provides a full summary of the debate. It is clear from the many regulations issued in connection with PL 98-457 and the earlier Baby Doe regulations that a major goal was to mandate aggressive care in nearly all cases of children with spina bifida.

20. I say "might be different" because such cases would force us to define whose preferences we are using when making this evaluation, the question raised above in note 14. The defender of aggressive therapy would do best, I think, to respond by saying "the preferences the child will probably develop." As problematic as that is, it is far less problematic, for reasons given in chapter 2, then attempting to develop some objective evaluation of consequences for use in the appeal to consequences.

21. It should be noted that the protocol in Gross, "Early Management," does just that. The children are fed on a regular schedule but are not given antibiotics.

22. It also poses no problems under PL 98-457, since aggressive care of this child would be virtually futile in terms of survival.

23. The issue of the moral licitness of artificial insemination of single women has been extensively discussed but will not be dealt with here.

24. Notice how the question is framed to make our deliberations consistent with the principle of consumer sovereignty in the evaluation of consequences. Notes 14 and 20 above should be consulted for purposes of comparison.

25. This is not a unique problem. Recent studies have shown that the final legacy of the dying child often is ruinous debt for the family. See, for example, B. Bloom, R. Knorr, and A. Evans, "The Epidemiology of Disease Expenses," *JAMA* 253 (April 26, 1985): 2393–97.

26. An excellent protocol which addresses these questions is R. N. Nitshke et al., "Therapeutic Choices Made by Patients with End-State Cancer," *Journal of Pediatrics* 101, no. 3 (1982): 471–76. One of the merits of their protocol is that it advocates honesty in communicating even with patients who are younger than J. It should be noted that the excessive encouragement I am criticizing is the hope of a cure or of a significant prolongation of life. One should always encourage the hope that the patient will be kept as comfortable as possible, and that hope may be far more important in these cases.

27. It is interesting to note here that recent natural-death acts, such as the Texas Natural Death Act of 1985, allow a child to override any parental decision to create a living will for the child. The thought seems to be that parents are not allowed to stop care when the child wants further care. No age limit is put on this authority of the child. Cases such as J's suggest that such an approach is mistaken.

28. See 45 CFR 46, subpart D. In fact, it might be argued that treating K experimentally without his assent is illegal under current law.

29. On this difference between the beliefs of a Jehovah's Witness and the beliefs of a Pentacostalist, see the appropriate chapters in R. Numbers and D. W. Amundsen, *Caring and Curing* (New York: Macmillan, 1986). The crucial point is that modern Pentacostalists, while accepting the value of prayer in response to illness, also respect the legitimacy of the physician's role.

30. For a discussion of relevant issues, see *Matter of Hamilton* 657 S.W. 2d. 425. That case, however, involved a 12-year-old.

31. Analogous but not exactly similar cases have given rise to conflicting court decisions about donations from minor donors. On this complex issue, see Holder, *Legal Issues,* pp. 167–78. I find that legal discussion unpersuasive, particularly in the case of a relatively benign bone-marrow transplant.

32. This was certainly the state of knowledge at the time this case occurred. Recent results of intensive chemotherapy, as an alternative to bone-marrow transplants, may mean that future cases will have a different moral structure because there will be an alternative available for the sibling. These recent results are found in G. Rivera et al., "Intensive Retreatment of Childhood ALL in First Bone Marrow Relapse," *NEJM* 315, no. 5 (July 31, 1986): 273–78.

33. I say "might not be justified" because there are significant arguments for accepting coerced donations to save lives. I am reminded here of the rabbinic dictum that all sins (including, presumably, accepting coerced donations) except for three (idolatry, adultery, and murder) are overruled by the necessity of saving lives.

# Index